Psychiatric Certification Review Guide for the Generalist and Clinical Specialist in Adult, Child, and Adolescent Psychiatric and Mental Health Nursing

Editor

Clare Houseman, Ph.D., R.N.,C.S.
Associate Professor
College of Health Sciences
Old Dominion University
Norfolk, Virginia

Health Leadership Associates
Potomac, Maryland

Health Leadership Associates

Sponsoring Editor: Virginia Layng Millonig, Ph.D., R.N.
Production Manager: Martha M. Pounsberry
Manuscript Editor: Cynthia L. Frazier
Cover Design: Frances R. Weber
Technical Support: Rebecca E. Grahl
Design and Production: Port City Press, Inc.

Printed in the United States of America

Health Leadership Associates, Inc. • P.O. Box 59153 • Potomac, Maryland 20859

Library of Congress Cataloging-in-Publication Data

Psychiatric certification review guide for the generalist and clinical specialist in adult, child, and adolescent psychiatric and mental health nursing / editor, Clare Houseman : contributing authors, Ivo L. Abraham . . . [et al.].
p. cm.
Includes bibliographical references and index.
ISBN 1-878028-11-1 : $43.95
1. Psychiatric nursing. 2. Psychiatric nursing—Examinations, questions, etc. I. Houseman, Clare. II. Abraham, Ivo Luc.
[DNLM: 1. Psychiatric Nursing—examination questions. WY 18 P9755 1994]
RC440.P72985 1994
610.73'68'076—dc20
DNLM/DLC
for Library of Congress 94-8830
CIP

To my son Greg whose presence brings joy to my life and to my parents Anthony and Phyllis Woodell for their continued unquestioning support of my efforts

Contributors

TEST TAKING STRATEGIES AND TECHNIQUES

Nancy Dickenson Hazard, M.S.N., C.P.N.P., F.A.A.N.
Executive Officer
Sigma Theta Tau International
Indianapolis, Indiana

Clare Houseman, Ph.D., R.N.,C.S.
Associate Professor
College of Health Sciences
Old Dominion University
Norfolk, Virginia

THE ESSENTIALS OF CARE

Clare Houseman, Ph.D., R.N.,C.S.
Associate Professor
College of Health Sciences
Old Dominion University
Norfolk, Virginia

MAJOR THEORETICAL FRAMEWORKS FOR PSYCHIATRIC NURSING

Joan Donovan, Ph.D., R.N.,C.S.
Private Practice
Richmond, Virginia

MENTAL DISORDERS DUE TO SUBSTANCE ABUSE

Therese K. Killeen, M.S.N., R.N.,C.S.
Clinical Nurse Specialist
Coordinator for Alcohol and Substance Abuse Program
Institute of Psychiatry
Medical University of South Carolina
Charleston, South Carolina

ANXIETY AND STRESS RELATED DISORDERS

Karma Castleberry, Ph.D., R.N.,C.S.
Associate Professor

School of Nursing
Radford University
Consultant
St. Albans Psychiatric Hospital
Radford, Virginia

SCHIZOPHRENIA AND OTHER PSYCHOTIC DISORDERS

Mary Fultz Spencer, M.N., R.N.,C.S.
Clinical Instructor
School of Nursing
University of North Carolina at Chapel Hill
Chapel Hill, North Carolina
Psychotherapist
Glenwood Psychiatric Associates
Raleigh, North Carolina

MOOD DISORDERS

Judith Haber, Ph.D., R.N.,C.S., F.A.A.N.
Family Therapist
Private Practice
Stamford, Connecticut

BEHAVIORAL SYNDROMES AND DISORDERS OF ADULT PERSONALITY

Richardean Benjamin-Coleman, Ph.D., M.P.H., R.N.,C.S
Assistant Professor
School of Nursing
Old Dominion University
Norfolk, Virginia

ORGANIC MENTAL DISORDERS

Anita Thompson-Heisterman, M.S.N., R.N.,C.S.
Clinical Nurse Specialist
Rural Elder Health Consortium
University of Virginia
Charlottesville, Virginia

Jane Neese, M.S.N., R.N.,C.S.
Research Associate
Rural Elder Health Consortium

University of Virginia
Charlottesville, Virginia

Ivo L. Abraham, Ph.D., R.N.
Director
Rural Elder Health Consortium
University of Virginia
Charlottesville, Virginia

BEHAVIORAL AND EMOTIONAL DISORDERS OF CHILDHOOD AND ADOLESCENCE

Michelle L. Zimmerman, M.A., R.N.,C.S.
Associate Professor
School of Nursing
Psychotherapist
Avery-Finney-Wald Associates
Norfolk, Virginia

THE LARGER MENTAL HEALTH ENVIRONMENT

Sherrill Marshall, M.S.N., R.N.,C.S.
Lecturer
Coordinator of Distance Learning
School of Nursing
Old Dominion University
Norfolk, Virginia

Reviewers

Carolyn V. Billings, M.S.N., R.N.,C.S.
Certified Specialist in
Adult Psychiatric-Mental Health Nursing
Private Practice
Raleigh, North Carolina

Anne D. Castillo, R.N.,C.
Clinical II
Mental Health Services
Intensive Treatment Area
Sentara Norfolk General Hospital
Norfolk, Virginia

Deane L. Critchley, Ph.D., R.N.,C.S., F.A.A.N.
Private Practice
Consultant
Albuquerque, New Mexico

Lois S. Walker, D.N.Sc., R.N.,C.S.
Private Practice of Psychotherapy
Consultant
Fairfax and Arlington, Virginia

Preface

This book has been developed especially for nurses preparing to take Certification Examinations offered by the American Nurses Credentialing Center (ANCC). The book is inclusive in that it contains both basic and advanced content so that nurses seeking certification as generalists as well as nurses seeking certification as clinical specialists in adult, child and adolescent psychiatric and mental health nursing will find the book useful for review.

Basic content has been highlighted in shaded blocks throughout the text (indicating content applicable for both the generalist and clinical specialist) whereas content areas not shaded are directed toward the clinical specialist. *The two exceptions are the Test Taking Strategies chapter which is essential information for all nurses who are taking certification examinations and the Childhood and Adolescence chapter which is directed exclusively toward the Clinical Specialist.*

The purpose of the book is twofold. This book will assist individuals engaged in self study preparation for Certification Examinations, and may be used as a brief reference guide in the practice setting.

Many nurses preparing for certification examinations find that reviewing an extensive body of scientific knowledge requires a very difficult search of many sources that must be synthesized to provide a review base for the examination. This publication provides a succinct, yet comprehensive review of the core material.

The book has been organized to provide the reader with test taking strategies and techniques. This is followed by chapters on The Essentials of Care, Major Theoretical Frameworks for Psychiatric Nursing, Mental Disorders Due to Substance Abuse, Anxiety and Stress Related Disorders, Schizophrenia and Other Psychotic Disorders, Mood Disorders, Behavioral Syndromes and Disorders of Adult Personality, Organic Mental Disorders, Behavioral and Emotional Disorders of Childhood and Adolescence and The Larger Mental Health Environment.

Following each chapter are test questions, which are intended to serve as an introduction to the testing arena. In addition a bibliography is included for those who need a more in depth discussion of the subject matter in each chapter. These references can serve as additional instructional material for the reader.

The editor and contributing authors are certified nurses who are respected experts in the field of psychiatric nursing. They have designed this book to assist potential examinees to prepare for success in the certification examination process.

It is assumed that the reader of this review guide has completed a course of study in psychiatric nursing. This Psychiatric Certification Review Guide for the Generalist and Clinical Specialist in Adult, Child, and Adolescent Psychiatric and Mental Health Nursing is not intended to be a basic learning tool.

Certification is a process that is gaining recognition both within and outside the profession. For the professional it is a means of gaining special recognition as a certified psychiatric nurse which not only demonstrates a level of competency, but may also enhance professional opportunities and advancement. For the consumer, it means that a certified nurse has met certain predetermined standards set by the profession.

Acknowledgments

As this text was being written the American Psychiatric Association was rewriting the Diagnostic and Statistical Manual, authors of this text received permission to utilize the American Psychiatric Association Diagnostic and Statistical Manual of Mental Disorders, Fourth Edition, Draft Criteria (March 1, 1993), in order to assure that the latest available material was included.

CONTENTS

Test Taking Strategies and Techniques

Nancy A. Dickenson Hazard
Clare Houseman

We all respond to testing situations in different ways. What separates the successful test taker from the unsuccessful one is knowing how to prepare for and take a test. Preparing yourself to be a successful test taker is as important as studying for the test. Each person needs to assess and develop their own test taking strategies and skills. The primary goal of this chapter is to assist potential examinees in knowing how to study for and take a test.

STRATEGY #1 Know Yourself

When faced with an examination, do you feel threatened, experience butterflies or sweaty palms, have trouble keeping your mind focused on studying or on the test question? These common symptoms of test anxiety plague many of us, but can be used advantageously if understood and handled correctly (Divine & Kylen, 1979). Over the years of test taking, each of us has developed certain testing behaviors, some of which are beneficial, while others present obstacles to successful test taking. You can take control of the test taking situation by identifying the undesirable behaviors, maintaining the desirable ones and developing skills to improve test performance.

Technique #1 From the following descriptions of test taking personalities, find yourself (Table 1). Write down those characteristics which describe you even if they are from different personality types. Carefully review the problem list associated with your test taking personality characteristics. Write down the problems which are most troublesome. Then make a list of how you can remedy these problems from the improvement strategies list. Be sure to use these strategies as you prepare for and take examinations.

STRATEGY #2 Develop Your Thinking Skills

Understanding Thought Processes: In order to improve your thinking skills and subsequent test performance, it is best to understand the types of thinking as well as the techniques to enhance the thought process.

Everyone has their own learning style, but we all must proceed through the same process to think.

Thinking occurs on two levels—the lower level of memory and comprehension and the higher level of application and analysis (ABP, 1989). Memory is the ability to recall facts. Without adequate retrieval of facts, progression through the higher levels of thinking can not occur easily. Comprehension is the ability to understand memorized facts. To be effective, comprehension skills must allow the person to translate recalled information from one context to another. Application, or the process of using information to know why it occurs, is a higher form of learning. Effective application relies on the use of understood memorized facts to verify intended action. Analysis is the ability to use abstract or logical forms of thought to show relationships and to distinguish the cause and effect between the variables in a situation.

Table 1

Test Taker Profile

Type	*Characteristics*	*Pitfalls*	*Improvement Strategies*
The Rusher	• Rushes to complete the test before the studied facts are forgotten • Arrives at test site early and waits anxiously • Mumbles studied facts • Tense body posture • Accelerated pulse, respiration and neuromuscular excitement • Answers questions rapidly and is generally one of the first to complete • Experiences exhaustion once test is over	• Unable to read question and situation completely • At high risk for misreading, misinterpreting and mistakes • Difficult items heighten anxiety • Likely to make quick, not well-thought-out guesses	• Practice progressive relaxation techniques • Develop a study plan with sufficient time to review important content • Avoid cramming and last minute studying • Take practice tests focusing on slowing down and reading and answering each option carefully • Read instructions and questions slowly
The Turtle	• Moves slowly, methodically, deliberately through each question • Repeated rereading, underlining and checking • Takes 60 to 90 seconds per question versus an average of 45 to 60 seconds	• Last to finish; often does not complete the exam • Has to quickly complete questions in last part of exam, increasing errors • Has difficulty completing timed examinations	• Take practice tests focusing on time spent per item • Place watch in front of examination paper to keep track of time • Mark answer sheet for where one should be halfway through exam based on total number of questions and total amount of time for exam • Study concepts not details • Attempt to answer each question as you progress through the exam

Type	*Characteristics*	*Pitfalls*	*Improvement Strategies*
The Personalizer	• Mature person who has personal knowledge and insight from life experiences	• Risk in relying on what has been learned through observation and experience since one may develop false understandings and stereotypes	• Focus on principles and standards that support nursing practice
		• Personal beliefs and experiences are frequently not the norm or standard tested	• Avoid making connections between patients in exam clinical situations and personal clinical experience
		• Has difficulty identifying expected standards measured by standardized examination	• Focus on generalities not experiences
The Squisher	• View exams as threat, rather than an expected event in education	• Procrastinates studying for exams	• Establish a plan of progressive, disciplined study
	• Preoccupied with grades and personal accomplishment	• Unable to study effectively since waits until last minute	• Use defined time frames for studying content and taking practice exams
	• Attempts to avoid responsibility and accountability associated with testing in order to reduce anxiety	• Increased anxiety over test since procrastinating study impairs ability to learn and perform	• Use relaxation techniques • Return to difficult items • Read carefully
The Philosopher	• Academically successful person who is well disciplined and structured in study habits	• Over analysis causes loss of sight of actual intent of question	• Focus on questions as they are written
	• Displays great intensity and concentration during exam	• Reads information into questions answering with own added information rather than answering the actual intent of question	• Work on self confidence and not on question. Initial response is usually correct
	• Searches questions for hidden or unintended meaning		• Avoid multiple rereadings of questions
	• Experiences anxiety over not knowing everything		• Avoid adding own information and unintended meanings
			• Practice, practice, practice with sample tests
The Second Guesser	• Answers questions twice, first as an examinee, second as an examiner	• Altering an initial response frequently results in an incorrect answer	• Reread only the few items of which one is unsure. Avoid changing initial responses

Type	*Characteristics*	*Pitfalls*	*Improvement Strategies*
	• Believes second look will allow one to find and correct errors	• Frequently changes answers because the pattern of response appears incorrect (i.e. too many "true" or too many correct responses)	• Take exam carefully and progressively first time, allowing little or no time for rereading • Study facts • Avoid reading into questions
	• Frequently changes initial responses (i.e. grades own test)		
The Lawyer	• Attempts to place words or ideas into the question (leads the witness)	• Veers from the obvious answer and provides response from own point of view	• Focus on distinguishing what patient is saying in question and not on what is read into question
	• Occurs most frequently with psychosocial or communication questions which ask for the most appropriate response	• Reads a question, jumps to a conclusion then finds a response that leads to predetermined conclusion	• Avoid formulating responses aimed at obtaining certain information
			• Choose responses that allow patient to express feelings which encourage hope, not catastrophe; those which are intended to clarify, which identify feeling tone of patient or which avoid negating or confronting patient feelings

From: "Making the grades as a test-taker," by N. Dickenson-Hazard, (1989) *Pediatric Nursing, 15,* p. 303. Adapted from: *Nurse's guide to successful test-taking* by M. B. Sides and N. B. Cailles, 1989. Philadelphia: J. B. Lippincott, Co., pp 59–70, 199–203. Copyright 1989 by A. J. Jannetti, Inc. Reprinted by permission.

As related to testing situations, the thought process from memory to analysis occurs quite quickly. Some examination items are designed to test memory and comprehension while others test application and analysis. An example of a memory question is as follows:

> Clients' initial response to learning that they have a terminal illness is generally:
>
> a) Depression
> b) Bargaining
> c) *Denial*
> d) Anger

To answer this question correctly, the individual has to retrieve a memorized fact. Understanding the fact, knowing why it is important or analyzing what should be done in this situation is not needed. An example of a question which tests comprehension is as follows:

> Shortly after having been informed that she is in the terminal stages of breast cancer, Mrs. Jones begins to talk about her plans to travel with her husband when he retires in two years. The nurse should know that:
>
> a) The diagnosis could be wrong and Mrs. Jones may not be dying
> b) *Mrs. Jones is probably responding to the news by using the defense mechanism of denial*
> c) Mrs. Jones is clearly delusional
> d) Mrs. Jones is not responding in the way most clients would

In order to answer this question correctly, an individual must retrieve the fact that Denial is often the first response to learning about a terminal illness and that Mrs. Jones' behavior is indicative of denial.

In a higher level of thinking examination question, individuals must be able to recall a fact, understand that fact in the context of the question, apply this understanding to explaining why one answer is correct after analyzing the answer choices as they relate to the situation (Sides & Cailles, 1989). An example of an application analysis question is as follows:

> Mr. Smith has just learned that he has an inoperable brain tumor. His comment when the nurse speaks to him later is ''This can't possibly be true. Mistakes are made in hospitals all the time. They might have mixed up my test results.'' The nurse's most appropriate response would be:
>
> a) Refer Mr. Smith for a psychiatric consultation
> b) *Neither agree nor disagree with Mr. Smith's comment*
> c) Confront Mr. Smith with his denial
> d) Agree with Mr. Smith that mistakes can happen and tell him you will see about getting repeat tests

To answer this question correctly, the individual must recall the fact that denial is often the initial response to learning about a terminal illness; understand that Mr. Smith's response in this case is evidence of the normal use of denial; apply this knowledge to each option, understanding why it may or may not be correct; and analyze each option for what action is most appropriate for this situation. Application/analysis questions require the examinee to use logical rationale, which demonstrates the ability to analyze a relationship, based on a well defined principle or fact. Problem solving ability becomes important as the examinee must think through each question option, deciding its relevance and importance to the situation of the question.

Building your thinking skills: Effective memorization is the cornerstone to learning and building thinking skills (Olney, 1989). We have all experienced ''memory power outages'' at some time, due in part to trying to memorize too much, too fast, too ineffectively. Developing skills to improve memorization is important to increasing the effectiveness of your thinking and subsequent test performance.

Technique #1: Quantity is NOT quality, so concentrate on learning important content. For example, it is important to know the various pharmacologic agents appropriate for the management of chronic obstructive pulmonary disease (COPD), not the specific dosages for each medication.

Technique #2: Memory from repetition, or saying something over and over again to remember it usually fades. Developing memory skills which trigger retrieval of needed facts is more useful. Such skills are as follows:

Acronyms: These are mental crutches which facilitate recall. Some are already established such as PERRL (pupils equal, round, reactive to light), or PAT (paroxysmal atrial tachycardia). Developing your own acronyms can be particularly useful since they are your own word association arrangements into a singular word. Nonsense words or funny, unusual ones are often more useful since they attract your attention.

Acrostics: This mental tool arranges words into catchy phrases. The first letter of each word stands for something which is recalled as the phrase is said. Your own acrostics are most valuable in triggering recall of learned information since they are your individual situation associations. An example of an acrostic is as follows:

Kissing **P**atty **P**roduces **A**ffection stands for the four types of nonverbal messages: **K**inesics, **P**aralanguage, **P**roxemics and **A**ppearance.

ABCs: This technique facilitates information retrieval by using the alphabet as a crutch. Each letter stands for a symptom, which when put together creates a picture of the clinical presentation of the disease. For example, the characteristics of the disease and symptoms of osteoarthritis using the ABC technique is as follows:

a) Aching or pain
b) Being stiff on awakening

c) Crepitus
d) Deterioration of articular cartilage
e) Enlargements of distal interphalangeal joints
f) Formation of new bone at joint surface
g) Granulation inflammatory tissue
h) Heberden's nodes

One letter: Recall is enhanced by emphasizing a single letter. The major symptoms of Schizophrenia are often remembered as follows:

Affect (flat)
Autism
Auditory hallucinations

Imaging: This technique can be used in two ways. The first is to develop a nickname for a clinical problem which when said produces a mental picture. For example, "a wane, wheezy pursed lip" might be used to visualize a patient with pulmonary emphysema who is thin, emaciated, experiencing dyspnea, with a hyperinflated chest, who has an elongated expiratory breathing phase. A second form of imaging is to visualize a specific patient while you are trying to understand or solve a clinical problem when studying or answering a question. For example, imagine an elderly man who is experiencing an acute asthma attack. You are trying to analyze the situation and place him in a position which maximizes respiratory effort. In your mind you visualize him in various positions of side lying, angular and forward, imaging what will happen to the man in each position. A second form of imaging is to visualize a specific situation while you are trying to answer a question. For example if you are trying to remember how to describe active listening or physical attending skills see yourself in a comfortable environment, facing the other person, with open posture and eye contact.

Rhymes, music & links: The absurd is easier to remember than the most common. Rhymes, music or links can add absurdity and humor to learning and remembering (Olney, 1989). These retrieval tools are developed by the individual for specific content. For example, making up a rhyme about diabetes may be helpful in remembering the predominant female incidence, origin of disease, primary symptoms and management as illustrated by:

There once was a woman
whose beta cells failed
She grew quite thirsty
and her glucose levels sailed
Her lack of insulin caused her to
increase her intake
And her increased urinary output
was certainly not fake
So she learned to watch her diet
and administer injections
That kept her healthy, happy
and free of complications.

Words which rhyme can also be used to jog the memory about important characteristics of phenomena. For example, the stages of group therapy can be remembered and characterized by the following according to Tuckman (1965):

Forming
Storming
Norming
Performing

Setting content to music is sometimes useful to remembering. Melodies which are repetitious jog the memory by the ups and downs of the notes and the rhythm of the music.

Links connect key words from the content by using them in a story. An example given by Olney (1989) for remembering the parts of an eye is IRIS watched a PUPIL through the LENS of a RED TIN telescope while eating CORN-EA on the cob.

Additional memory aids may also include the use of color or drawing for improving recall. Use different colored pens or paper to accentuate the material being learned. For example, highlight or make notes in blue for content about respiratory problems and in red for cardiovascular content. Drawing assists with visualizing content as well. This is particularly helpful for remembering the pathophysiology of the specific health problem.

The important thing to remember about remembering is to use good recall techniques.

Technique #3: Improving higher level thinking skills involves exercising the application and analysis of memorized fact. Small group review is particularly useful for enhancing these high level skills. It allows verbalization of thought processes and receipt of input about content and thought process from others (Sides & Cailles, 1989). Individuals not only hear how they think, but how others think as well. This interaction allows individuals to identify flaws in their thought process as well as to strengthen their positive points.

Taking practice tests are also helpful in developing application/analysis thinking skills. They permit the individual to analyze thinking patterns as well as the cause and effect relationships between the question and its options. The problem solving skills needed to answer application/analysis questions are tested, giving the individual more experience through practice (Dickenson-Hazard, 1990).

STRATEGY #3 Know The Content

Your ability to study is directly influenced by organization and concentration (Dickenson-Hazard, 1990). If effort is spent on both of these aspects of exam preparation, examination success can be increased.

Preparation for studying: Getting organized. Study habits are developed early in our educational experiences. Some of our habits enhance learning while others do not. To increase study effectiveness, organization of study materials and time is essential. Organization decreases frustration, allows for easy resumption of study and increases concentrated study time.

Technique #1: Create your own study space. Select a study area that is yours alone, free from distractions, comfortable and well lighted. The ventilation and room temperature should be comfortable since a cold room makes it difficult to concentrate and a warm room makes you sleepy (Burkle & Marshak, 1989). All your study materials should be left in your study space. The basic premise of a study space is that it facilitates a mind set that you are there to study. When you interrupt study, it is best to leave your materials just as they are. Don't close books or put away notes as you will just have to relocate them, wasting your study time, when you do resume study.

Technique #2: Define and organize the content. From the test giver, secure an outline or the content parameters which are to be examined. If the test giver's outline is sketchy, develop a more detailed one for yourself using the recommended text as a guideline. Next, identify your available study resources: class notes, old exams, handouts, textbooks, review courses, or study groups. For national standardized exams, such as initial licensing or certification, it is best to identify one or two study resources which cover the content being tested and stick to them. Attempting to review all available resources is not only mind boggling, but increases anxiety and frustration as well. Make your selections and stay with them.

Technique #3: Conduct a content assessment. Using a simple rating scale of

1 = requires no review
2 = requires minimal review
3 = requires intensive review
4 = start from the beginning

Read through the content outline and rate each content area (Dickenson-Hazard, 1990). Table 2 provides a sample exam content assessment. Be honest with your assessment. It is far better to recognize your content weaknesses when you can study and remedy them, rather than thinking during the exam how you wished you had studied more. Likewise with content strengths: if you know the material, don't waste time studying it.

Technique #4: Develop a study plan. Coordinate the content which needs to be studied with the time available (Sides & Cailles, 1989). Prioritize your study needs, starting with weak areas first. Allow for a general review at the end of the study plan. Lastly, establish an overall goal for yourself; something that will motivate you when it is brought to mind.

Table 3 illustrates a study plan developed on the basis of the exam content assessment in Table 2. Conducting an assessment and developing a study plan should require no more than 50 minutes. It is a wise investment of time with potential payoffs of reduced study stress and exam success.

Technique #5: Begin now and use your time wisely. The smart test taker begins the study process early (Olney, 1989). Sit down, conduct the content assessment and develop a study plan as soon as you know about the exam. DON'T PROCRASTINATE!

Getting Down To Business: The Actual Studying. There is no better way to prepare for an examination than individual study (Dickenson-Hazard, 1989). The responsibility to achieve the goal you set for this exam lies with you alone. The means you employ to achieve this goal do vary and should begin with identifying your peak study times and using techniques to maximize them.

Table 2

Sample Content Assessment

Category: Provided by Test Giver	*Exam Content: Theories & Skills* — *Rating: Provided by Examinee*
Group dynamics	2
Group process	2
Behavior modification	1
Crisis intervention	4
Reality therapy	3
Communication process	3
Interviewing skills	4
Self-care	3
Decision-making	1
Legal/ethical issues	2
Cognitive techniques	1
Mental status evaluation	2
Problem solving	2
Community resources evaluation	1
Nursing process	4
Nursing theory	4
Role therapy	3
Change theory	4
Communication theories	1
Organizational theory	2
Research design	2
Research evaluation	4
Research application	3
Team building	3
Conflict management	1
Teaching/learning skills	2
Supervisory skills	4
Observation skills	3
Evaluation skills	4
Nursing diagnosis	4
DSM III-R	1
Grief and loss theory	2
Death and dying	3
Stress management theory	2
Stress management skills	4
Family dynamics	1
Assertiveness training skills	2
Motivation skills	2

Technique #1: Study in short bursts. Each of us have our own biologic clock which dictates when we are at our peak during the day. If you are a morning person, you are generally active and alert early in the day, slowing down and becoming drowsy by evening. If you are an evening person, you don't completely wake up

Table 3

Sample Study Plan

Goal: Achieve a passing grade on the certification exam. Time Available: 2 Months

Objective	*Activity*	*Date Accomplished*
Understand elements of milieu therapy	Read section in Chapter 2	Feb 5 & 6, 1 hour each day
	Read notes from review class and combine with notes taken from text	Feb 7, 1 hour
	Review combined notes and sample test questions	Feb 8, 1 hour
Master social/cultural/ethnic factors	Read section in Chapter 2. Take notes on chapter content	Feb 9 & 10, 1 hour each day
	Read notes from review class and combine with notes taken from text	Feb 11, 1 hour
	Review combined notes and sample test questions	Feb 12, 1 hour
Know material contained in Code for Nurses with Interpretive Statements	Read ANA Pub. No. G-56, 1985. Take notes on content	Feb 13 & 14, 1 hour each day

until late morning and hit your peak in the afternoon and evening. Each person generally has several peaks during the day. It is best to study during those times when your alertness is at its peak (Dickenson-Hazard, 1990).

During our concentration peaks, there are mini peaks, or bursts of alertness (Olney, 1989). These alertness peaks of a concentration peak occur because levels of concentration are at their highest during the first part and last part of a study period. These bursts can vary from ten minutes to one hour depending on the extent of concentration. If studying is sustained for one hour there are only two mini peaks; one at the beginning and one at the end. There are eight mini peaks if that same hour is divided into four, 10-minute intervals. Hence it is more helpful to study in short bursts (Olney, 1989). More can be learned in less time.

Technique #2: Cramming can be useful. Since concentration ability is highly variable, some individuals can sustain their mini-peaks for 15, 20 or even 30 minutes at a time. Pushing your concentration beyond its peak is fruitless and verges on cramming, which in general is a poor study technique. There are, however, times when cramming, a short term memory tool, is useful. Short term memory generally is at its best in the morning. A quick review or cram of content in the morning can be useful the day of the exam (Olney, 1989). Most studying, however, is best accomplished in the afternoon or evening when long term memory functions at its peak.

Technique #3: Give your brain breaks. Regular times during study to rest and absorb the content is needed by the brain. The best approach to breaks is to plan them and give yourself a conscious break (Dickenson-Hazard, 1990). This approach eliminates the ''day dreaming'' or ''wandering thought'' approach to breaks that many of us use. It is better to get up, leave the study area and do something non-study related for longer breaks. For shorter breaks of 5 minutes or so, leave your desk, gaze out the window or do some stretching exercises. When your brain says to give it a rest, accommodate it! You'll learn more in less stress free time.

Technique #4: Study the correct content. It is easy for all of us to become bogged down in the detail of the content we are studying. However, it is best to focus on the major concepts or the ''state of the art'' content. Leave the details, the suppositions and the experience at the door of your study area. Concentrate on the major textbook facts and concepts which revolve around the subject matter being tested.

Technique #5: Fit your studying to the test type. The best way to prepare for an objective test is to study facts, particularly anything printed in italics or bold. Memory enhancing techniques are particularly useful when preparing for an objective test. If preparing for an essay test, study generalities, examples and concepts. Application techniques are helpful when studying for this type of an exam (Burkle & Marshak, 1989).

Technique #6: Use your study plan wisely. Your study plan is meant to be a guide, not a rigid schedule. You should take your time with studying. Don't rush through the content just to remain on schedule. Occasionally study plans need revision. If you take more or less time than planned, readjust the plan for the time gained or lost. The plan can guide you, but you must go at your own pace.

Technique #7: Actively study. Being an active participant in study rather than trying to absorb the printed word is also helpful. Ways to be active include: taking notes on the content as you study; constructing questions then answering them; taking practice tests or; discussing the content with yourself. Also using your individual study quirks are encouraged. Some people stand, others walk around and some play background music. Whatever helps you to concentrate and study better, you should use.

Technique #8: Use study aids. While there is no substitute for individual studying, several resources, if available, are useful in facilitating learning. Review courses are an excellent means for organizing or summarizing your individual study. They generally provide the content parameters and the major concepts of the content which you need to know. Review courses also provide an opportunity to clarify not-well-understood content, as well as to review known material (Dickenson-Hazard, 1990). Study guides are useful for organizing study. They provide detail on the content which is important to the exam. Study groups are an excellent resource for summarizing and refining content. They provide an opportunity for thinking through your knowledge base, with the advantage of hearing another person's point of view. Each of these study aids increases understanding of content and when used correctly, increase effectiveness of knowledge application.

Technique #9: Know when to quit. It is best to stop studying when your concentration ebbs. It is unproductive and frustrating to force yourself to study. It is far better to rest or unwind, then resume at a later point in the day. Avoid studying outside your A.M. or P.M. concentration peaks and focus your study energy on your right time of day or evening.

STRATEGY #4 Become Test-wise

Most nursing examinations are composed of multiple choice questions (MCQs). This type of question requires the examinee to select the best response(s) for a specific circumstance or condition. Successful test taking is dependent not only on content knowledge but on test taking skill as well. If you are unable to impart your knowledge through the vehicle used for its conveyance, i.e., the MCQ, your test taking success is in jeopardy.

Technique #1: Recognize the purpose of a test question. Most test questions are developed to examine knowledge at two separate levels: memory (or recall) and comprehension (or application). A memory question requires the examinee to recall facts from their knowledge base while an application question requires the examinee to use and apply the knowledge (ABP, 1989). Memory questions test recall while application questions test synthesis and problem-solving skills. When taking a test you need to be aware of whether you are being asked a fact or to use that fact.

Technique #2: Recognize the components of a test question. Multiple choice questions may include the basic components of a background statement, a stem and a list of options. The background statement presents information which facilitates the examinee in answering the question. The stem asks or states the intent of the question. The options are 4 or 5 possible responses to the question. The correct option is called the keyed response and all other options are called distractors (ABP, 1989). Knowing the components of a test question helps you sift through the information presented and focus on the question's intent (see Table 4).

Table 4

Anatomy Of A Test Question

Background Statement:	A woman brings her 65 year old mother in to see a clinical nurse specialist because she is concerned that it is now a month since her mother was widowed and she continues to be tearful when talking about the loss and wants to visit the grave regularly.
Stem:	Which of the following initial approaches would most likely result in compliance with your nursing recommendations?
Options:	(A) Three or four short questions followed by requesting a psychiatrist to prescribe an antidepressant (B) Immediate Reassurance only *(C) Careful listening and open-ended questions* (D) Refer the mother to a support group

Table 5

Test Question Key Words And Phrases

First	Priority	True Statements
Best	Advice	Correct Statements
Most	Approach	Contributing to
Initial	Consideration	Of the following
Important	Management	Which of the following
Major	Expectation	Each of the following
Common	Intervention	
Least	Assessment	
Except	Contraindication	
Not	Evaluation	
Greatest	Counseling	
Earliest	Facilitative	
Useful	Indicative	
Leading	Suggestive	
Significant	Appropriate	
Immediate	Accurately	
Helpful	Likely	
Closely	Characteristics	

From ''Anatomy of a test question'' by N. Dickenson-Hazard, 1989, *Pediatric Nursing 15,* p. 395. Copyright 1989 by A. J. Jannetti, Inc. Reprinted by permission.

Technique #3: Identify the key word(s) in a test question. Key words are generally included in the stem of a test question, whereas key concepts or conditions appear in the background statement. You should pay particular attention to the key words in the stem and their impact on the intent of the question (See Table 5).

Technique #4: Recognize the item types. Basically two styles of MCQs are used for examinations. One requires the examinee to select the one best answer; the other requires selection of multiple correct answers. Among the one best answer styles there are 3 types. The A type requires the selection of the best response among those offered. The B type requires the examinee to match the options with the appropriate statement. C type items require the examinee to compare or contrast two related conditions. The X type asks the examinee to respond either true or false to each option (ABP, 1989). Table 6, on the following page illustrates these item types. **Most standardized tests, such as those used for nursing licensure and certification, are composed of four or five option-A type questions.**

Technique #5: Read the directions to the questions carefully. Since an examination may have several types of questions, it is imperative to read the directions carefully. If different item types are used on an exam, they are generally grouped together by type and marked clearly with directions. Be on the lookout for changing item types and be sure you understand the directions on how you are to answer before you begin reading the question.

Technique #6: Apply the basic rules of test taking. Examination candidates can avert many problems associated with test taking if they give thought to the mechanics of sitting down, reading the question and noting their answers. Timing yourself to avoid spending too much time on a question, returning to difficult questions, and not changing your answers are all techniques that can improve performance. Table 7 provides helpful hints for the basic rules of test-taking. Review these and apply them to the testing situation.

Technique #7: Practice, practice, practice. Taking practice tests can improve performance. While they can assist in evaluation of your knowledge, their primary benefit is to assist you with test taking skills. You should use them to evaluate your thinking process, your ability to read, understand and interpret questions, and your skills in completing the mechanics of the test.

Technique #8: Be prepared for exam day. It is important to familiarize yourself with the test site, the building, the parking and travel route prior to the exam day. If you must travel, arrive early to allow time for this familiarization. It is helpful to make a list of things you need on the exam day: pencils, admission card, watch and a few pieces of hard candy as a quick energy source. On exam day allow yourself plenty of time to arrive at the site. Wear comfortable clothes and have a good breakfast that morning. The night before the exam, go to bed at a reasonable hour; avoid last minute cramming; and avoid excessive drinking or eating (Sides & Cailles, 1989). The idea is to arrive on time at the test site, prepared and as rested as possible.

TABLE 6

Item Type Examples

A TYPE

Directions for One Best Choice Items: This item-type requires that you indicate the one best answer from the lettered alternatives offered for each item. After you have decided on the one BEST answer, completely blacken the corresponding lettered circle on the answer sheet.

#1 Sally is a 28 year old client with Schizophrenia. One day she says to the nurse: "I see you are wearing black shoes today. That means you have it in for me." Sally is experiencing:

(A) A delusion
(B) A hallucination
(C) *An idea of reference*
(D) An imaginary fantasy

B TYPE

Directions: Each group of questions below consists of five lettered headings followed by a list of numbered words or statements. For each numbered word or statement, select the one lettered heading that is most closely associated with it and fill in the circle beneath the corresponding letter on the answer sheet. Each lettered heading may be selected once, more than once, or not at all.

#2-4

Laboratory test:

(A) Lithium level
(B) Dexamethasone Suppression Test
(C) MAOI level
(D) Benzodiazepine level

Related to the treatment of:

#2. Depression (B)
#3. Manic Depression (A)
#4. Substance Abuse (D)

C TYPE

Directions: Each set of lettered headings below is followed by a list of numbered words or phrases. For each numbered word or phrase fill in the circle on the answer sheet under:

a. If the item is associated with (A) only,
b. If the item is associated with (B) only,
c. If the item is associated with both (A) and (B),
d. If the item is associated with neither (A) nor (B).

(A) Antipsychotic medication
(B) Antidepressant medication
(C) Both
(D) Neither

#5 — Dry mouth (C)
#6 — Hypertensive crisis (B)
#7 — Sedation (C)
#8 — Extrapyramidal side effects (A)
#9 — Urinary frequency (D)

X TYPE

Directions: Each of the questions or incomplete statements below is followed by five suggested answers or completions. For EACH lettered alternative completely blacken one lettered circle in either column T or F on the answer sheet.

#10 True statements about developmental processes according to theorists include:

(A) According to Freud, from birth to 18 months the infant is learning muscle control, especially that related to defecation (F)
(B) According to Erikson the task of Adulthood is Generativity vs Stagnation (T)
(C) According to Sullivan the task of late adolescence is developing an enduring relationship with members of the same sex (F)
(D) According to Piaget from ages 7 to 12 the child learns to reason systematically and use abstract thought (T)
(E) According to most theorists, children begin to learn socially acceptable behavior when they can delay gratification and incorporate the demands of significant others (T)

From "Anatomy of a test question." by N. Dickenson-Hazard, 1989, *Pediatric Nursing 15,* p. 396. Copyright 1989 by A. J. Jannetti, Inc. Adapted by permission.

TABLE 7

Basic Rules For Test Taking

Basic Rule	Helpful Hints
Use time wisely and effectively	Allow no more than 1 minute per question —If you can't answer question, make an intelligent guess
Know the parts of a question Background statement: Informational scenario Stem: Specific question or intent statement	Select the option that best completes question or solves the problem Relate options to question and balance against each other Cnsider all options
Read question carefully	Understand stem first, then look for answer Underline key words in background information and stem (i.e. first, best, initial, early, most, appropriate, except, least, not).
Identify intent of item based on information given	Don't assume any information not given Don't read in or add any information not given Actively reason through question
Answer difficult questions by eliminating obviously incorrect options first	Select the best of the viable, available options using logical thought Reread stem; select strongest option Skip difficult questions and return to them later or make an educated guess
Select responses guided by principles of communication	Choose therapeutic, respectful, communication enhancing options Avoid inappropriate, punitive responses
Know the principles of nursing practice	Select options that relate to common need or the population in general Select options that are correct without exception Select options which reflect nursing judgement
Know and use test-taking principles	Avoid changing answers without good reason Attempt every question Don't rely on flaws in test construction Be systematic and use problem-solving technique in answering questions

From ''Making the grade as a test-taker'' by N. Dickenson-Hazard, 1989. *Pediatric Nursing 15,* p. 304. Adapted from *How to take tests.* (pp 15-57) by J. Millman and W. Paul, 1969, New York: McGraw-Hill Co. and from *Nurses's guide to successful test taking.* (pp 43-53) by M.B. Sides and N.B. Cailles, 1989, Philadelphia: J. B. Lippincott Co. Copyright 1989 A.J. Jannetti, Inc. Reprinted and adapted by permission.

STRATEGY #5 Psych Yourself Up: Taking tests is stressful

While a little stress can be productive, too much can incapacitate you in your studying and test taking (Divine & Kylen, 1979). Your attitude and approach to test taking and studying can influence the results you achieve. Psyching yourself up can have a positive affect and make examinations a non-anxiety laden experience (Dickenson-Hazard, 1990). The following techniques are based on the principles of successful test taking as presented by Sides & Cailles (1989). Incorporation of these techniques can improve response and performance in examination situations.

Technique #1: Adopt an ''I can'' attitude. Believing you can succeed is the key to success. Self belief inspires and gives you the power to achieve your goals. Without a success attitude, the road to your goal is much harder. We all stand an equal chance of success in this world. It is those who believe they can who achieve it. This "I can" attitude must permeate all your efforts in test taking, from studying, to improving your skills, to actually writing the test.

Technique #2: Take control. By identifying your goal, deciding how to accomplish it and developing a plan for achieving it, you take control. Do not leave your success to chance; control it through action and attitude.

Technique #3: Think positively. Examinations are generally based on a standard which is the same for all individuals. Everyone can potentially pass. Performance is influenced not only by knowledge and skill but by attitude as well. Those individuals who regard an exam as an opportunity or challenge will be more successful.

Technique #4: Project a positive self-fulfilling prophecy. While preparing for an examination, project thoughts of the positive outcomes you will experience when you succeed. Self-talk is self-fulfilling. Expect success, not failure, of yourself.

Technique #5: Feel good about yourself. Without feeling a sense of positive self worth, passing an examination is difficult. Recognize your professional contributions and give yourself credit for your accomplishments. Think "I will pass", not "I suppose I can".

Technique #6: Know yourself. Focus exam preparation and test taking on your strengths. Try to alter your weaknesses instead of becoming hung up on them. If you tend to overanalyze, study and read test questions at face value. If you're a speed demon when taking a test, slow down and read more carefully.

Technique #7: Failure is a possibility. We all have failed at something at some point in our lives. Rather than dwelling on the failure, making excuses and believing you'll fail again, recognize your mistakes and remedy them. Failure is a time to begin again; use it as a motivator to do better. It is not the end of the world unless you allow it to be. It is best to deal with the failure and move on, otherwise it interferes with your success.

Technique #8: Persevere, persevere, persevere! Endurance must underlie all your efforts. Call forth those reserve energies when you've had all you think you can take. Rely upon yourself and your support systems to help you maintain a sense of direction and keep your goal in the forefront.

Technique #9: Motivation is muscle. Most individuals are motivated by fear or desire. The fear in an exam situation may be one of failure, the unknown or discovery of imperfection. Put your fear into perspective; realize you are not the only one with fear and that all have an equal opportunity for success. Develop strategies to reduce fear and use fear to your advantage by improving the imperfections. Desire is a powerful motivator and you should keep the rewards of your desire foremost in your mind. Whatever motivates you, use it to make you successful. Reward yourself during your exam preparation and once the exam has been completed. You alone hold the key to success; use what you have wisely.

This chapter has provided concepts, strategies and techniques for improving study and test taking skills. Your first task in improvement is to know yourself: how you study and how you take a test. You should use your strengths and remedy the weaknesses. Next you need to develop your thinking skills. Work on techniques to improve memory and reasoning. Now you need to organize your study and concentrate on using your strengths and these new and improved skills to be successful. Create a study space, develop a plan of action, then implement that plan during your periods of peak concentration. Before taking the exam be sure you understand the components of a test question, can identify key words and phrases and have practiced. Apply the test taking rules during the exam process. Finally, believe in yourself, your knowledge and your talent. Believing you can accomplish your goal facilitates the fact that you will.

BIBLIOGRAPHY

American Board of Pediatrics. (1989). *Developing questions and critiques.* Unpublished material.

Burke, M. M., & Walsh, M. B. (1992). *Gerontologic nursing*, St. Louis: Mosby Year Book.

Burkle, C.A., & Marshak, D. (1989). *Study program: Level 1.* Reston, Va: National Association of Secondary School Principals.

Conaway, D. C., Miller, M. D., & West, G. R. (1988). *Geriatrics.* St. Louis: Mosby Year Book.

Dickenson-Hazard, N. (1989). Making the grade as a test taker. *Pediatric Nursing*, *15*, 302–304.

Dickenson-Hazard, N. (1989). Anatomy of a test question. *Pediatric Nursing*, *15*, 395–399.

Dickenson-Hazard, N. (1990). The psychology of successful test taking. *Pediatric Nursing*, *16*, 66–67.

Dickenson-Hazard, N. (1990). Study smart. *Pediatric Nursing*, *16*, 314–316.

Dickenson-Hazard, N. (1990). Study effectiveness: Are you 10 a.m. or p.m. scholar? *Pediatric Nursing*, 16, 419–420.

Dickenson-Hazard, N. (1990). Develop your thinking skills for improved test taking. *Pediatric Nursing*, 16, 480–481.

Divine, J. H., & Kylen, D. W. (1979). *How to beat test anxiety.* New York: Barrons Educational Series, Inc.

Millman, J., & Pauk, W. (1969). *How to take tests.* New York: McGraw-Hill Book Co.

Millonig, V. L. (Ed.). (1991). *The adult nurse practitioner certification review guide* (rev. ed). Potomac, MD: Health Leadership Associates.

Olney, C. W. (1989). *Where there's a will, there's an A.* New Jersey: Chesterbrook Educational Publishers.

Sides, M., & Cailles, N. B. (1989). *Nurse's guide to successful test taking.* Philadelphia: J. B. Lippincott Co.

Essentials of Care

Clare Houseman

Mental Health

- Definition: Traditionally, to both love and work successfully; some definitions also include happiness.
- Components according to Johnson (1993):
    1. Self-governance—autonomy, guidance from values within; functions dependently, interdependently or independently as needed
    2. Growth orientation—strives for self-realization, androgyny,and maximization of capacities
    3. Tolerance of uncertainty—uses faith and hope to face life and death
    4. Self-esteem—built on awareness of abilities and limitations
    5. Environmental mastery—creative and effective in influencing and reacting to surroundings
    6. Reality orientation—tells fact from fantasy and responds accordingly
    7. Stress management—experiences appropriate depression, anxiety, tolerates stress as temporary and can tolerate failure; flexible and copes with crises with help from friends and family
- Absence of mental health may be perceived as uncomfortable to the individual and/or his significant others and result in the perception of a need for change.

Change

- Definition: Process resulting in transformation
- Planned change—deliberate, goal directed effort to solve problems; applicable to any system (individual, family, organization)
- Process involves the following responses according to Huelskoetter and Romano (1991):
    1. Feelings of tension, anxiety, and fear
    2. A sense of need
    3. Feelings of hope
    4. A search
    5. Decision and goal setting

6. Commitment to goals and change
7. Creative behavior
8. Changes in behavior

- Success of change dependent on the change agent's ability to facilitate a helping relationship and collaborate with the individual, group, family, or organization
- Change involves risk and resistance. It cannot be rushed.
- Change is effected by nurses within the nursing process.

The Nursing Process—involves the following:

- Assessment—data are collected in a continuous, comprehensive, accurate, and systematic manner. Interviews are usually conducted with clients and others to complete the nursing history. Relevant data include:
    1. Appearance
    2. Presenting problem
    3. Personal and family history
    4. Medical and psychiatric history
    5. Physical status
    6. Mental status
        a. Reaction to interview
        b. Behavior (Speech, ADL, etc)
        c. Level of consciousness
        d. Orientation
        e. Intellect
        f. Thought content and process
        g. Judgment
        h. Affect
        i. Mood
        j. Insight

k. Memory

l. Comprehension

7. Sociocultural status

   a. Socioeconomic status

   b. Life values and goals

   c. Social habits—including drinking and drug use

   d. Sexual behavior

   e. Social support network

8. Spiritual status

   a. Philosophy and meaning of life

   b. Sense of oneness or spiritual integrity

   c. Relatedness to God or higher power

   d. Relatedness to people and nature

- Diagnoses are made according to:

  1. North American Nursing Diagnosis Association (NANDA)

  2. Standard classification of mental disorders, i.e., The American Psychiatric Association's Diagnosis and Statistical Manual (DSM IV) or International Classification of Disease (ICD10)

- Planning provides goals and actions that are:

  1. Specific

  2. Individualized

  3. Collaborative

- Intervention—treatment according to diagnoses and care plan should be based on scientific theory and includes:

  1. Psychotherapeutic interventions—may be talking, poetry writing, social skills training, cooking, modeling assertiveness, or expression of feelings

  2. Health teaching—about medication, nutrition, sleep hygiene

  3. Self-care activities—i.e., relaxation, exercise, spirituality

  4. Somatic therapies—i.e., nursing care of clients receiving ECT

5. Therapeutic environment—milieu
6. Psychotherapy (Clinical Nurse Specialist role)
7. Interventions can be interdependent (other team members must collaborate) or independent (discussed and determined with client)

- Evaluation of client responses to nursing action is based on client changes in the following:
  1. Cognition
     a. Giving up irrational beliefs
     b. Making positive self-statements
     c. Improved ability to problem solve
  2. Affect
     a. Decreased anxiety
     b. Decreased depression
     c. Decreased loneliness
  3. Behavior
     a. Adaptive responses
     b. Improved coping skills
     c. Improved social skills
- Revisions to plan of care are made as needed and the process continues.
- The nursing process and all nursing interventions occur within the context of the nurse-client relationship.

Nurse-Client Relationship

- Definition: A dynamic, collaborative, therapeutic, interactive process between the nurse and the client
- Purpose—to create a safe climate wherein clients feel free to reveal themselves and their concerns and feel comfortable to try out new ideas and behaviors
- Phases of nurse-client relationship according to Peplau (1952):
  1. Orientation—begin as strangers

a. Client—seeks or is brought in for help; communicates needs and expectations

b. Nurse—responds to client; explains parameters of relationship; gathers data; listens and clarifies areas of concern; establishes rapport; negotiates contract which establishes frequency and duration of sessions, specifies type of work to be done, clarifies fees if any, and lays groundwork for termination

2. Identification

   a. Client—responds to help offered by nurse, explores deeper feelings, identifies with nurse and may be dependent, active, and compliant

   b. Nurse—structures relationship to focus on client and facilitates expression of problems and feelings; avoids fostering unnecessary dependency; encourages self-care

3. Exploitation—working

   a. Client—more independent in accessing services and working in partnership to interpret behaviors; begins to try out new behaviors

   b. Nurse—supports client and explores feelings and problems at client's pace; deals with resistances, encourages risk taking and facilitates achievement of goals

4. Resolution—termination

   a. Client—engages in new problem-solving skills and coping behaviors; views self positively and plans for future; may decompensate when anticipating separation

   b. Nurse—reviews goals and accomplishments; shares own feelings and assists client to express feelings about relationship and separation

- Phenomena that occur in nurse-client relationships

  1. Therapeutic use of self—application of nurse's own personality characteristics within the interaction to facilitate healing

  2. Transference—client experiences emotional reaction towards nurse based on unconscious feelings that originated in past relationships. Nursing response is to confront distortions of reality gently to facilitate client self-awareness.

3. Countertransference—nurse responds to client with feelings from own earlier conflicts. Nurse must increase self-awareness and access supervision to assist in dealing with client more effectively.
4. Resistance—attempts to keep anxiety-provoking thoughts and feelings out of awareness by disrupting the interactional process with avoidance, acting out, forgetting, silence, lateness, etc. Nursing response is to make observations and support client in dealing with anxiety.
5. Testing behaviors according to McMahon (1992)
   a. Attempting a social relationship
   b. Casting nurse into parental role
   c. Assessing whether nurse trusts them
   d. Attempting to take care of nurse
   e. Avoiding discussion of problems
   f. Asking for personal data
   g. Violating personal space
   h. Seeking attention from nurse
   i. Assessing nurse's commitment
   j. Revealing information to shock nurse
   k. Touching nurse inappropriately

   Nurse must set limits and encourage client to discuss meaning of behavior.

- Psychotherapy—use of relationship and communication to change feelings, attitudes, and behaviors
  1. Supportive—express feelings, explore choices
  2. Re-educative—learn new ways of belief and behavior
  3. Reconstructive—deep emotional and cognitive restructuring

Communication

- Definition: Continuous process by which information is transmitted between people and their environment
- Goal—understanding

- Process of communication:

Figure 1: Process of Communication

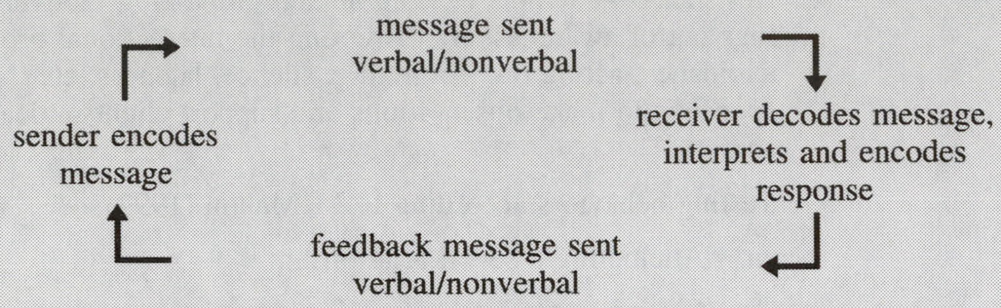

- All behavior communicates some message.
- Verbal messages include the written and spoken word.
- Nonverbal messages are observed by the receiver in four ways:
  1. Kinesics—body motion, i.e., facial expression, posture, position of arms and legs, eye contact, touch
  2. Paralanguage—tone of voice, inflection, emphasis, pauses, sighs, laughter
  3. Proxemics—use of personal space, territoriality, i.e., backing away or moving closer, selection of a particular seating arrangement
  4. Appearance—personal image, i.e., clothing, makeup, hair, beard
- Nonverbal messages may be congruent with verbal messages or they may conflict with them
- Culture and social class influence perceptions and values which influence how communication is transmitted and received.
- Type of relationship also influences type of communication.
  1. Therapeutic communication takes place between the nurse and client and focuses on the client's thoughts, feelings, behavior, and roles with the expectation that the active listening of the nurse will help the client explore, understand, and change.
  2. Social communication is less goal oriented, more superficial and does not necessarily involve the expectation of help.

- Although nurse-client relationships may involve some social communication, the main component is therapeutic communication.

Therapeutic communication includes:

- Active listening or physical attending skills:
    1. Comfortable environment—privacy, low noise, soft light
    2. Facing the other person and leaning towards him/her
    3. Open, relaxed posture
    4. Eye contact
- Attitude
    1. Non-judgmental
    2. Positive regard
    3. Acceptance and confirmation
    4. Respect
    5. Genuineness
    6. Empathy
- Communication techniques
    1. Using broad openings and open-ended questions
    2. Clarifying content and feelings
    3. Reflecting content and feelings
    4. Confronting content and feelings
    5. Verifying perceptions
    6. Giving information
    7. Providing feedback
    8. Stating observations
    9. Silence
    10. Directing
    11. Focusing
    12. Questioning

13. Connecting information
14. Summarizing

- Barriers to therapeutic communication
    1. Advice
    2. Reassurance
    3. Being judgmental
    4. Changing the subject
    5. Excessive questioning/ closed-ended questions
    6. Challenging
    7. Stereotypical comments
    8. Self-focusing behavior
    9. Using emotionally charged words
- Communication with children
    1. Introduce to play materials
    2. Encourage to verbalize at own pace
    3. Ask questions that are relevant to developmental age
- Result of therapeutic communication is enhanced client self-disclosure
- Nurse self-disclosure can enhance or inhibit therapeutic communication depending on its use. Like all interventions, it requires timing and judgment. Its use, according to Auvil and Silver (1984) depends on:
    1. Nurse's theoretical framework—i.e., more likely to occur if working from a humanist perspective than from a psychoanalytic or behaviorist approach
    2. Stage of the relationship:
        a. Orientation—nurse self-disclosure that occurs early in the relationship more likely to meet nurses' needs
        b. Working phase—appropriate if used by the nurse to help client cooperate within the relationship, learn about themselves and others, encourage their catharsis of feelings and support their goals

c. Termination—expression of feelings about end of relationship to model appropriate behaviors for client

Cultural and Ethnic Factors

- Definitions
  1. Culture—patterns of knowledge, belief, behavior, and custom that are learned by members of a particular society
  2. Ethnicity—membership in diverse groups according to race, birthplace, language, culture, or religion
  3. Ethnocentric—judging others' behavior by the values of our own culture
  4. Culturally relativistic—attempting to understand the behavior of others within the context of their own culture
  5. Stereotype—overgeneralizations based on culture or ethnicity; may occur unconsciously
- Impact of culture on mental health nursing
  1. Influences client coping behaviors
  2. Defines what symptoms are labelled as illness
  3. Prescribes taboo topics and behaviors
  4. Determines how mentally ill are perceived
  5. Prescribes health-seeking behaviors and attitudes to health care providers
  6. Determines types of acceptable treatment approaches
- Cultural differences according to Tripp-Reimer and Lively (1993):
  1. Time—emphasis on present (predominant in African American, Native American and Hispanic culture) vs. future (predominant in U.S. and other highly industrialized nations which also value schedules)
  2. Success—doing: people valued for accomplishments (Predominant U.S.) vs. being: people valued for being themselves (Chinese)
  3. Relational—collectivist: individual goals are subordinate to group goals (African and Native American and Hispanic) vs. individualistic: individual goals are more important than group goals (Predominant U.S.)

4. Nature—people dominant to nature(Middle class U.S.) vs. live in harmony with nature (Native American), vs. subjugated to nature (Moslem cultures)
5. Verbal Communication—volume (Asians speak softly), speed and directness (Asians value indirectness); silence interpreted differently by various cultures
6. Privacy—personal space (arabic:closer vs. U.S.: further); eye contact (Native American prefer less than predominant U.S.)

- Nursing approaches
  1. Have a clear understanding of the client's culture
  2. Know the role expectations of the nurse in that group, e.g., white middle class client might expect the nurse to be democratic and non-directive. Hispanic, Asian, or Native American clients may view nurse as an authority figure who gives suggestions.
  3. Adapt your activity level, tone of voice, and remarks to the cultural background of the client.
  4. Show respect and acceptance to clients in ways they understand.

Interdisciplinary Treatment and the Health Care Team

- Components
  1. Interdisciplinary treatment utilizes members of different professions who come together to plan and evaluate the treatment of individual clients.
  2. Each member is considered to have vital input to the treatment plan based on his/her particular area of expertise.
  3. The client is also considered to be a member of the team.
- Goal—targeted interventions, consistently implemented and evaluated by everyone involved with the client
- Attributes of mental health team
  1. Strong team commitment
  2. Shared responsibility, control, and decision making
  3. Common goals and philosophy of intervention
  4. Flattened heirarchy of authority

5. Decision making by consensus
6. Open communication
7. Examination of roles and relationships
8. Setting limits on own and others' behavior in a nonpunitive way
9. Flexibility, versatility, creativity, and optimism

- Professions involved with mental health team
    1. Diet therapy—provides culturally relevant, attractive, nourishing foods with awareness of psychological importance of food, conflicts about eating (Eating Disorders) and drug interactions with certain foods (MAO Inhibitors)
    2. Expressive therapies
        a. Art—uses art work of clients to express underlying feelings and conflicts
        b. Music—vicarious listening stimulates the expression of ideas and emotions verbally. Active production of music allows for nonverbal expression
        c. Psychodrama—exploration of psychological conflicts through enactment rather than verbalization
    3. Nursing—establishes and maintains milieu; responsible for 24-hour care, activities of daily living and safety. Clinical Nurse Specialists may perform individual, family, or group psychotherapy.
    4. Ministry—assists with spiritual care of client and family; may provide marital therapy or pastoral counseling
    5. Psychiatry—diagnoses and treats conditions amenable to medical treatment; responsible for admission and discharge; may provide individual, group, or family therapy
    6. Occupational Therapy—involves clients in meaningful activities and provides vocational rehabilitation if needed
    7. Psychology—performs diagnostic testing, and provides plans for treatment based on causative factors; may implement individual, group, or family therapy
    8. Social Work—evaluates family, social, and environmental contributions to problem; may provide family, group, or individual psychotherapy

- Nurses may be case managers for clients or client advocates at all levels within the health care system.

Client Advocacy

- Definition: Interceding on behalf of clients who are unable to speak or act for themselves or are unaware of available options
- Examples
  1. Informing clients about treatment alternatives
  2. Presenting information to the treatment team
  3. Helping clients enter and navigate the health care system
  4. Testifying on behalf of clients in court
  5. Promoting respect for mentally ill in policy and law
- Guidelines for advocacy according to Boyd and Luetje (1991)
  1. Make sure client has need for advocacy.
  2. Check plans with clients and others regarding support system.
  3. Get support and information from others with similar goals.
  4. Present data clearly.
  5. Include all pertinent information.
  6. Don't use more power than is necessary.
  7. Be patient and persistent.

Case Management

- Definition: Assessment for, and coordination of, individualized, culturally appropriate mental health, and other health and social services, for clients and their families or residential care groups
- Goal—improved functioning and empowerment for clients and cost containment and provider accountability for third party payers
- Types
  1. Rehabilitative—refers to time-limited services provided as part of a private benefit plan with emphasis on returning client to productivity

2. Supportive—refers to services provided to chronically mentally ill clients for as long as necessary

Psychiatric Liason Nursing

- Providing and coordinating psychiatric care and maintaining a therapeutic environment for clients admitted with a physical symptom or dysfunction
- Clinical Nurse Specialist, as member of the health care team, provides direct care, including psychotherapy, to individuals, groups, and families as well as consultation to nursing and other hospital staff, around client, unit, or institutional issues.
- Staff may accept or reject suggestions of Clinical Specialist Liason Nurse since this role is a consultative one which does not involve administrative authority.
- Liason nurses use knowledge about "systems, change, organizations, problem solving, stress, crisis, interpersonal relationships, communication, and sociocultural concepts" (Walker and Price-Hoskins, 1992, p. 267).

Milieu

- Definitions
  1. Therapeutic environment—physical and psychosocial surroundings as an integrated, interrelated whole are seen as the treatment agent in a variety of settings (Watson, 1992)
  2. Milieu therapy—scientific planning of the social and physical environment so that every interaction and activity is therapeutic
  3. Therapeutic community—a structured environment with an established philosophy of care
  4. Token community—therapeutic community drawn from behavior modification theory; uses tokens to reinforce adaptive behavioral responses; clients can then exchange tokens for privileges.
- Structured aspects of milieu
  1. Community meetings
  2. Daily schedule
  3. Physical environment
  4. Rules and regulations

5. Classes, activities, and groups

- Unstructured aspects of milieu
  1. Daily interactions among clients
  2. Interactions between clients and staff
- Characteristics of successful milieu
  1. Effective interaction between and among staff and clients
  2. Norms which provide predictability and security
  3. Patient government using democratic process
  4. Patient's active responsibility for own treatment and for treatment of others
  5. Fosters growth in direction of increased recognition of strengths and personal empowerment
  6. Encourages self awareness, risk taking, and change
  7. Confronts misperceptions, destructive behavior, and poor judgment
  8. Links with client's family and significant others
  9. Links with community
- Nurses' role in milieu
  1. Creation and maintenance of milieu
  2. Physical care and assurance of safety
  3. Medication administration and education
  4. Attitude therapy—active friendliness, passive friendliness, kind firmness, no demand
  5. Model healthy behavior as participant in community
  6. Intervene to influence attitudes, behaviors, and relationships in therapeutic way as described by Greene (1993):
     a. Clarify and correct perceptions of current stressors.
     b. Identify thoughts and feelings evoked by stressors.
     c. Examine how thoughts and feelings influence behavior.
     d. Evaluate the extent to which coping behaviors are adaptive or effective.

e. Identify alternative adaptive coping strategies.

f. Test identified alternative coping stragegies in milieu.

Group dynamics and group process theory

- Background
  1. Groups are complex human systems whose whole is greater than the sum of their parts.
  2. Individuals can learn, grow, and change more in groups due to opportunities for feedback and consensual validation.
  3. Nurses who participate in groups or Clinical Nurse Specialists who serve as group therapists are aware of the powerful forces harnessed by group work.
- Curative factors of groups (Yalom, 1985)
  1. Imparting information
  2. Instillation of hope
  3. Universality
  4. Altruism
  5. Imitative behaviors
  6. Interpersonal learning
  7. Catharsis
  8. Corrective recapitulation of primary family group
  9. Development of socializing techniques
  10. Group cohesiveness
  11. Existential factors
- Descriptors of groups
  1. Homogeneous—members chosen for preselected criteria, i.e., sexually abused women.
  2. Heterogeneous—mix of individuals regarding diagnosis, but vary sex, age, etc.
  3. Mixed—share essential feature, i.e., same diagnosis but vary sex, age, etc.

4. Closed—after group begins, no new members are added.
5. Open—members and leaders change.

- Types of groups
  1. Task—emphasis on accomplishing what needs to be done
  2. Teaching—impart information, i.e., orient to unit
  3. Supportive/therapeutic—help others who share same experience cope with stress and overcome dysfunction, i.e., bereavement, weight loss.
  4. Psychotherapy—emphasis is on person reducing intrapsychic stress, changing behavior, ideas, etc. Clinical Nurse Specialist role.
  5. Psychoeducational—structured group involving teaching, with member disclosure of related thinking and behavioral problems, and homework to put learned information and skills into practice, e.g., groups for family members of the chronically mentally ill and assertiveness training groups
  6. Peer support group—share stresses related to common situation, e.g., hospice nurses
  7. Multiple family—teach about disease process and utilize group process to understand mental health issues; may also refer to a group modality in which the therapist works with one family while other families watch and learn vicariously
- Group dynamic issues according to Long and McMahon (1992)
  1. Rank—position member holds in relation to other members of the group; members who participate frequently and actively usually rank high in the group and thus have greater influence on group behavior.
  2. Status—prestige given to certain positions or individuals in a group; members vie for status in group; may be due to member characteristics or behavior
  3. Group content—what is said in a group, i.e., information discussed
  4. Group process—activities in a group, i.e., how interactions occur among members, timing of interactions, roles of members, seating arrangements, tone of voice of members, and nonverbal behaviors
  5. Sociogram—method of recording group process

- Group process issues
    1. Style of leader
        a. Autocratic—leader is in charge and controls.
        b. Democratic—leader shares responsibility with members.
        c. Laissez Faire—leader is nondirective.
    2. Roles of members
        a. Building or maintenance roles—contribute to group process and functioning, e.g., encourager, gatekeeper, harmonizer.
        b. Task roles—emphasize completing the task, e.g., initiator, opinion giver, evaluator, energizer, information seeker
        c. Individual roles—not related to group tasks or maintenance and may inhibit group, e.g., aggressor, dominator, help-seeker, playboy, special-interest pleader, blocker.
- Group development stages (Tuckman, 1965)
    1. Forming—(orientation)—group leader more directive and active, members look to leader for structure and approval. Leader describes group contract (i.e., goals, confidentiality, and communication rules), encourages interaction among group, and maintains working level of anxiety. Members develop initial roles.
    2. Storming—conflict regarding control, power, and authority. Anxiety increases and resistance may occur as evidenced by client absence, shared silence, excessive dependency on leader, scapegoating, excessive hostility toward the leader, forming subgroups and acting out. Leader encourages healthy expression of anger.
    3. Norming—(cohesiveness stage)—members express positive feelings toward one another and feel strongly attracted to the group. Self-disclosure occurs and new roles are adopted.
    4. Performing—(working phase)—leader's activity decreases and usually consists of keeping the group on course or dealing with resistance of group and individuals within. Responsibility for group is more equally shared. Anxiety of group is decreased and energy is channeled to completing tasks.
    5. Mourning—(termination)—begins during first phase but is most acutely felt in closed group when it approaches end and in open

group when members or leaders leave. Leaders encourage discussion of ending and expression of pain and loss experienced in grieving process. Members may try to avoid, experience anxiety, anger, or regression; they should also be encouraged to reminisce, evaluate, and experience sense of accomplishment and give feedback to one another (Lasalle and Lasalle, 1991).

- Transference and countertransference also occur in groups and may be dealt with by group members as well as leaders.

Family Therapy

- Background
  1. Treatment modality which theorizes that the presenting problem displayed by the client with psychiatric symptoms (identified patient) is of the result of pathology throughout the entire family system.
  2. This family dysfunction is due to imbalances in the system, generally caused by conflict between the marital partners. This conflict is expressed unconsciously by the following behaviors:
     a. Triangling—another family member is brought in, in order to stabilize the emotional process.
     b. Scapegoating—another family member is blamed.
  3. Result of these behaviors is psychiatric symptoms.
- Therapeutic goals
  1. Assist family members to identify and express their thoughts and feelings.
  2. Resolve conflict between marital partners to decrease need for triangling and scapegoating.
  3. Assist parents to work together and strengthen their parental authority.
  4. Clarify family expectations and roles.
  5. Practice different, more constructive methods of interacting.
- Techniques used in family therapy according to Hogarth (1993)
  1. Joining—finding similarities and matching family's behaviors; respecting their values and hierarchies
  2. The family history

a. Data are gathered beginning with the parents' initial relationship and include each family member in chronological order.

b. Information may be recorded in a genogram which maps out significant events and relationships over three generations of the family.

c. History taking takes focus off identified patient and emphasizes the family as a whole.

3. Encouraging interactions and relationships

   a. The family, or specific family members, are instructed to discuss a pertinent issue.

   b. Therapist clarifies and interprets the family's communication.

   c. Individuals required to speak for themselves in expressing feelings and concerns rather than allowing others to speak for them

   d. Family members asked to share responsibility for resolution of problems instead of laying blame

4. Experiential activities

   a. Homework—tasks assigned by the therapist, which when enacted by the family members further the therapeutic process; completion or failure to complete the task is discussed at the next session.

   b. Paradoxical prescription—instructions to perform the opposite of what is intended in order to produce change

   c. Sculpting—enactment of an experience with words omitted that when "frozen" is a symbolic representation of the family members' relationships; by asking a family member to rearrange the "sculpture," change is modeled.

5. Results in family therapy are measured by the degree to which families are moved from dysfunctional to functional patterns. Optimal family functioning according to Hogarth (1993) includes:

   a. Open systems orientation

   b. Clear boundaries

   c. Positive links to society

   d. Contextual clarity

e. Clear and congruent communication

f. Strong parental coalition

g. Appropriate power distribution

h. Autonomous persons

i. Warm, caring affective tone

j. High self-esteem of members

k. Efficient negotiation and task performance

l. Transcendent values of hope and altruism

Ethical Aspects

- Ethics—branch of philosophy that deals with morality
- Ethical theories or perspectives according to Sellin (1991):
  1. Egoism—the right act is the one best for oneself.
  2. Utilitarianism—the right act promotes the greatest good for the greatest number.
  3. Deontology or formalism—the right act is established by use of ethical principles as follows:
     a. Autonomy—individuals are respected for themselves and should have control over their own choices whether or not these are in their best interest or agree with our opinions. If someone decides what is best for another it is termed paternalism. Children, the mentally retarded, and the mentally ill are often thought not to be competent enough to be autonomous.

     b. Beneficence—promoting the good of others and preventing them from harm

     c. Nonmaleficence—responsibility to do no harm; many suggest that it is more important to avoid harm than to do good. Some interpret it as a person's duty to prevent someone else from harming a third person.

     d. Justice—distribution of resources, benefits and burdens fairly among members of a society

e. Ethical principles may conflict with one another so that it is difficult to determine which act produces the most good.

f. From ethical principles client rights have been specified.

Right—a just claim that is due an individual or group; rights may be established by policies and/or protected by laws. Important patient rights in psychiatric nursing include:

- Right to privacy
  1. Confidentiality—no information shared about client, including fact of hospitalization or whether in therapy
  2. Privileged communication—in five states court may not legally mandate nurses to give information obtained in a professional capacity (Stuart and Sundeen, 1991); does not apply to patient records
  3. Exceptions:
     a. Tarasoff—therapist reasonably certain that a client is going to harm someone, must breach confidentiality and inform potential victim
     b. Possible child abuse—many states mandate that cases be reported to authorities
     c. Guardianship or involuntary commitment hearings—clinical information must be shared.
- Right to treatment—patients cannot be held against their will without an individualized treatment plan and certain other standards of care specified by law.
- Right to treatment in least restrictive setting
  1. Clients who are not dangerous cannot be hospitalized against their will.
  2. Clients capable of functioning on an open ward should not be held in a locked ward.
  3. Clients can wear their own clothes and keep their own personal effects excluding dangerous objects and valuables that cannot be protected.
  4. Clients who with support can live in the community should be discharged to outpatient care.

5. Seclusion and restraint can only be utilized when therapeutically necessary and all other methods have failed to control violent behavior to self or others.

- Right to informed consent
    1. Voluntary permission given by a competent client after procedures to be performed have been explained and are understood
    2. Clients often sign forms on admission which cover psychiatric treatment.
    3. Commitment procedure gives hospital the right to treat involuntary patients.
    4. Written consent for ECT and experimental drugs
- Right to refuse treatment
    1. Clients, including committed patients in nonemergencies, may not be forcibly medicated.
    2. Guardians can give permission or a court order can be sought for incompetent clients.
    3. If patient is violent to self or others and all less restrictive methods have failed, patients (including those who have been voluntarily admitted) may be forcibly medicated.
    4. Nurses must know the laws in their state and assure adequate written documentation.
- Right to habeas corpus—committed clients may at any time petition the court for release on the grounds that they are sane.
- Right to independent psychiatric examination—clients may demand evaluation by physician of own choice and must be released if determined to be not mentally ill.
- Right to outside communication
    1. Clients may have visitors, write and receive letters, make and receive phone calls, including those to judges and lawyers.
    2. The hospital can limit times for phone and visitors and deny access when they could cause harm to clients or staff.
- Right to be employed if possible—clients cannot be forced to work, and if they choose to as part of therapy, must be paid minimum wage.

Malpractice

- Definition: Failure of professionals to provide acceptable standards of care which results in harm to the client
- Nurses should be familiar with the following resources which help define standards of care:
  1. Code for Nurses with Interpretive Statements
  2. Standards of Psychiatric and Mental Health Nursing Practice of the American Nurses Association
  3. Standards of Child and Adolescent Psychiatric and Mental Health Nursing Practice of the American Nurses Association
  4. Standards of Psychiatric Consultation-Liaison Nursing Practice
  5. Documents published by the Joint Commission on Accreditation of Health Care Organizations (JCAHO)
  6. Statements from the American Hospital Association
  7. Policies and Procedures of the employing agency
  8. Nurse practice statutes of the state
- If standards are not clear in a particular instance, a lawyer should be consulted.

Mental Health Education

- Definition: Imparting of knowledge to clients and families
- Goals according to Walker and Price-Hoskins (1992)
  1. Offering information about the illness and interventions
  2. Helping people recognize symptoms
  3. Teaching people when and how to intervene for themselves
  4. Offering relief from blame and guilt
  5. Clarifying family expectations
  6. Instilling confidence that change can occur
  7. Developing an objective perspective and balance
- Methods of Learning
  1. Lecture

2. Discussion
3. Modeling
4. Observation
5. Experiential
    a. Role playing
    b. Behavioral rehearsal
6. Coaching
7. Audio or videotaped presentation
8. Self-instruction
    a. Keeping a diary
    b. Monitoring thoughts, feelings, and behaviors

- Guidelines for teaching adult learners
    1. Assess knowledge base.
    2. Increase awareness of need for learning.
    3. Encourage self-direction.
    4. Encourage learners to apply material to what they already know.
    5. Use mode of learning most useful to the learner, i.e., auditory, visual, or kinesthetic.
    6. Repeat as often as necessary changing and combining methods and modes as required.
    7. Accommodate teaching to the client's capacity for learning and attention span both of which may be affected by illness.

QUESTIONS
select the best answer

1. According to traditional definitions of mental health, which of the following would the nurse be most likely to describe as mentally healthy?
   a. Jerry Jones, a VietNam veteran with no family ties, who has been unemployed for 10 years
   b. Tom Sarris, a CEO, who spends 14 hours at work each day and is too tired to do anything with his family on weekends
   c. George Connors, a shoe salesman who delights in playing affectionately with his children but has been unable to hold a steady job since they were born
   d. Sam Thomas, a restaurateur who loves his work, but sets limits on the hours he spends there in order to enjoy his family and friends

2. Which of the following would be described as a component of mental health according to Johnson?
   a. Refusing to be involved in any relationship that limits independence
   b. Absence of anxiety under any circumstances
   c. Dependence on friends and family to assist with crises
   d. Ignoring cues from the environment when deciding what to do

3. In helping a client change, the nurse should:
   a. Encourage the client to move rapidly to avoid delay
   b. Realize that the problems the client is facing will make him or her eager to change
   c. Encourage feelings of hope
   d. Understand that change is a natural process which never involves anxiety and fear

4. In facilitating change the nurse should:
   a. Avoid deliberate goal-directed activity since this will inhibit the process
   b. Restrict clients to few choices to avoid overwhelming them
   c. Give up if resistance is encountered
   d. Form a helping relationship and collaborate with clients

5. John Korman is a 36-year-old male recently admitted to a psychiatric unit. The nurse taking his history observes that his speech is slurred, and he states that he cannot remember where he has been for the past 12 hours, but the police

who brought him in stated that he was arrested driving the wrong way on a one-way street. Which of the following items on the mental status exam would the nurse mark "impaired"?

a. Behavior
b. Judgment
c. Memory
d. All of the above

6. Which of the following is NOT necessary for the nurse to make a spiritual assessment?

a. Assure that the client has a religious affiliation
b. Determine if client believes in a higher power
c. Evaluate the client's relationship to others
d. Determine the client's philosophy of life

7. Which of the following interventions would be labeled as an independent nursing intervention on a psychiatric unit?

a. Giving medications
b. Making discharge plans
c. Deciding privileges
d. Assuring safety

8. The staff of a day treatment program have determined that all clients must participate in a group outing to a local museum because all of the staff want to see the exhibit. Two women clients in the group voice their opposition to visiting the museum because they do not wish to risk being identified as psychiatric clients by others in the community. The staff refuse to listen to their concerns and insist that they go on the trip, but do not describe any particular reason. Which adjective describes the type of goal planning evident in this situation?

a. Specific
b. Individualized
c. Collaborative
d. None of the above

9. Which of the following behaviors would indicate a good client response to a nursing action?

a. The client's body is noticably less tense and he or she has stopped pacing.

b. The client stops interacting with others on the unit.
c. The client states "If I don't do what people want they won't like me."
d. The client refuses to listen to feedback from other members of the community.

10. A nurse brings a client the Clozapine medication that she has been taking. The client doesn't look well and complains of a sore throat. The nurse notes that her temperature is elevated and concludes that the client has an upper respiratory infection. After giving the client the medication, she states that she will ask the doctor for a PRN aspirin order. The doctor orders a CBC and determines that the client has agranulocytosis. At which step of the Nursing Process did this nurse's problem begin?

    a. Assessment
    b. Diagnosis
    c. Planning
    d. Intervention

11. Which of the following is NOT true of the Resolution or Termination Phase of the Nurse-Client relationship?

    a. Preliminaries for this phase are introduced in the Orientation phase.
    b. Talk about the impending separation should be avoided so that the client does not decompensate.
    c. The client should be encouraged to review his progress and goals.
    d. The nurse should model appropriate expression of feelings.

12. Which of the following statements would the nurse NOT make in negotiating a contract with the client within the Nurse-Client Relationship?

    a. "I would like to meet with you on a once a week basis while we are trying to resolve this crisis."
    b. "We need about 10 sessions to work on this problem."
    c. "I have malpractice insurance in case there is any problem"
    d. "We will not be exploring your past, but only looking at things that are going on now."

13. In a session with the nurse, the client begins to whine about his inability to complete his assigned task from the previous session. The nurse responds by scolding him for his failure. This is an example of:

    a. Transference
    b. Countertransference

c. Both of the above
d. Neither of the above

14. Sarah has been at least 10 minutes late for each of her previous sessions. Today she arrives 20 minutes late. The nurse should:

    a. Express anger towards Sarah
    b. Confront Sarah firmly and set limits on her behavior
    c. Discuss terminating their sessions if she continues this pattern
    d. Comment on her observations and assist Sarah to understand her behavior

15. Jim, a 14-year-old client, is discussing his drug abuse problem with his nurse. When she asks him to clarify the types of substances he routinely uses, he responds by saying "How about you, have you ever used Marijuana?" How should the nurse respond?

    a. "That's none of your business, Jim, now let's get back to your problem."
    b. "Why, yes I have, but I was older and more responsible."
    c. "As you recall, Jim, we agreed to work on your problems with drugs in our sessions. I wonder what concerns you about whether I have used drugs."
    d. "That's an inappropriate question. I don't have to answer that and wonder why you'd even ask it."

16. According to the Communication Process, at the end of the feedback loop, the sender becomes the receiver

    a. True
    b. False

17. Which of the following statements is true concerning communication?

    a. Some behavior is random and does not communicate a message
    b. The message sent by the sender is obvious and does not have to be interpreted by the receiver
    c. The main goal of communication is understanding
    d. The only real form of communication is the verbal message, either written or spoken

18. Sobbing and grunting would be forms of what kind of nonverbal messages?

    a. Kinesics
    b. Paralanguage
    c. Proxemics

d. Appearance

19. Terry Barr is describing to the nurse that he sees himself as extremely patient and laid back. As he speaks, he drums his fingers on the arm of the chair. What can the nurse infer from this communication?

  a. Terry is obviously lying and trying to fool the nurse
  b. Terry's verbal and non-verbal communications are not congruent
  c. Terry is in touch with his feelings and expressing them openly and honestly
  d. Terry's culture is interfering with his ability to communicate

20. As they are walking down the hall the nurse and client are discussing their favorite movies. This is an example of:

  a. Social communication
  b. Therapeutic communication
  c. Inappropriate communication
  d. Lack of communication

21. Which of the following would be the best example of an open ended question?

  a. How did you come to be in the hospital?
  b. Did your husband bring you over to the hospital?
  c. Who brought you to the hospital?
  d. All of the above

22. Adrienne has just finished describing how devastated she was at the recent loss of her mother. Which of the following responses by the nurse would NOT be a barrier to therapeutic communication?

  a. "I know how you feel. I lost my mother recently too."
  b. "Well, it's better to have loved and lost, if you know what I mean."
  c. "When did she die? Of what? Does anyone else in your family have that problem?"
  d. "It sounds like it's been a really tough period for you."

23. Timmy, a six-year-old, is accompanying his parents to a family therapy session to deal with his school phobia. Which of the following behaviors by the nurse would NOT constitute therapeutic communication skills with a child?

  a. "Let's pick out some toys from the closet to play with while I talk to your Mom and Dad?"
  b. "What do you like best about school, Timmy? What do you like least?"

c. "Tell me about the picture you drew of your family."
d. "Is there something that makes you anxious about going to school, Timmy?"

24. In a peer supervision group a nurse is discussing a recent self-disclosure to a client. What questions might the group ask to assist the nurse in determining whether the intervention was appropriate?

    a. What theoretical approach have you been using?
    b. In what phase have you and your client been working?
    c. What was your purpose in sharing this information with your client?
    d. All of the above

25. Susan, a new graduate, has recently joined the staff of an inner-city Mental Health Clinic. She is shocked at some of the parenting behaviors of her initial client and tells other clinicians that she thinks her client should know better. How could her attitude be labeled?

    a. Stereotyping
    b. Culturally relativistic
    c. Ethnocentric
    d. Culturally deprived

26. Susan finds herself frustrated when her client uses some money she receives to buy winter coats for her nephews instead of saving it to buy a car so she could commute to a better job. Susan's client is demonstrating which cultural values?

    a. Present oriented, individualistic
    b. Future oriented, individualistic
    c. Present oriented, collectivist
    d. Future oriented, collectivist

27. A Middle Eastern client comes to the nurses station and stands face to face less than a foot away from the nurse. The nurse should be aware that:

    a. The client is becoming aggressive and trying to intimidate the nurse.
    b. The client has a different sense of personal space than the predominant American culture.
    c. The client is testing the nurse and needs to be confronted.
    d. The client is being seductive with the nurse.

28. An Asian American client arrives for her first session with the nurse. She speaks softly and avoids discussion of her problem directly. The nurse should:

a. Understand that she has low self-esteem and suggest that they work on this problem
b. Realize that this behavior is due to extreme guilt and shame and indicates a secret that needs disclosing
c. Be aware that this is defensive behavior and probably foreshadows a great deal of resistance
d. Understand that this is culturally appropriate behavior and should be respected and mirrored

29. In a well functioning mental health team who is the most important member?

 a. The doctor
 b. The nurse
 c. The psychologist
 d. None of the above

30. Which of the following characteristics are most indicative of success in a mental health team?

 a. A team leader with a decisive authoritarian approach
 b. A set of firm rules and regulations to cover most situations that could arise
 c. Many diverse philosophies of treatment
 d. None of the above

31. The goal of Art Therapy and Music Therapy is:

 a. To assist clients in passing time in the hospital productively
 b. To teach clients a new skill or hobby
 c. To evaluate clients for possible job training
 d. To stimulate the expression of feelings

32. Which of the following is not a responsibility of the generalist nurse?

 a. Psychotherapy
 b. 24 hour care
 c. Milieu management
 d. Safety

33. Which of the following is most true about a Clinical Nurse Specialist who testifies in court on behalf of a child who has been sexually abused?

 a. The nurse is functioning as an advocate for the child
 b. The nurse is functioning as a case manager for the child

c. The nurse is exceeding her capabilities as a Clinical Nurse Specialist
d. The nurse is functioning as a Psychiatric Liason Nurse

34. Of the following advocacy guidelines which is true?

a. All clients are in need of advocacy as provided by the nurse.
b. Joining forces with other groups with similar goals should be avoided since this leads to a large group which is difficult to handle.
c. The maximum power possible should be brought to the task to ensure the maximum benefit.
d. Patience and persistence are important characteristics of successful client advocates.

35. Jerry Coleman is a 46-year-old client with Manic Depressive illness who has recently had an exacerbation of his Manic symptoms. He has been referred for appropriate services to a Clinical Nurse Specialist by his disability insurance company. What kind of services might he expect to receive from his case manager?

a. A thorough evaluation of his case and coordination of all services
b. Referral for medication evaluation and maintenance
c. Referral for vocational rehabilitation if necessary
d. All of the above

36. Sharon Getty has been admitted to a neurological unit with a complaint of chronic pain. She has been referred to the Clinical Nurse Specialist who functions as the Psychiatric Liason Nurse for that unit. Which might be a response of the Liason Nurse?

a. Discussion with R.N.s on the unit about the need for them not to talk with the client about the emotional components of her pain
b. Avoid talking with the client's family because they will probably be upset to learn that they might be contributing to the client's problems with pain
c. Realize that individual psychotherapy with the client is the role of the psychiatrist
d. Referring the client to occupational therapy if appropriate

37. Which of the following is NOT true?

a. Milieu therapy implies that all activity is therapeutic.
b. A therapeutic environment cannot exist without community meetings.
c. Token communities use privileges to reward appropriate behavior.
d. The physical environment is an important part of the Milieu.

38. To which of the following values would the nurse working within the therapeutic milieu probably NOT subscribe?

    a. The need for accessible team members and cooperative working relationships
    b. Empowerment of clients and staff to make decisions that affect the group
    c. Emphasis on the individual at the expense of the group
    d. Encouragement of risk taking and growth

39. Carmine d'Angelo is a 29-year-old client with a diagnosis of Schizophrenia, Paranoid Type. When he is denied off unit privileges at a community meeting he becomes hostile and accuses certain community members of ''having it in for him.'' What would be the most appropriate response of the nurse?

    a. Ignore the behavior because it is inappropriate
    b. Confront Mr. D'Angelo with his inappropriate behavior and put him in seclusion
    c. Meet with him at their usual time and clarify his misperceptions
    d. Ask the community members that he accused to have nothing more to do with him

40. What types of things would the nurse be expected to work on with Mr. d'Angelo over the next few sessions?

    a. How his thoughts and feelings influence his behavior
    b. Whether or not his behavior at the previous community meeting achieved his purpose
    c. What other coping strategies might be more effective
    d. All of the above

41. In a therapy group, a client makes inappropriate demands of the Clinical Nurse Specialist who is the group therapist. The Clinical Nurse Specialist responds assertively and effectively resolves the problem to the satisfaction of all concerned. What curative factor, according to Yalom does this situation exemplify?

    a. Altruism
    b. Catharsis
    c. Interpersonal Learning
    d. Universality

42. Mrs. C.S. is an extremely shy individual who was admitted to the hospital with

a Depressive Disorder. What characteristics of therapy groups will best serve her needs?

a. The realization that no one else in the group has anything like the problem she has
b. The fact that two members of the group are talking constantly without interuption will protect her from feeling like she must participate
c. The experience of being left alone by other group members will protect her autonomy and decrease her performance anxiety
d. The fact that others support one another in learning to change will encourage her to take the risks needed to grow.

43. A Clinical Nurse Specialist is called in as a consultant to a nursing home seeking to enhance the morale of its residents. The Clinical Nurse Specialist decides to begin an ongoing Resocialization Group since many of the clients have been pretty much isolated from others in their previous living situations. How would such a group be classified?

a. Homogeneous, closed ended
b. Heterogeneous, open ended
c. Open ended, task
d. Closed ended, psychotherapy

44. Ann and John lose their first child to Sudden Infant Death Syndrome. They decide to attend a hospital-sponsored group for people who have had this experience. What type of group will they be attending?

a. Teaching group
b. Psychotherapy group
c. Task group
d. Supportive/Therapeutic group

45. A Clinical Nurse Specialist working as a group psychotherapist makes observations about the effective way members handled a participant who was acting out in the group. What type of leadership style does this nurse exhibit?

a. Autocratic
b. Democratic
c. Laissez Faire
d. None of the above

46. After a particularly difficult community meeting, the staff of a unit sit down

and begin to talk about which clients were seated in close proximity and who agreed with whom on the issues that came up. What is the staff discussing?

a. Gossip
b. Rank and Status
c. Group Content
d. Group Process

47. A nursing group has convened to make decisions about renovation plans for a psychiatric unit. One of the members is discussing how little the hospital ever pays attention to input from nursing staff. Which member role is this participant exhibiting?

a. Maintenance role
b. Task role
c. Individual role
d. All of the above

48. A Clinical Nurse Specialist has had several meetings with a therapy group. On this particular occasion it is noted that members seem angry with the nurse and each other. They seem to be competing with each other to see who can refrain from breaking the silence longest. Which stage of group development do these behaviors signify?

a. Storming
b. Norming
c. Performing
d. Mourning

49. A Clinical Nurse Specialist notes that members of her therapy group have become most supportive of one another and very attached to the group. Which stage of group development do these behaviors signify?

a. Forming
b. Storming
c. Norming
d. Performing

50. Whose responsibility is it to deal with transference issues in group therapy?

a. The nurse
b. The group members
c. Both
d. Neither

51. How should a member terminating be handled in groups?

    a. Little attention should be paid to it since this person is now ready to leave and other members are more in need of assistance
    b. Members may discuss it if they wish, but should be allowed to avoid it if it causes anxiety
    c. Members should be encouraged to focus only on the positive aspects of the leaving so that negative feelings don't arise
    d. Members should be encouraged to express whatever feelings arise in the process of leaving*

52. Which of the following best summarizes the family therapist's position on how mental illness occurs?

    a. The symptomatic person is the innocent victim of other members of the family.
    b. If other family members are given education and support, they can help the symptomatic person.
    c. The symptomatic person is the result of pathology throughout the entire family system.
    d. If other family members set limits and confront the symptomatic person with reality, they can help him or her.

53. A Clinical Nurse Specialist is the family therapist for a family whose youngest child is the identified patient. The child has been brought in for therapy because he has been doing poorly and acting out at school. How will the nurse begin the initial session with the family?

    a. By asking the child why he is doing poorly in school
    b. By asking the parents why they think he is doing poorly at school
    c. By asking each family member how they did in school
    d. By asking questions about the family in general

54. In working with the family, the nurse finds that the child is waking many times during the night and climbing into the parents' bed. Which of the following would the nurse probably NOT use as an intervention in this situation?

    a. Suggesting that one of the parents sleep in the child's room so everyone can get a good night's sleep
    b. Encouraging the parents to work together to set limits on the child's sleeping in their bed
    c. Asking the parents to talk together about how they will handle the situation when the child wakes up in the night

d. Encouraging each member of the family to talk about his/her feelings in the matter

55. The nurse suggests that if the child can't sleep that he/she play a cassette tape on his recorder and try to listen to as many cassettes as he can, making sure that he gets out of bed, so that he doesn't fall asleep in the process. This intervention is known as:

a. Homework
b. Paradoxical prescription
c. Sculpting
d. Triangling

56. The nurse also asks the parents to keep a record of the number of nights the child stays in his own room and to reward him with a treat if he can do it three nights in a row. This intervention is known as:

a. Homework
b. Paradoxical prescription
c. Sculpting
d. Triangling

57. A family with extremely rigid boundaries will probably NOT have:

a. Positive links to society
b. Clear boundaries
c. Strong parental coalition
d. Efficient negotiation and task performance

58. Members of a therapeutic community decide at a community meeting that it is not right for two extremely demanding clients to determine the activities for the entire group. This decision can best be classified under which ethical perspective?

a. Egoism
b. Utilitarianism
c. Deontology
d. Formalism

59. When the nurse asks potentially suicidal clients to relinquish any sharp objects they have in their possession, which ethical principle is being utilized?

a. Autonomy
b. Beneficence

c. Nonmaleficence
d. Justice

60. A government agency doing a security check on an individual calls a Clinical Nurse Specialist seeking information about any mental health problems that the individual might have. What response is the best for the Clinical Nurse Specialist?

    a. Turn all written records over to the investigators
    b. Submit a treatment summary describing the client's problems
    c. Write a report that describes the client's problems in the least damaging way possible
    d. Refuse to acknowledge that the client is in therapy until a release of information form is signed by the client

61. A Clinical Nurse Specialist has been treating a client for several months. Recently the client has become increasingly agitated and expressed a great deal of hostility towards his ex-wife. At their last session, the client described a detailed plan to kill her and kidnap his children. What is the Clinical Nurse Specialist's response?

    a. Call the client's ex-wife and inform her that she may be in danger
    b. Call the police and discuss the case with them
    c. Consult a lawyer about the case
    d. Preserve the client's right to confidentiality

62. A mother brings her adolescent son in to be seen by a Clinical Nurse Specialist. The mother wishes to hospitalize the boy. She indicates that she can no longer control his behavior and that he is dating girls of whom she does not approve and staying out past his curfew. Based on the boy's right to treatment in the least restrictive setting, what is the Clinical Nurse Specialist's best response?

    a. Determine the most secure facility to hospitalize the child because he is probably a "run risk"
    b. Seek a Day Treatment Program since the child's behavior is not dangerous.
    c. Offer to work with the mother and son in regard to appropriate expectations and discipline.
    d. Tell the mother that all adolescents act that way and that she is wrong to be upset about this normal behavior.

63. Leroy Jones was committed to an inpatient psychiatric unit because of hallucinations which have not been controlled by oral medications prescribed on an outpatient basis. In the hospital, Mr. Jones has been prescribed I.M. Prolixin. When the nurse brings the first injection, Mr. Jones refuses the medication. What is the nurse's best immediate response in this situation?

    a. Talk with Mr. Jones about his objections to the medication
    b. Tell Mr. Jones that he cannot refuse the medication since it is necessary for his treatment
    c. Call his doctor and tell him/her that Mr. Jones has refused the medication
    d. Call an emergency team to restrain Mr. Jones while the medication is being given

64. Which of the following is NOT an accurate statement regarding client rights?

    a. Committed clients may petition the courts for release
    b. Committed clients may demand an evaluation by any physician
    c. Committed clients may not have letters restricted
    d. Committed clients may not be hospitalized involuntarily

65. A nurse who is unaware of standards of care and fails to provide care which results in harm to the client is not subject to being charged with Malpractice.

    a. True
    b. False

66. The parents of an autistic child consult a Clinical Nurse Specialist about their failure to relate to their child. The nurse decides that some education would be helpful to this family in dealing with the problem. What could the family NOT expect to receive as a result of the nurse's teaching intervention?

    a. An objective perspective
    b. Decreased blame and guilt
    c. Clarification of expectations
    d. A solution to their problems

67. In an assertiveness group, a nurse encourages a client to act out a distressing interaction she has had repeatedly with her mother-in-law. The nurse has the client play herself while the nurse plays the mother-in-law. Which methods of learning are exemplified in this situation?

    a. Lecture
    b. Experiential
    c. Self-instruction

d. All of the above

68. Alice Walsh is a 46-year-old admitted to a psychiatric unit with a Major Depressive Disorder. Her doctor prescribes an MAO inhibitor which she will be taking when she leaves the hospital in four days. Her nurse wants to teach her about the side effects of her medication, particularly the dietary restrictions. She prepares a 45-minute presentation which covers everything about the medication. Afterwards Mrs. Walsh seems confused and still cannot relate several essential facts about the medication. What is the best nursing response to the situation?
    a. Phone the doctor and suggest that Mrs. Walsh be placed on another medication with fewer restrictions
    b. Realize that Mrs. Walsh will probably not be able to understand the essentials regarding her medication and teach a relative instead
    c. Realize that Mrs. Walsh's depression is probably inhibiting her ability to learn and repeat the presentation in a few days when she is a little better
    d. Break down the essential facts into a few brief sessions that can be repeated over the next several days and assess Mrs. Walsh's knowledge of the previous session before proceeding

ANSWERS

1. d
2. c
3. c
4. d
5. d
6. a
7. d
8. d
9. a
10. b
11. b
12. c
13. c
14. d
15. c
16. a
17. c
18. b
19. b
20. a
21. a
22. d
23. d
24. d
25. c
26. c
27. b
28. d
29. d
30. d
31. d
32. a
33. a
34. d
35. d
36. d
37. b
38. c
39. c
40. d
41. c
42. d
43. b
44. d
45. b
46. d
47. c
48. a
49. c
50. c
51. d
52. c
53. d
54. a
55. b
56. a
57. a
58. b
59. b
60. d
61. a
62. c
63. a
64. d
65. b
66. d
67. b
68. d

BIBLIOGRAPHY

Auvil, C. A. & Silver, B. W. (1984). Therapist self-disclosure: When is it appropriate? *Perspectives in Psychiatric Care, 22*(2), 57–64.

Boyd, M. A. & Luetje, V. M. (1991). Nursing advocacy in mental health settings. In R. B. Murray & M. M Huelskoetter (Eds.) *Psychiatric mental health nursing: Giving emotional care* (pp. 731–748). Norwalk, CT: Appleton and Lange.

Greene, J. (1993). Milieu therapy. In B. S. Johnson (Ed.), *Psychiatric-mental health nursing: Adaptation and growth* (183–193). Philadelphia: J.B. Lippincott.

Hogarth, C. R. (1993). Families and family therapy. In B. S. Johnson (Ed.), *Psychiatric-mental Health Nursing: Adaptation and Growth* (pp. 233–256). Philadelphia: J. B. Lippincott.

Huelskoetter, M. M. & Romano, E. (1991). The change process. In R. B. Murray & M. M. Huelskoetter (Eds.) *Psychiatric mental health nursing: Giving Emotional care* (pp. 191–204). Norwalk, CT: Appleton and Lange.

Johnson, B. S. (1993). Introduction to psychiatric-mental health nursing. In B. S. Johnson (Ed.), *Psychiatric-mental health nursing: Adaptation and growth* (pp. 3–22). Philadelphia: J. B. Lippincott.

Lasalle, P. C. & Lasalle, A. J. (1991). Small groups and their therapeutic forces. In G. W. Stuart and S. J. Sundeen (Eds.), *Principles and practice of psychiatric nursing* (pp. 809–826). St. Louis: Mosby Year Book.

Long, P. & McMahon, A. L. (1992). Working with groups. In J. Haber, A. McMahon, P. Price-Hoskins and B. Siedeleau (Eds.), *Comprehensive psychiatric nursing* (pp. 324–346). New York: Mosby-Year Book.

McMahon, A. L. (1992). Nurse-client relationship. In J. Haber, A. McMahon, P. Price-Hoskins and B. Siedeleau (Eds.), *Comprehensive psychiatric nursing* (pp. 159–176). New York: Mosby-Year Book.

Peplau, H. (1952). *Interpersonal relations in nursing.* New York: G. P. Putnam.

Sellin, S. R. (1991). Ethical issues in psychiatric mental health nursing. In G. K. McFarland & M. D. Thomas (Eds.), *Psychiatric mental health nursing* (pp. 943–949). Philadelphia: J. B. Lippincott.

Shanks, S. R. (1991). Legal issues in psychiatric mental healh nursing. In G. K. McFarland & M. D. Thomas (Eds.), *Psychiatric mental health nursing* (p. 933–942). Philadelphia: J. B. Lippincott.

Stuart, G. W. & Sundeen, S. J. (1991). Legal and ethical aspects of psychiatric care.

In G. W. Stuart and S. J. Sundeen (Eds.), *Principles and practice of psychiatric nursing* (pp. 205–236). St. Louis: Mosby Year Book.

Tripp-Reimer, T., & Lively, S. H. (1993). Cultural considerations in mental health-psychiatric nursing. In R. P. Rawlins, S. R. Williams, & C. K. Beck (Eds.), Mental Health-Psychiatric Nursing: *A holistic life-cycle approach* (pp. 166–179). New York: Mosby-Year Book.

Tuckman, B. W. (1965). Developmental sequences in small groups. *Psychology Bulletin, 63,* 384–389.

Walker, M., & Price-Hoskins, P. (1992). Role of the nurse in psychiatric settings. In J. Haber, A. McMahon, P. Price-Hoskins and B. Siedeleau (Eds.), *Comprehensive Psychiatric Nursing* (pp. 267–287). New York: Mosby Year Book.

Watson, J. (1992). Maintenance of therapeutic community principles in an age of biopharmacology and economic restraints. *Archives of Psychiatric Nursing, 6*(3), 183–188.

Yalom, I. D. (1985). *The theory and practice of group psychotherapy.* New York: Basic Books.

[illegible]

Webb [illegible]

[illegible]

Major Theoretical Frameworks for Psychiatric Nursing

Joan Donovan

Theory

- Definition: A set of concepts, definitions, and propositions, used to describe, explain, predict, or control a phenomenon
- Characteristics
  1. Can interrelate concepts in such a way as to create a different way of looking at a phenomenon
  2. Must be logical in nature
  3. Should be relatively simple, yet generalizable
  4. Can be the bases for hypotheses that can be tested
  5. Contribute to and assist in increasing the general body of knowledge within the discipline through the research implemented to validate them
  6. Can be utilized by the practitioners to guide and improve their practice
  7. Must be consistent with other validated theories, laws and principles, but will leave open unanswered questions that need to be investigated (George, 1990)

Theory and Research

1. Theory is constructed through deductive or inductive approaches:
   a. Deductive theory construction proceeds from the general to the specific. The theorist or investigator borrows concepts from other bodies of knowledge and tests the concepts and relationships in nursing practice. An example is Rogers' Theory of Nursing.
   b. Inductive theory construction proceeds from the specific to the general. The theorist or investigator immerses himself/herself in the data and attempts to generate theoretical statements. An example is Orem's theory of Self Care (Riehl & Roy, 1980).
2. Theory serves to:
   a. Guide research—the theory sets limits on questions to ask and methods to pursue in research.
   b. Guide practice—after validation from research, theory can give direction to practice.

c. Provide a common language between practitioners and researchers.

d. Enhance professional autonomy and accountability—theory, supported by research, allows nurse to predict consequences of care, contributing to autonomous nursing practice (Meleis, 1985).

Research

Systematic method of gathering data which provides means of developing and testing theories as well as measuring outcomes of nursing interventions in the clinical area. Participation in research is an ANA Psychiatric Mental Health Standard of Practice.

- Research Process
  1. Determine problem.
  2. Review relevant literature.
  3. Identify a theoretical framework.
  4. Determine the research variables.
  5. Formulate hypothesi(e)s.
  6. Select research instruments.
  7. Collect data.
  8. Analyze data.
  9. Determine results and conclusions.
- Types of Research
  1. Experimental—experimenter uses random sampling, manipulates the independent variable and uses control and experimental groups.
  2. Quasiexpermental—variable may be manipulated but subjects not assigned randomly to control and treatment groups.
  3. Nonexperimental—researcher measures variables as they occur naturally; uses correlations to determine nature and extent of relationship between and among variables; includes prospective and retrospective.

4. Qualitative—researcher makes observations or interviews participants. Data used to describe process or phenomena—most common forms are Phenomenological and Ethnographic.
5. Case Study—researcher describes and analyzes one or a small number of cases.

- Research Instruments—may measure physical or psychological characteristics. Often questionnaires are used which must be evaluated for
  1. Reliability—ability to measure the same trait repeatedly
  2. Validity—ability to measure what it is supposed to be measuring
- Statistical Data Analysis (Polit and Hungler, 1991)
  1. Descriptive—Means, Medians, Modes, Standard deviation
  2. Inferential Statistics—used to test hypotheses and decide if relationship between variables is supported
     a. Testing differences between two group means
        (1) t-Tests for independent samples
        (2) Paired t-Tests
     b. Testing differences between three or more groups
        (1) ANOVA
        (2) Kruskal-Wallace test
        (3) Mann Whitney U
        (4) Friedman test
     c. Comparing differences between cases that fall into categories—Chi Square Test
     d. Testing the relationshp between two variables
        (1) Pearson product moment correlation (r)
        (2) Spearman's rho
        (3) Kendall's tau
     e. Multivariate statistics
        (1) Multiple regression analysis—used to understand the effects of two or more independent variable on a dependent measure

(2) Stepwise multiple regression—all potential predictors considered simultaneously to determine the combination of variables providing the most predictive power

(3) Analysis of Covariance—used statistically to control one or more extraneous variables; useful to adjust for initial differences in situations where random assignment is impossible

(4) Factor Analysis—reduces a large set of variables into a smaller set of related variables

3. Level of Significance—describes the probability of a particular result occurring by chance

- Protection of Human Subjects
  1. Right to Informed Consent—may be more complicated with psychiatric clients due to nature of illness
  2. Right to Confidentiality (privacy of data) and Anonymity (privacy of source of information)
  3. Right to Refuse to Participate or Withdraw at Anytime

Nursing Theoretical Models

Developed around four core concepts:

- Individual—the person or client in need of nursing care
- Environment—the combination of all forces that affect an individual
- Health—a state of well being
- Nursing—the discipline and practice of assisting others to maintain or recover health (George, 1990; Fawcett, 1984)

Nursing Theories

- The Theory of Self-Care (Dorothea Orem)
  1. Self-care—an individual's activities to maintain life, health, and well being. Self-care requisites are actions directed toward the provision of self-care. The three categories of self-care requisites are:
     a. Universal—activities of daily living

   b. Developmental—specialized activities related to a developmental task or an event

   c. Health deviation—activities required by illness, injury, or disease

2. Self-care deficit—the inability to provide complete self-care; the need for nursing care. Nursing care includes the following:

   a. Entering into and maintaining nurse-patient relationships

   b. Assessing how patients can be helped

   c. Responding to patients' requests and needs

   d. Prescribing, providing, and regulating direct help

   e. Coordinating and integrating nursing with other services

3. Nursing systems refer to the amount of nursing care a patient requires. Categories are as follows:

   a. Wholly compensatory—the nurse provides all care.

   b. Partly compensatory—the nurse and patient provide care.

   c. Supportive-educative—the patient provides care. The nurse promotes the patient as a self-care agent (Foster & Janssens, 1990).

- Theory of Goal Attainment (Imogene King)

  King describes her theory of goal attainment within an open systems framework.

  1. The three systems in the framework are as follows:

     a. Personal systems—each individual is a personal system.

     b. Interpersonal systems—the interaction among human beings

     c. Social systems—an organized boundary system of roles, behaviors, and practices

  2. The theory of goal attainment states that people come together to help and be helped to maintain health. Concepts of the theory are as follows:

     a. Interaction—goal-directed communication

     b. Perception—organizing, processing, storing, and exporting information

c. Communication—information is given from one person to another.

d. Transaction—observable behaviors of people interacting with their environment

e. Role—set of behaviors expected of a person occupying a certain position

f. Stress—an energy response to a stressor

g. Growth and development—continuous changes that take place in life

h. Time—a sequence of events moving to the future

i. Space—physical area; territory (George, 1990)

- Theory of Nursing (Martha Rogers)

1. The phenomenon central to nursing is the life process of human beings.

2. Assumptions of Rogers' Theory:

   a. The human being is a unified whole possessing his/her own integrity and manifesting characteristics that are more than and different from the sum of his/her parts.

   b. The person and environment are continually exchanging matter and energy with each other.

   c. The life process revolves irreversibly and unidirectionally along the space-time continuum.

   d. Pattern and organization identify individuals and reflect their wholeness.

   e. The human being is characterized by the capacity for abstraction and imagery, language and thought, sensation and emotion.

3. Building blocks of Rogers':

   a. Energy field—an electrical field in a continuous state of flux

   b. Openness—energy fields are open to exchange with other energy fields.

   c. Pattern—energy fields have patterns that change as required.

d. Four dimensionality—energy fields are embedded in a four-dimensional space-time matrix.

4. Principles of homeodynamics are built upon the five assumptions and four building blocks.

   a. Integrality—the continuous, mutual, simultaneous interaction between human and environmental fields

   b. Resonancy—the identification of human and environmental fields by changing wave patterns

   c. Helicy—the evolving innovative repatterning growing out of the mutual interaction of man and environment (Rogers, 1983; Falco & Lobo, 1990)

- The Adaptation Model (Sister Callista Roy)

  There are five essential elements of the model:

  1. Each person is an adaptive system with input, internal processes, adaptive modes, and output.

     a. Input—internal or external stimuli

     b. Internal processes—coping mechanisms

        (1) Regulator subsystem—chemical, neural, and endocrine transmitters

        (2) Cognator subsystem—perception, information processing, judgment, emotion

     c. Adaptive modes or system effectors

        (1) Physiological function mode—identifies patterns of physical functioning

        (2) Self-concept mode—identifies patterns of values, beliefs, and emotions

        (3) Role function mode—identifies patterns of social interactions

        (4) Interdependence mode—identifies patterns of human value, affection, love, and affirmation

     d. Output:

        (1) Adaptive response, or

        (2) Ineffective response

2. The goal of nursing—the promotion of adaptive responses in relation to the adaptive modes
3. Health—a process of being and becoming an integrated person
4. Environment—conditions, circumstances, and influences affecting the growth and the behavior of a person
5. The Nursing Process:
   a. First-level assessment—behavioral assessment; assessment of four adaptive modes
   b. Second-level assessment:
      (1) Identification of focal, contextual, and residual stimuli
      (2) Identification of ineffective responses
   c. Identification of nursing diagnosis
   d. Goal setting with the client
   e. Implementation—manipulating focal, contextual, or residual stimuli
   f. Evaluation—assessment of goal behaviors and possible readjustment of goals and interventions (Galbreath, 1990)

- Theory of Culture Care Diversity and Universality (Madeleine Leininger)
  1. The main tenet of the theory is that ''care is the essence of nursing and the central, dominant, and unifying focus'' (Leininger, 1991, p. 35).
  2. Other concepts include:
     a. Culture—the learned, shared, and transmitted values, beliefs, norms, and lifeways of a group that guide their actions and decisions
     b. Cultural care diversity—differences in meanings, patterns, values, or symbols of care, within or between collectivities related to human care expressions
     c. Cultural care universality—uniform meanings, patterns, or symbols that are manifest in many cultures and reflect ways to help people
     d. Cultural and social structure dimensions—patterns of structural and organizational factors of a particular culture, including:

(1) Religious factors

(2) Social and kinship factors

(3) Political and legal factors

(4) Economic factors

(5) Educational factors

(6) Technological factors

(7) Cultural values

(8) Ethnohistorical factors

e. Ethnohistory—past facts, events, and experiences of individuals, groups, cultures, or institutions which are people-centered and which describe, explain, and interpret human lifeways within a certain culture

f. Cultural care preservation or maintainance—actions and decisions that help people retain relevant cultural care values to maintain well-being, recover from illness, and face handicaps or death

g. Cultural care accommodation or negotiation—actions and decisions to help people of a designated culture negotiate for a beneficial outcome with health caregivers

h. Cultural care repatterning or restructuring—actions and decisions to help clients modify their lifeways for beneficial health care, while respecting their cultural values and beliefs

i. Cultural congruent nursing care—actions and decisions tailored to fit cultural values and beliefs (Leininger, 1991)

Personality Theories (Object Relations)

- Psychoanalysis (Sigmumd Freud)

  Concepts in the theory of Freud include the following:

  1. Levels of awareness

     a. Conscious—thoughts, feelings, and desires a person is aware of and able to control

     b. Preconscious—thoughts, feelings, and desires that are not in immediate awareness but can be recalled to consciousness

   c. Unconscious—thoughts, feelings, and desires that are not available to the conscious mind

2. Stages of development—according to Freud, each person passes through the following stages of psychosexual development. A person can get stuck in any stage.
   a. Oral—the focus is on sucking and swallowing, gratification of oral needs
   b. Anal—focus on spontaneous bowel movements, control over impulses
   c. Phallic—focus on genital region, identification with parent of the same gender
   d. Latency—sexual impulses are dormant; focus is on coping with the environment.
   e. Genital—focus on erotic and genital behavior, developing mature sexual and emotional relationships
3. Personality structure—the personality has three main components:
   a. Id—the pleasure principle; unconscious; desire for immediate and complete satisfaction; disregard for others
   b. Ego—the reality principle; rational and conscious; weighs actions and consequences
   c. Superego—the censoring force of the personality; conscious and unconscious; evaluates and judges behavior (Scroggs, 1985)
4. Several terms common to psychiatric nursing originated with Freud, including:
   a. Oedipus Complex or Electra Conflict—at the age of four or five, the child falls in love with the parent of the opposite sex and feels hostility toward the parent of the same sex.
   b. Defense mechanisms—conscious or unconscious actions or thoughts to protect the ego from anxiety (See Table 1).

Table 1

Defense Mechanisms

Type	Definition	Example
Compensation	An individual makes up for a felt lack in one area by emphasizing strengths in another	A student who feels devoid of athletic ability becomes an outstanding member of the debating team
Denial	Failure to acknowledge the reality of an anxiety-producing situation	A woman ignores behavior changes in her husband that would indicate to others that he is having an affair
Displacement	Shifting of feelings from an emotionally charged person or object to a substitute, less threatening, person or object	A nurse becomes angry with a second nurse, later, the second nurse berates a family member for asking too many questions
Dissociation	Temporary but drastic modification of character or sense of personal identity to avoid emotional distress	A soldier, fearful of leading his patrol into enemy territory and not wanting to acknowledge cowardice,
Fantasy	Symbolic wish fulfillment with nonrational thought	A young boy, unable to protect his mother from his father's abuse, daydreams of singlehandedly killing a herd of wild animals that surround his home, thereby saving the family
Identification	Internalizing the characteristics of an idealized person	A young woman has high regard for her aunt and chooses to become a nurse just like her
Intellectualization	Reasoning or logic is used in an attempt to avoid confrontation with an objectionable impulse or affect	A man deals with intellectual formulations about the nature of death and the thoughts of various philosophers and scientists on the subject rather than the personally relevant feelings about his father's recent death
Introjection	Taking on another person's ego and becoming like that other person	A young child incorporates the personality of an adult and actually behaves like one
Isolation	Splitting of affect from the rest of a person's thinking	When a man who had been angry with his father (yet also loved him) hears of his father's death, he acknowledges the death, but deals with it in a mechanical way—he prevents himself from having feelings about the event
Projection	False attribution of the person's own undesirable feelings, thoughts, and impulses to others	A client states that a coworker does not like her, as a projection of her own dislike for the coworker
Rationalization	Finding logical or acceptable, but incorrect, reasons or excuses for behavior that is unacceptable to one's self-image	A college student who has low grades because of careless study habits rationalizes that he could have good grades if he had different instructors
Reaction formation	Substitution of behavior, thoughts and feelings diametrically opposed to unacceptable ones	A man who finds his sexual impulses unacceptable adopts puritanical beliefs and totally devotes himself to fighting pornography
Regression	Return to an earlier, more comfortable level of development	A child upset by the arrival of a new sibling may return to thumb-sucking or bed-wetting
Repression	Involuntary exclusion from consciousness of those ideas, feelings, and situation that are unacceptable to the self	After a painful interpersonal experience, the individual involved cannot recall his part in the interaction
Sublimation	Establishment of a secondary goal that an individual can satisfy in place of a primary goal that is socially unacceptable or physically impossible	A teenager with strong aggressive tendencies gains social acceptance through sports
Suppression	Voluntary exclusion from level of thought those feelings and situations that produce discomfort and some anxiety	A student with a poor report card "forgets" to give it to his parents for their signature
Undoing	A person symbolically acts out in reverse something unacceptable that has already been done	A man, raised to believe sex is immoral and dirty, relieves his sexual desires from time to time by masturbating; afterward, feeling tremendous guilt, he tries to undo the way he has fouled his hands (by touching his genitals) and develops a compulsion to wash his hands over and over

Note. From "Defensive Coping" by M. I. Fitch and L. L. O'Brien-Pallas in G. K. McFarland and M. O. Thomas, 1991, *Psychiatric Mental Health Nursing*, (p. 202), Philadelphia: J. B. Lippincott. Copyright 1991 by J. B. Lippincott Company. Reprinted by permission.

c. Freudian slips—also known as parapaxes—overt actions with unconscious meanings

d. Free association—a method for discovering the contents of the unconscious by associating words with other words or emotions

e. Transference—feelings, attitudes, and wishes linked with a significant figure in one's early life are projected onto others in one's current life

f. Countertransference—feelings and attitudes of the therapist are projected onto the patient inappropriately

g. Resistance—anything that prohibits a person from producing material from the unconscious

h. Fixation—getting stuck in one stage of development (Scroggs, 1985; Drapela, 1987)

5. Treatment—psychoanalysis:

   a. Daily therapy sessions for several years

   b. The patient reveals thoughts, feelings, dreams, etc.

   c. The therapist reveals no personal information, functioning primarily as a shadow figure. The therapist interprets the patient's behavior for him or her.

- Psychoanalysis (Carl Jung)

  The major concepts of Jung's theory are as follows:

1. Archetype—unconscious, intangible collective idea, image, or concept; Scroggs (1985) defines the main archetypes identified by Jung:

   a. The Way—the image of a journey or voyage through life

   b. The Self—the aspect of mind that unifies and orders experience

   c. Animus and Anima—the image of gender

   d. Rebirth—the concept of being reborn, resurrected, or reincarnated

   e. Persona—the role or mask one shows to others

   f. Shadow—the dark side of one's personality

g. Stock characters—dramatic roles that appear over and over in folktales

(1) Hero—the character who vanquishes evil and rescues the downtrodden

(2) Trickster—the character who plays pranks or works magic spells

(3) Sage—the wise old person

h. Power—symbol, such as the eagle or the sword

i. Number—certain numbers reappear throughout history and across cultures.

2. Psychological types—Jung described two attitudinal and four functional types of personalities:

a. Attitudinal types

(1) Introvert—one oriented toward the inner, subjective world

(2) Extrovert—one oriented toward the outer, external world

b. Functional types

(1) Thinking—intellectual process involving ideas

(2) Feeling—evaluative function involving value or worth

(3) Sensing—function involving recognition that something exists, without categorizing or evaluating it

(4) Intuiting—function involving creative inspiration, knowing without having the facts (Scroggs, 1985)

3. Collective unconscious

- Theory of Individual Psychology (Alfred Adler)

Adler saw individuals in a social context; he is considered a social -interpersonal theorist by some. Key ideas include:

1. Inferiority feelings are the source of all human strivings.

2. Personal growth results from the attempts to compensate for inferiority.

3. Complexes:

a. Inferiority complex—an inability to solve life's problems

b. Superiority complex—an exaggerated opinion of one's abilites and accomplishments, a result of the attempt to overcompensate for an inferiority complex

4. The goal of life—to strive for superiority

5. Lifestyle—the unique set of behaviors created by each individual to compensate for inferiority and achieve superiority

6. The influence of birth order:

   a. First-born—happy and secure, the center of attention, until dethroned by the second child; develops interest in authority and organization

   b. Second-born—born into a more relaxed atmosphere; has the first-born as a model, or a threat to compete with; develops interest in competition

   c. Youngest child—pet of the family; may retain dependency (Schultz, 1987; Adler, 1983)

- Theory of Basic Anxiety (Karen Horney)

  Because of her focus on family, some consider Horney a social/interpersonal theorist. Concepts include:

  1. A child has two basic needs—safety and satisfaction.
  2. When those needs are not met, the child feels hostility.
  3. The child represses the hostility, and this leads to basic anxiety.
  4. Basic anxiety—a pervasive feeling of being lonely or helpless in a hostile world
  5. Protective mechanisms against basic anxiety in relationships:
     a. Moving toward people
     b. Moving against people
     c. Moving away from people
  6. Neurosis—compulsive and unconscious extension of maladaptive childhood mechanisms (Scroggs, 1985; Wilson & Kneisl, 1992)

Theories of Growth and Development

- Theory of Psychosocial Development (Erik Homburger Erikson)
  1. The term used in naming each stage identifies the conflict to be resolved during that stage.
  2. In each stage, the individual has a particular focus and a task.
  3. The stages of development, approximate ages, foci, and tasks are as follows:
     a. Trust vs. mistrust—0 to 2 years—focus on oral needs, acquisition of hope
     b. Autonomy vs. shame—1.5 to 3 years—focus on anal needs, acquisition of will
     c. Initiative vs. guilt—3 to 6 years—focus on genital needs, acquisition of purpose
     d. Industry vs. inferiority—6 to 12 years—focus on socialization, acquisition of competence
     e. Identity vs. identity diffusion—13+—focus on search for self, acquisition of fidelity
     f. Intimacy vs. isolation—adulthood—focus on human closeness, sexual fulfillment, acquisition of love
     g. Generativity vs. self absorption—middle-age—focus on productivity, creativity, acquisition of care
     h. Integrity vs. despair—old age—focus on philosophy, acquisition of wisdom (Erikson, 1963)
- Theory of Cognitive Development (Jean Piaget)

  Piaget's stages of development are:
  1. Sensory-Motor Period—0 to 2 years
     a. Stage I—0 to 1 month—no distinction between self and outer reality; characterized by reflexive, uncoordinated body movements
     b. Stage II—1 to 4 months—response patterns begin to be formed; the baby's fist finds its way into his or her mouth.
     c. Stage III—4 to 8 months—response patterns are coordinated and repeated intentionally.

d. Stage IV—8 to 12 months—more coordinated responses ensue; child pushes obstacles aside, searches for vanished objects.

e. Stage V—12 to 18 months—behavior patterns are deliberately varied, as if to observe different results; groping toward a goal emerges.

f. Stage VI—18 months to 2 years—behavior patterns are internalized; symbolic representation emerges.

2. Pre-operational Period—2 to 7 years—characterized by egocentric thinking expressed in artificialism, realism, and magic omnipotence

   a. Pre-conceptual Stage—2 to 4 years—conceptualization begins to emerge, represented in language, drawings, dreams, and play.

   b. Perceptual or Intuitive Stage—4 to 7 years—prelogical reasoning appears, based on appearances; trial and error may lead to discovery of correct relationships.

3. Concrete Operations Period—7 to 11 years—characterized by thought that is logical and reversible; the child understands classes, relationships, and part-whole relationships dealing with concrete things.

4. Formal Operations Period—11 years to adulthood—characterized by the development of logic and reasoning and second-order thoughts, that is, thinking about thoughts (Pulaski, 1971).

- Theory of Moral Development (Lawrence Kohlberg)

  The stages of moral development are:

1. Level I—external standards

   a. Stage 1—avoidance of punishment; the punishment or power of others determines what is right and wrong.

   b. Stage 2—desire for reward or benefit; action is based on getting something in return, in satisfying gratification. There is a sense of fairness and reciprocity, but not a sense of loyalty, gratitude, or justice.

2. Level II—conventional order.

a. Stage 3—anticipation of disapproval of others, or "good boy-nice girl" orientation; there is conformity to expectations of appropriate behavior, seeking approval.

b. Stage 4—anticipation of dishonor; behavior is oriented toward respecting authority, maintaining social order, and obeying social rules for their own goodness.

3. Level III—Principled Morality.

a. Stage 5—social contract, legalistic orientation; behavior is oriented toward the belief that justice flows from a social contract that assures equality for all. Behavior is geared toward rules and legalities.

b. Stage 6—universal ethical principles orientation. Behavior is oriented toward universal, ethical abstract principles (Kohlberg, 1984).

- Theory of Moral Development (Carol Gilligan)

Moral development of women is based more upon an ethic of caring and attachment (Gilligan, 1982). Gilligan has not yet described stages of development in females.

Personality Theories (Social/Interpersonal)

- Theory of Interpersonal Development—Harry Stack Sullivan

Sullivan focuses on behavior as interpersonal. Major concepts include:

1. Self-system—a construct built from the child's experience, made up of reflected appraisals from the approval or disapproval of significant others

2. Two basic drives that underlie behavior:

a. The drive for satisfaction—basic physiological drives, e.g., hunger

b. The drive for security—a sense of well being and belonging

3. Anxiety—any painful feeling or emotion that arises from social insecurity or blocks to satisfaction; characteristics of anxiety are:

a. Interpersonal

b. Can be described; can be observed in behavior

c. Individuals try to reduce anxiety.

4. Security operations—measures taken by individuals to reduce anxiety, e.g., selective inattention
5. Mental illness—self-system interferes with ability to attend to basic drives.
6. Therapy is based upon the belief that by experiencing a healthy relationship with the therapist, the patient can learn to build better relationships. Therapy is an active partnership based on trust (Sullivan, 1953).

Personality Theories (Existential/Humanistic)

The theorists focus on experience in the here and now, with little attention to the past.

- Client Centered Therapy (Carl Rogers)

  The key idea is that people can become fully functioning persons when they are unconditionally valued. Rogers described:

1. The attributes of the therapist:
   a. Congruence—inner feelings match outer actions.
   b. Unconditional positive regard—the therapist sees the client as a person of intrinsic worth, likes the client, and treats the client non-judgmentally.
   c. Empathic understanding—the therapist is an empathetic, sensitive listener.
2. The goal of therapy is to help the client become a fully functioning person. The client reaches this goal by:
   a. Relinquishing facades
   b. Banishing ''oughts''
   c. Moving away from cultural expectations and becoming nonconformist
   d. Pleasing oneself, as opposed to pleasing others; being self directed
   e. Opening up and dropping defenses
   f. Trusting his or her inner self, his or her intuition
   g. Becoming willing to be a complex process

h. Accepting others (Rogers, 1961; Scroggs, 1985)

- Gestalt (Frederick (Fritz) Perls)

1. Here-and-now therapy of immediate experiencing, attained by removing masks and facades
2. Involves a creative interaction between therapist and client to gain ongoing awareness of what is being felt, sensed, and thought
3. Describes boundary disturbance—lack of awareness of the immediate environment, which takes the following forms:

   a. Projection—fantasy about what another person is experiencing

   b. Introjection—accepting the beliefs and opinions of others without question

   c. Retroflection—turning back on oneself that which is meant for someone else

   d. Confluence—merging with the environment

   e. Deflection—a method of interfering with contact, used by receivers and senders of messages

4. Goal of therapy—integration of self and world awareness
5. Techniques of therapy include:

   a. Playing the projection—taking and experiencing the role of another

   b. Making the rounds—speaking or doing something to other group members to experiment with new behavior

   c. Sentence completion—e.g., ''I take responsibility for. . . .''

   d. Exaggeration of a feeling or action

   e. Empty chair dialogue—having an interaction with an imaginary provocateur

   f. Dream work—describing and playing parts of a dream (Hardy, 1991)

- Humanistic/Holistic (Abraham Maslow)

1. When basic needs are met, health and growth will naturally follow.
2. Best known for his description of a heirarchy of basic needs:

   a. Physiological needs

   b. Safety needs
   c. Love and belongingness needs
   d. Self esteem needs
   e. Self-actualization needs (Drapela, 1987; Scroggs, 1985)

- Rational Emotive Therapy (Albert Ellis)

  Some consider this an existential theory while others refer to it as a "cognitive" theory, because the focus is on changing thinking, rather than on feeling or experiencing. Assumptions and key concepts include:

  1. People largely control their own destinies.
  2. People act on their basic values and beliefs.
  3. People interpret events according to their basic values or beliefs and the interpretation can change.
  4. A-B-C of therapy:
     a. Activating event
     b. Belief
     c. Consequences—emotional and/or behavioral
  5. Irrational beliefs have four basic forms:
     a. Something should, ought, or must be different.
     b. Something is awful, terrible, or horrible.
     c. One cannot bear, stand, or tolerate something.
     d. Something or someone is damned, as a louse, rotten person, etc.
  6. "Musturbatory" ideologies have three forms:
     a. I must do well and win approval or I am a rotten person.
     b. You must act kindly and justly toward me or you are a rotten person.
     c. My life must remain comfortable and easy or the world is damnable and life hardly seems worth living.
  7. Therapy consists of detecting and eradicating irrational beliefs and musturbatory ideologies by:

a. Disputing—detecting irrationalities, debating against them, discriminating between logical and illogical thinking, and defining what helps to create new beliefs

b. Debating—questioning and disputing the irrational beliefs

c. Discriminating—distinguishing between wants and needs, desires and demands, and rational and irrational ideas

d. Defining—define words and re-define beliefs

Personality theories (Behavioral)

The behavioral theories are generally not concerned with thoughts, feelings, or unconscious phenomena, except to view them as "behaviors." The focus of behavioral therapy is on replacing maladaptive behaviors with more effective behaviors.

- Behavior Therapy (Burrhas Frederic Skinner)

  All behavior is determined by contingencies of reinforcement (Scroggs, 1985). Important concepts include:

  1. Operant conditioning (also called instrumental learning)—the individual performs a behavior which leads to a positive or negative reinforcement, making it either more or less likely that the behavior will be repeated.
  2. Schedules of reinforcement—Skinner found that different schedules of reinforcement had different effects on supporting or extinguishing particular behaviors.

     a. Fixed ratio schedule—behaviors are rewarded or reinforced every time they are repeated.

     b. Variable ratio schedule—behaviors are rewarded randomly.

     c. Fixed interval schedule—behaviors are rewarded at specific time intervals.

     e. Random interval schedule—behaviors are rewarded at random time intervals (Skinner, 1974; Scroggs, 1985).

- Reciprocal Inhibition (Joseph Wolpe)

  A "process of relearning whereby in the presence of a stimulus a non-anxiety producing response is continually repeated until it extinguishes the old, undesirable reponse'' (Wolpe, 1968, p. 234). Types of reciprocal inhibition include:

1. Systematic desensitization—used primarily in the treatment of phobias—the following steps comprise the most common mode of systematic desensitization:
    a. Training in deep muscle relaxation
    b. Listing examples of phobic reactions; arranging them in descending order of intensity
    c. Desensitization:
        (1) Fantasy desensitization—while the client relaxes as deeply as possible, the examples are presented to his or her imagination. They are repeated until the anxiety is eliminated.
        (2) In vivo desensitization—in addition to fantasy desensitization, the client actually faces the feared object or situation.
2. Avoidance (aversive) conditioning is the application of the reciprocal inhibition principle to overcome undesirable responses. An example of avoidance conditioning is the use of the drug antabuse to overcome an alcoholic's undesirable response of drinking (Wolpe, 1968; Charron, 1990).

- Reality Therapy (William Glasser)

Focuses on changing present behavior—the basic premise is that everyone who seeks psychiatric treatment is unable to fulfill his or her basic needs and is denying the reality of the world around him or her. Major concepts include:

1. Each person has two basic needs:
    a. The need to love and be loved—each person needs to be involved with at least one other person who is in touch with reality and able to fulfill his/her own basic needs.
    b. The need to feel worthwhile to himself and others—to be worthwhile, one must maintain a satisfactory standard of behavior.
2. Responsibility—the ability to fulfill one's needs in a way that does

not deprive others of the ability to fulfill their needs; the cause of all psychiatric problems is irresponsibility.

3. Role of the therapist:
    a. Become so involved with the patient that the patient can face reality.
    b. Reject the behavior which is unrealistic while accepting the patient and maintaining involvement.
    c. Teach the patient better ways to fulfill his needs.
    d. Emphasize behavior, not attitude or emotions.
    e. Emphasize responsibility and planning to change inappropriate behavior.

Cognitive Theories

- Cognitive Therapy (Aaron Beck)

While practicing psychoanalysis, Beck discovered that, in addition to the thoughts verbalized during ''free association,'' his patients had a concurrent, second set of thoughts. He called these ''automatic thoughts.'' Automatic thoughts were those that labelled, interpreted, and evaluated, according to a personal set of rules. Beck called dysfunctional automatic thoughts ''cognitive distortions.'' Concepts in cognitive therapy include:

1. The relationship between therapist and client:
    a. The relationship is a collaborative partnership.
    b. Therapist and client determine the goal of therapy together.
    c. The therapist encourages the client to verbalize disagreement with the therapist when appropriate.
2. The process of therapy:
    a. The therapist explains to the client that:
        (1) Perception of reality is not reality.
        (2) Interpretation of sensory input depends on cognitive processes.
    b. Recognize maladaptive ideation—the client is trained to observe his cognitive and emotional reactions to events, identifying:

(1) The observable behavior

(2) The underlying motivation

(3) His thoughts and beliefs

c. Distance and decenter—the client practices distancing the maladaptive thoughts.

d. Authenticate conclusions—the client explores his conclusions and tests them against reality.

e. Change the rules.

(1) The client makes the rules less absolute and extreme.

(2) The client drops false rules from the repertoire and substitutes adaptive rules.

- Social Learning Theory (Albert Bandura)

Combines cognitive and behavioral theories—the key concept of the theory is modeling, also called imitating or learning by observation. Other concepts include:

1. Retention process—verbally encoding an observed behavior
2. Motor Reproduction Process—practicing the motor skills of the observed behavior
3. Reinforcement and Motivational Process—receiving reward or reinforcement for the behavior (Scroggs, 1985)

Theories of Communication

Theories of communication focus upon the process of verbal and nonverbal communication between and among people.

- Neurolinguistic Programming (NLP) (Richard Bandler & John Grinder)

The assumption behind NLP is that we all create personal models or maps of the world and use language to represent our models. People ''get stuck,'' not by their situation, but by the choices they perceive are available to them because of their maps. Concepts include:

1. Representational Systems—sensory modalities through which people access information

a. Auditory

b. Visual

c. Kinesthetic

2. Cues to representational systems—patterns that are associated with representational systems and can be heard or observed

a. Preferred predicates—e.g., the word "view" suggests a visual system.

b. Eye-Accessing cues—e.g., looking upward suggests a visual system.

c. Gross hand movements—e.g., pointing toward the ear suggests an auditory system.

d. Breathing patterns—e.g., deep abdominal breathing suggests a kinesthetic system.

e. Speech pattern and voice tone—e.g., quick bursts of high pitched words suggest a visual system.

3. Language structure

a. Surface structure—the sentences that native speakers of a language speak and write

b. Deep structure—the full linguistic representation from which the surface structures of a language are derived

c. Ambiguity—a surface structure may represent more than one deep structure

4. Human modeling—the process of representing something, e.g., the world of experience is represented in language. Modeling involves the following processes:

a. Generalization—a specific experience comes to represent the entire category of which it is a member.

b. Deletion—selected portions of the world are excluded from the representation created by an individual.

c. Distortion—the relationships among the parts of the model differ from the relationships they are supposed to represent (Bandler & Grinder, 1975, 1976; Wilson & Kneisl, 1992).

- Transactional Analysis (TA) Eric Berne

The focus is on the interaction between persons. Concepts include:

1. Ego State—frame of mind
   a. Parent—exhibits feelings and behaviors learned from parents and authorities; the parent may be nurturing or critical.
   b. Adult—exhibits feelings and behaviors of a mature adult, e.g., analysis, perception, and sociability
   c. Child—exhibits feelings and behaviors natural to children under seven years old; the child may be natural or adapted. The adapted child is acting under parental influence.
2. Transaction—verbal and non-verbal communication between two people
   a. Complementary transactions
      (1) A message sent *from* the ego state of Person A is responded to in that ego state.
      (2) A message sent *to* an ego state in Person B is responded to from that ego state.
   b. Crossed transactions
      (1) A message sent *from* the ego state of Person A is responded to in another ego state.
      (2) A message sent *to* an ego state in Person B is responded to from another ego state.
   c. Ulterior transactions—messages that occur on two levels
      (1) The social or overt level
      (2) The hidden or psychological level
3. Games—recurring sets of ulterior transactions with a concealed motive, e.g., "Why don't you . . . Yes, but."
4. Script—an unconscious life plan
5. Therapy using TA may be done in conjunction with other modes of therapy, e.g., psychoanalysis. Therapy consists of:
   a. Explaining TA to the client
   b. Structural analysis of the client's ego states
   c. Transactional analysis of the client's interactions

d. Game analysis

e. Script analysis (Berne, 1961, 1964; Wilson & Kneisl, 1992)

Theories of Group Behavior and Therapy

Many theories already described in this chapter have been applied to group behavior and group therapy, including theories of psychoanalysis, personality and communication. The theory considered basic to all groups is systems theory.

- Systems Theory (Von Bertalanffy)

  According to Von Bertalanffy (1934) the world consists of entities called "systems." The theory has frequently been used to explain group behavior. Selected concepts include:

  1. All systems are hierarchically arrayed.
     a. Suprasystem
     b. System
     c. Subsystem
  2. A system has three functions:
     a. Meet its purpose
     b. Self maintainance
     c. Adaptation
  3. The whole is more than the sum of the parts.
  4. A change in one part affects other parts and/or the whole system.
  5. There is feedback or input and output:
     a. Within the system
     b. Between the system and the environment (Von Bertalanffy, 1934; Van Servellen, 1984)

- Psychodrama (J. L. Moreno)

  Psychodrama is a here-and-now action psychotherapy, a therapeutic drama, used primarily in group settings. The therapist functions as the "Director" of the drama chosen by the client. Psychodrama consists of a three-part process:

1. Warm up—the protaganist chooses the time, place, scene, and auxiliary egos for his production.
2. Action—the issue or conflict is acted out or re-lived.
3. Post-action Sharing—group members discuss their identification with the subject (Moreno, 1964).

Family Theories

Family therapies focus on the family as a whole. The family member who has a problem to be dealt with in therapy is known as the ''identified patient.''

- Family Systems Theory (Murray Bowen)

  Bowen applied systems theory to the treatment of dysfunctional families, developing a ''transgenerational'' therapy. The main concepts of the theory are:

  1. Differentiation of self—the lower the level of self-differentiation, the less adaptive one is under stress. There are two types of differentiation of self:
     a. Differentiating thought from emotion
     b. Differentiating oneself from one's ''family ego mass''
  2. Triangles—when a two-member alliance, or dyad, becomes emotionally stressed, the members pull in a third member to reduce anxiety. Bowen considers a triangle the basic building block of any emotional system.
  3. Nuclear family emotional system—patterns of emotional interaction among family members
  4. Multigenerational transmission process—relationship patterns and anxiety about specific issues that have been transmitted through the generations
  5. Family projection process—assignment of characteristics to certain family members
  6. Sibling position—birth order and gender
  7. Emotional cutoff—distancing to deal with intense unresolved emotional issues
  8. Therapy—consists of role modeling and guiding family members to:

a. Increase differentiation of self from a ''pseudoself'' consisting of beliefs and values acquired in the family to a highly differentiated self

b. Detriangle—observe one's own effect and control one's participation in the triangle, while maintaining emotional contact (Bowen, 1978; Stuart & Sundeen, 1991; Kerr & Bowen, 1988)

- Structural Family Therapy (Salvador Minuchin)

In this theory, the therapist joins the family and works to modify the family structure. Concepts in Structural Family Therapy include:

1. The family in transition—the family is considered a social system in transformation that must maintain its continuity and adapt to internal and external stressor.
2. Stages of family development—each stage requires restructuring. The stages are:

   a. Courtship period—when the young person reaches adulthood and seeks a mate

   b. Marriage—when one member moves from the family of origin to create a new family

   c. Middle years of marriage—when parents must wean themselves from their children

   d. Retirement and old age—one spouse may die; adult children may assume care provider role.
3. Family structure, which consists of:

   a. Power and influence—the hierarchy of power and authority; parental authority is advocated.

   b. Subsystems—sets of relationships or dyads formed by generation, gender, interest, or function

   c. Boundaries—rules of who participates with whom—boundary problems include:

      (1) Enmeshment—weak or absent boundaries between individuals and/or subsystems; perceptions of self and others are poorly differentiated.

      (2) Disengagement—rigid boundaries between individuals

and/or subsystems; communication and contact is minimal.

4. Tasks of the therapist include:
   a. Joining and accommodation—tasks include:
      (1) Maintainance—e.g., join the family and maintain family strengths by pointing them out.
      (2) Assessment—e.g., assess the family structure and transaction patterns.
   b. Restructuring
      (1) Actualize family transactional patterns—e.g., re-create communication channels.
      (2) Mark boundaries—delineate individual and subsystem boundaries.
      (3) Escalate stress—e.g., block transactional patterns.
      (4) Assign tasks within and between sessions.
      (5) Utilize symptoms—e.g., exaggerate, de-emphasize or relabel symptoms; move to new symptoms.
      (6) Support, educate, and guide (Minuchin and Nichols, 1993; Helm, 1991).

- Strategic Family Therapy (Madanes and Haley)

Strategic Family Therapy, also known as Problem Solving Therapy, is brief therapy that focuses on solving the presenting problem(s) (Haley, 1987; Madanes, 1981). Concepts include:

1. Symptom—a behavior that analogically or metaphorically expresses a family problem
2. Problem—part of a sequence of acts between people; the way one person communicates with another
3. Focus of therapy—changing analogies and metaphors
4. Goal—prevent repetition of problem sequences; introduce more complexity and alternatives
5. Hierarchy—parents are considered responsible for and in charge of children.
6. Interventions:

a. Decide which family members are involved.

b. Design and implement a strategy to shift the family organization so the present problems are not necessary.

c. Directives—the therapist tells the family members to do something. Directives may be:

   (1) Straightforward—e.g., the mother is directed to assume a parental role.

   (2) Paradoxical, e.g.—a spouse is directed to encourage the other spouse to have the ''symptom'' more frequently.

d. Changes are planned in stages so that changes in one situation or relationship will lead to changes in another. The therapist may even create another problem and shift to another abnormal hierarchy before shifting to a normal hierarchy.

e. If the strategy does not work within a few weeks, the therapist plans and implements another strategy (Madanes, 1981; Haley, 1987).

Miscellaneous theories

- The medical model

In the medical model, a cognitive, emotional, or behavioral disturbance is considered a medical illness that can be located in some part of the body or central nervous system. The illness can be diagnosed, classified, and labelled according to the biochemical and mental symptoms. Medical focus is on the diagnosis and treatment of the illness. Much of modern psychiatric care is dominated by the medical model (Wilson & Kneisl, 1992). The Medical Model consists of the following sequence of steps:

1. Assessment—physical examination, history of the present illness, past history, family and social history, medical history, review of symptoms, mental status examination, and laboratory tests

2. Diagnosis—diagnosis is made, according to the categories of the *Diagnostic and Statistical Manual,* (DSM-IV). The DSM-IV specifies diagnostic criteria along five axes:

   a. Axis I—clinical syndromes: other conditions that may be a focus of clinical attention

   b. Axis II—personality disorders

c. Axis III—general medical conditions
d. Axis IV—psychosocial and environmental problems
e. Axis V—global assessment of functioning

3. Treatment—treatment may entail pharmacotherapy, nursing care, individual or group counseling or psychotherapy, and treatments for specific diseases—e.g., Electroconvulsive Therapy for depression.
4. Evaluation—evaluation of treatment is based upon observation of symptoms (Stuart & Sundeen, 1991).

- Crisis Intervention (Donna Aguilera)
  1. Types of crises:
     a. Situational—external events that cause unusual stresses, e.g., hospitalization or divorce
     b. Maturational—normal processes of growth and development in which there is difficulty with maturation, e.g., adolescence and adulthood
     c. Adventitious—accidental, uncommon, and unexpected events, e.g., fire, earthquake, or flood (Aguilera, 1990)
  2. Phases of crisis intervention:
     a. Assessment—assessing the precipitating event and the client's perceptions of the event
     b. Planning of the intervention—evaluating strengths, coping skills, support systems, and alternative methods of coping
     c. Intervention—treatment lasting one to six weeks, with the goal of returning the individual to his previous level of functioning
        (1) Helping the person gain an intellectual understanding of the crisis
        (2) Helping the person express feelings
        (3) Exploring coping mechanisms
        (4) Reopening the social world
     d. Resolution and anticipatory planning—reinforcing adaptive mechanisms, summarizing the process of intervention and planning for future coping (Aguilera, 1990)

- Theory of Self-Concept (John Hattie)

  The attributes of self-concept include:

  1. A cognitive appraisal consisting of beliefs about self
  2. Three aspects of self-concept are:
     a. Expectations from self and others—high expectations in a dimension or a task can lead to low self concept and vice-versa. For example, if an average high school athlete expects to become a professional basketball star, his or her high expectation may lead to low self-concept.
     b. Descriptions of oneself which are:
        (1) Hierarchical—from a description of a simple, isolated characteristic to a general, all-inclusive description of self
        (2) Multi-faceted—having numerous dimensions
     c. Prescriptions—standards of correctness
  3. Integrated across various dimensions by means of
     a. Self-verification—soliciting feedback to confirm the view of self
     b. Self-consistency—internal harmony among opinions, attitudes, and values
     c. Self-complexity—viewing self as complex and multi-faceted
     d. Self-enhancement—viewing self's positive qualities as more important than self's negative qualities
  4. Subject to confirmation from self and others
  5. Implicit and culturally bound (Hattie, 1991)

- Theory of Self-disclosure (Richard L. Archer)

  Summarizing the research and definitions of self-disclosure, Archer (1987) focused on the orientations and functions of self-disclosure which are as follows:

  1. The self-orientation—disclosures are concerned with exploring the nature and contents of oneself, for oneself.
  2. The self-to-other orientation—disclosures are concerned with locating oneself in relation to others by getting feedback.

3. The other-to-self orientation—disclosures are used as a means of social control or of obtaining benefits from others.
4. The other orientation—disclosure is geared toward obtaining reciprocal disclosure.
5. The self-and-other orientation—disclosure is concerned with interdependence of participants in a relationship (Archer, 1987).

- Stress Theory (Hans Selye)

Selye developed a theory of the physical response to stress called the General Adaptation Syndrome (GAS). The stages of the GAS are as follows:

1. Alarm stage—a threat is perceived, and the endocrine system and the immune system respond, creating physical and mental alertness.
2. Resistance Stage—the threat continues, and attempts are made to adapt.
3. Exhaustion Stage—if the threat continues, the adaptive hormones are depleted and the body succumbs to illness (Selye, 1976; Wilson & Kneisl, 1992).

- Role Theory (Hardy and Conway)

According to Hardy and Conway (1988), Role Theory ''represents a collection of concepts and a variety of hypothetical formulations that predict how actors will perform in a given role, or under what circumstances certain types of behavior can be expected'' (p.63). Concepts include:

1. Approach to studying roles:
   a. Structural approach—roles are fixed positions with certain expectations and demands, enforced by societal sanctions.
   b. Symbolic Interactionist approach—behavior is a response to the symbolic acts (primarily gestures and speech) of others.
2. Role making—a process of modifying a role; phases of role making include:
   a. Initiator behavior
   b. Other response
   c. Interpretation

   d. Altered response
   e. Role validation
3. Role taking—the proces of imagining oneself in the place of another
4. Socialization—the process of learning the social roles, skills, and knowledge that prepare one for role performance
5. Role stress—a condition in which role obligations are unclear, conflicting or impossible to meet
6. Role strain—a subjective state of frustration or distress in meeting role expectations
7. Stratification—a hierarchical ranking of people according to wealth, status, power, or occupation (Hardy & Conway, 1988)

QUESTIONS
Select the best answer

1. The purpose of a theory is to:
   a. Describe, explain, predict or control a phenomenon
   b. Encourage the development of more research
   c. Prove that there can be one way to describe a phenomenon
   d. All of the above

2. Characteristics of theories include:
   a. They provide laws by which to govern practice.
   b. They have little in common with practice.
   c. They can guide and improve practice.
   d. They need not be logical.

3. Inductive theory construction:
   a. Consists largely of concepts borrowed from other disciplines
   b. Validates deductive theory construction
   c. Proceeds from the general to the specific
   d. Proceeds from the specific to the general

4. Theories serve to:
   a. Guide practice
   b. Guide research
   c. Provide a common language for practitioners and researchers
   d. All of the above

5. The concepts central to the discipline of nursing are:
   a. Self-care, self-care deficit, and nursing systems
   b. Caring and curing
   c. Assessment, diagnosis, intervention, and evaluation
   d. Person, environment, health, and nursing

6. The central focus in Dorothea Orem's theory of nursing is:
   a. Behavioral systems
   b. Self-care
   c. The environment
   d. Adaptation

7. In Orem's theory, Nursing Systems are described as:

   a. Desciptions of a variety of ideal hospital staffing models
   b. The theories that she drew from
   c. Simple, complex, and combined
   d. Wholly compensatory, partly compensatory, and supportive-educative

8. Nurse A, who utilizes Orem's theory, is caring for Patient B. Patient B requires a complete bed bath. When charting, Nurse A will describe the Patient B's inability to provide complete self-care as:

   a. A health deviation
   b. Illness
   c. A self-care deficit
   d. A diagnostic indication

9. Imogene King's theory of nursing is:

   a. A theory of personal systems
   b. A theory of goal attainment
   c. A theory of adaptation
   d. A behavioral systems theory

10. In King's theory, a set of behaviors expected of a person occupying a certain position is called a:

    a. Role
    b. Perception
    c. Transaction
    d. Developmental position

11. One of the basic assumptions in the theory of Martha Rogers is:

    a. People come together to help and be helped to maintain health.
    b. The universe is a continuously expanding, evolving, growing field of energy.
    c. The person and environment are continually exchanging matter and energy with each other.
    d. Energy fields are four dimensional, unidirectional expanding sources of knowledge.

12. Rogers describes the human being as:

    a. Characterized by the capacity for abstraction and imagery

b. Characterized by the capacity for language and thought
c. Characterized by the capacity for sensation and emotion
d. All of the above

13. The building blocks of Rogers' theory are:

    a. Energy, openness, pattern and four-dimensionality
    b. Person, life process, pattern and organization, energy
    c. Person, environment, health, nursing
    d. All of the above

14. Sister Callista Roy's theory of nursing is:

    a. The Interpersonal Relations Model
    b. The Problem Solving Model
    c. The Communication Model
    d. The Adaptation Model

15. Roy's adaptive modes are:

    a. Physiological function, self-concept, role function, and interdependence
    b. Regulator, cognator, external, and informational
    c. Value, belief, thought, and emotion
    d. All of the above

16. The nurse who utilizes Roy's model in providing nursing care would first:

    a. Identify focal stimuli
    b. Manipulate focal stimuli
    c. Identify input and internal processes
    d. Conduct a first-level assessment

17. The nurse who utilizes Roy's model in providing nursing care will include in the second-level assessment:

    a. Identification of ineffective responses
    b. Identification of nursing diagnosis
    c. Identification of goals
    d. Patterns of physical functioning

18. The main concept in Leininger's Theory of Culture Care Diversity and Universality is that:

a. Culture is the learned, shared, and transmitted values, beliefs, norms, and lifeways of a group
b. Care is the essence of nursing
c. There is diversity and universality in every culture
d. Nurses should seek to know the universality of Transcultural nursing

19. According to Leininger, the important factors to study in cultural care include:

    a. Religious factors
    b. Nutritional factors
    c. Rest patterns
    d. Prenatal care

20. Cultural care accommodation refers to:

    a. Actions and decisions to help people of a given culture negotiate for a beneficial outcome with health caregivers
    b. Actions and decisions to help a client modify their lifeways for beneficial health care, while respecting their cultural values and beliefs
    c. Actions and decisions that help people retain relevant cultural care values
    d. Actions and decisions that are based on universal cultural care

21. The two most famous psychoanalytic theorists are:

    a. Horney and Adler
    b. Freud and Jung
    c. Kohlberg and Gilligan
    d. Adler and Sullivan

22. According to Freudian theory, unconscious actions or thoughts to protect the ego from anxiety are called:

    a. Freudian slips
    b. Unconscious motivation
    c. Defense mechanisms
    d. Transference

23. According to Freudian theory, thoughts, feelings, and desires that are not in immediate awareness, but can be recalled to consciousness, are considered:

    a. Conscious
    b. Preconscious
    c. Subconscious
    d. Unconscious

24. According to Freudian theory, the personality has three main components. The component characterized by the desire for immediate and complete satisfaction is the:

    a. Reality principle
    b. Id
    c. Ego
    d. Superego

25. Freud posits that children of four or five fall in love with the parent of the oppostie sex. This is known as:

    a. Projection
    b. Transference
    c. The pleasure principle
    d. The oedipus complex

26. According to Freud, whatever inhibits a person from producing material from the unconscious is considered:

    a. Resistance
    b. Transference
    c. Counter-transference
    d. Fixation

27. In Jungian theory, the unconscious collective intangible idea, image, or concept is the:

    a. Persona
    b. Shadow
    c. Archetype
    d. Rebirth

28. Jung's archetypes include:

    a. The animus
    b. The shadow
    c. Stock characters
    d. All of the above

29. The functional types described by Jung include:

    a. Extrovert and introvert
    b. The hero, the trickster, and the sage

c. Thinking, feeling, sensing, intuiting
d. All of the above

30. Adler developed the Theory of Individual Psychology. The main concern of Adler's theory is:

    a. The individual going through the stages of development
    b. Personal growth through compensating for inferiority
    c. Providing client-centered therapy
    d. The effect of relationships on unconscious behaviors

31. Adler identified effects of the birth order of siblings. According to his theory, the child most likely to be interested in authority and organization is:

    a. The first-born
    b. The second-born
    c. The middle child in a large family
    d. The youngest child

32. The key concept in the personality theory of Horney is:

    a. Neurosis
    b. Hostility
    c. Basic anxiety
    d. Satisfaction of needs

33. According to Horney, people protect themselves by:

    a. Moving toward other people
    b. Moving against other people
    c. Moving away from other people
    d. All of the above

34. Erikson identified eight stages of growth and development. The stage characterized by a focus on genital needs and the acquisition of a purpose is:

    a. Trust vs. mistrust
    b. Autonomy vs. shame
    c. Initiative vs. guilt
    d. Industry vs. inferiority

35. If a child's activities are primarily social interaction, doing homework and practicing basketball, then according to Erikson, he is in the following stage of development:

a. Trust vs. mistrust
b. Autonomy vs. shame
c. Initiative vs. guilt
d. Industry vs. inferiority

36. According to Erikson, the stage of development characterized by the acquisition of wisdom is:

a. Identity vs. Identity diffusion
b. Intimacy vs. Isolation
c. Generativity vs. self-absorption
d. Integrity vs. despair

37. Jean Piaget developed a theory of:

a. Psychosexual development
b. Cognitive development
c. Moral development
d. Social development

38. In the developmental theory of Piaget, the period characterized by egocentric thinking, expressed in artificialism, realism and magical thinking is the:

a. Sensory motor period
b. Pre-operational period
c. Concrete operations period
d. Formal operations period

39. In the developmental theory of Piaget, the period characterized by the development of logic and reasoning, and second-order thoughts, that is, ''thinking about thoughts,'' is

a. Sensory motor period
b. Pre-operational period
c. Concrete operations period
d. Formal operations Period

40. The nurse is working with Mrs. L. who has been sexually promiscuous and manipulative with her family. While developing a treatment plan for Mrs. L, the nurse recognizes that her behavior is consistent with the behavior in Stage 2 of Kohlberg's theory of moral development. Mrs. L. will be motivated by:

a. Avoidance of punishment
b. Desire for reward or benefit

c. Anticipation of disapproval of others
d. Anticipation of dishonor

41. If Mrs. L.'s behavior was consistent with the behavior of Stage 4 of Kohlberg's theory of moral development, she would be motivated by:

    a. Anticipation of disapproval of others
    b. Anticipation of dishonor
    c. A legalistic orientation
    d. Belief in universal ethical principles

42. In Kohlberg's theory of moral development, behavior in Stage 6 is motivated by:

    a. Anticipation of disapproval of others
    b. Anticipation of dishonor
    c. A legalistic orientation
    d. Belief in universal ethical principles

43. According to the work of Gilligan on moral development:

    a. In applying Kohlberg's theory, women are generally more moral than men.
    b. Most women achieve the moral reasoning in Stage 6 of Kohlberg's theory.
    c. Women and men have the same moral reasoning.
    d. The moral development of women is based on different motivations than that of men.

44. The main focus of the social-interpersonal theories of personality is:

    a. Neurosis
    b. Anxiety about relationships
    c. The effects of interactions with others
    d. Inferiority and superiority feelings

45. In the interpersonal theory of Harry Stack Sullivan, the ''self-system'' is:

    a. The part of the personality that satisfies the drive for security,
    b. A construct to describe the narcissism inherent in all interpersonal relationships
    c. A construct built from the child's experience, made up of reflected appraisals by significant others
    d. All of the above

46. According to Sullivan, the basic drives that underlie human behavior are:

    a. The drive to reduce anxiety and the drive to avoid fear
    b. The drive for satisfaction and the drive for security
    c. The drive to fulfill basic physical needs and the drive to fulfill sexual needs
    d. All of the above

47. The existential theories of personality focus on:

    a. The meaning of life for the individual
    b. Present experience, with little attention to the past
    c. One's philosophy of life
    d. All of the above

48. According to Carl Rogers, the important attributes of the therapist are:

    a. Congruence, unconditional positive regard and empathetic understanding
    b. Knowledge of Rogers' theory, patience, and ability to interpret dreams
    c. Knowledge of Rogers' theory, congruence, and interest in human development
    d. Willingness to drop facades, openness to individual meanings, and compassion

49. For the therapist who utilizes Rogerian therapy, the main goal of therapy is for the client to become a fully functioning person. The client reaches this goal in therapy by:

    a. Relinquishing facades
    b. Moving away from cultural expectations and becoming non-conformist
    c. Trusting their inner self, their intuition
    d. All of the above

50. The therapist utilizing Gestalt therapy recognizes that introjection is:

    a. A fantasy about what another person is experiencing
    b. Accepting the beliefs and opinions of others without question
    c. Turning back on oneself that which is meant for someone else
    d. Merging with the environment

51. The main goal of Gestalt Therapy is;

    a. Dropping facades
    b. Differentiating between self and others

c. Integration of self and world awareness
d. All of the above

52. Techniques in Gestalt therapy include:

    a. Playing the projection
    b. Making the rounds
    c. Exaggeration of a feeling or action
    d. All of the above

53. Maslow's hierarchy of basic needs include:

    a. Safety and satisfaction, health and growth
    b. Physiological needs, safety, love and belongingness, self esteem, and self-actualization
    c. Physical, biological, psychological, sociological, and spiritual needs
    d. Food, fluid, activity, meaning and purpose, and self-actualization

54. The A-B-Cs of Ellis's Rational Emotive Therapy are:

    a. Action, behavior, congruence
    b. Anticipation, belief, consequence
    c. Acceptance, behavior, caring
    d. Activating behavior, belief, consequence

55. According to Ellis's Rational Emotive Therapy, a basic form of irrational beliefs is that:

    a. One cannot meet one's goals.
    b. Life is difficult.
    c. Something is awful, terrible, or horrible.
    d. All of the above

56. For the nurse who uses Rational Emotive Therapy in practice, the focus of treatment is on:

    a. Behavior rather than beliefs
    b. Accepting the beliefs of others
    c. Disputing, debating, discriminating, and defining
    d. Anticipating, acting, and accepting

57. Behavioral theories of personality are concerned with:

    a. Unconscious phenomena

b. Cognition
c. Emotions
d. Reinforcement

58. One concept of Skinner's theory is that an individual performs a behavior which leads to a positive or negative reinforcement, making it either more or less likely that the behavior will be repeated. This is called:

a. A schedule of reinforcement
b. A fixed ratio
c. A variable interval
d. Operant conditioning

59. In a variable ratio schedule of reinforcement, behaviors are rewarded:

a. Each nth they are performed
b. Every time they are repeated
c. At specific time intervals
d. At random time intervals

60. Mrs. J. seeks treatment for her fear of automobiles. After the initial assessment, the nurse decides to use systematic desensitization. The first step in systematic desensitization is to:

a. Help Mrs. J. get a prescription for valium and take her for an automobile ride
b. Explore other means of transportation
c. Train Mrs. J. in deep muscle relaxation
d. Show Mrs. J. a picture of an automobile and ask how she feels

61. The two types of systematic desensitization are:

a. Automatic desensitization and standard desensitization
b. Fantasy desensitization and in vivo desensitization
c. Desensitization with medication and desensitization without medication
d. Reciprocal inhibition and aversive conditioning

62. According to the Reality Therapy of William Glasser, each person has the following two basic needs:

a. Psychological needs and spiritual needs
b. Physiological needs and psychological needs
c. The need to love and be loved, and the need to be productive
d. The need to love and be loved, and the need to feel worthwhile

63. According to Glasser, the cause of all psychiatric problems is:

    a. Neurosis
    b. Irresponsibility
    c. Childhood training
    d. Irrational beliefs

64. The therapist who is utilizing Glasser's therapy will emphasize:

    a. Unconscious motivation
    b. Dream interpretation
    c. Changing behavior
    d. Rexperiencing traumatic childhood events

65. Aaron Beck developed a theory of cognitive therapy after he discovered that his clients had ''automatic thoughts.'' The automatic thoughts:

    a. Came from too much free association
    b. Labelled, interpreted, and evaluated situations according to a personal set of rules
    c. Indicated to the client that he should not trust the therapist
    d. Warned clients of any physiological needs

66. The therapist who utilizes Beck's therapy will warn the client:

    a. To try to ignore or suppress his automatic thoughts
    b. That emotionally healthy individuals do not have automatic thoughts
    c. That automatic thoughts are deeply imbedded and cannot be changed
    d. That a perception of reality is not necessarily reality

67. The therapist utilizing Beck's therapy will help the client to:

    a. Recognize and change his automatic thoughts
    b. See reality as the therapist sees it
    c. Change his reality by changing his environment
    d. Recognize and accept that automatic thoughts suggest delusional thinking

68. In the Social Learning Theory of Alfred Bandura, the key concept is:

    a. Modeling
    b. Encoding a behavior
    c. Rewarding behavior appropriately
    d. Rewarding behavior on a ratio interval scale

69. In the Neurolinguistic Programming (NLP) of Bandler and Grinder, the "representational systems" are:

    a. Auditory, visual and kinesthetic
    b. Methods of analyzing communication
    c. Right brain and left brain
    d. Parent, adult and child

70. An assumption behind NLP is that:

    a. We all have irrational beliefs
    b. We all create models of the world, and use language to represent them
    c. We are all philosophers
    d. Verbal and non-verbal communication is important in nursing

71. In NLP, the sentences which native speakers of a language speak and write are called:

    a. Deep structure
    b. Surface structure
    c. Multi-model sentences
    d. Cues to beliefs

72. In NLP, human modeling involves:

    a. Generalization
    b. Deletion
    c. Distortion
    d. All of the above

73. In Transactional Analysis (TA), the theory by Eric Berne, ego states include:

    a. Sane, neurotic, and psychotic
    b. Rational and irrational
    c. Parent, adult, and child
    d. Manic, depressive, and schizophrenic

74. In TA, when a message is sent from an ego state of Person A and is responded to in that ego state, there is a:

    a. Crossed transaction
    b. Ulterior transaction
    c. Complementary transaction
    d. All of the above

75. In TA, a message that occurs on two levels is:

    a. A crossed transaction
    b. An ulterior transaction
    c. A Complementary transaction
    d. All of the above

76. Concepts in Systems theory include:

    a. Systems are designed to serve people
    b. Systems are by nature complex
    c. All systems are hierarchically arrayed
    d. All of the above

77. According to Systems Theory, the functions of a system include:

    a. Cooperation
    b. Conflict
    c. Adaptation
    d. All of the above

78. The originator of Psychodrama was:

    a. Moreno
    b. Minuchin
    c. Beck
    d. Adler

79. In Psychodrama, the therapist functions as a:

    a. Protagonist
    b. Auxiliary ego
    c. Director
    d. Partner

80. The nurse utilizing Bowen's theory in family therapy will observe the patterns of emotional interaction within a family. Bowen calls these patterns:

    a. Triangles
    b. The family projection process
    c. The nuclear family emotional system
    d. The family differentiation process

81. In Bowen's Family Systems Therapy, the multigenerational family transmission process refers to:

    a. Genetic traits
    b. Relationship patterns and anxiety about specific issues that have been transmitted through the generations
    c. Relationships between grandparents and grandchildren
    d. Hereditary disorders

82. The nurse practicing Bowen's Family Systems Therapy will guide family members to:

    a. Use their sibling position to their advantage
    b. Periodically cut off other family members emotionally
    c. Create specific triangles
    d. Increase differentiation of self

83. When the nurse using Minuchin's Structural Family Therapy observes that a mother holds a 7-year-old child in her lap, answers questions for the child, and describes protecting the child from siblings and neighbors, the nurse will suspect.

    a. Accommodation
    b. Enmeshment
    c. Disengagement
    d. An unusual transaction

84. In Minuchin's Structural Family Therapy, the main tasks of the therapist are:

    a. Joining and restructuring
    b. Clarifying the family structure and explaining it
    c. Identifying family communication patterns and maintaining family strengths
    d. Enacting the family structure and delineating boundaries

85. A therapist who utilizes Minuchin's Structural Family Therapy will probably:

    a. Point out family strengths
    b. Identify multigenerational transactions
    c. Maintain his position of authority
    d. All of the above

86. In the Structural Family Therapy of Minuchin, when the therapist blocks the

usual transactional patterns or emphasizes differences among family members, he is probably trying to:

a. Accommodate the family
b. Identify the true patient
c. Escalate stress
d. Identify the executive subsystem

87. A therapist who utilizes the Structural Family Therapy of Minuchin might utilize symptoms by:

a. Moving to new symptoms
b. De-emphasizing symptoms
c. Exaggerating symptoms
d. All of the above

88. The focus of Strategic Family Therapy is to:

a. Emphasize symptoms
b. Change analogies and metaphors in the family
c. Help the family to be more democratic
d. Identify and solve all family problems

89. After identifying the symptom and the problem, the nurse who is practicing Strategic Family Therapy will:

a. Identify the family structure
b. Work to detriangle all family members
c. Design a strategy to shift the family organization
d. Mark subsystem boundaries

90. In the medical/biological model, the emphasis is upon:

a. Diagnosing and treating the illness
b. Understandng the meaning of childhood experiences
c. Utilizing group therapy and social support
d. Changing behavior

91. In the Diagnostic and Statistical Manual, Third edition, Revised (DSM-IV), Axis I contains the:

a. Clinical syndromes; other conditions that may be a focus of clinical attention
b. Developmental disorders and personality disorders

c. Physical disorders
d. Severity of psychosocial stressors

92. According to the Crisis Intervention Theory of Aquilera, types of crises are:

a. Familial, academic, and social
b. Major disasters and daily events
c. Situational, maturational, and adventitious
d. Growth inducing and growth hindering

93. Crisis Intervention Therapy usually lasts:

a. From one to six weeks
b. From one to six months
c. From three months to one year
d. More than one year

94. The main goal of Crisis Intervention is to:

a. Assist the client in identifying his strengths
b. Assist the client to gain insight as to why he reacted as he did
c. Help the client to return to his previous level of functioning
d. Help the client to prevent another crisis

95. According to the Self-Concept Theory of Hattie, the first attribute of self-concept is:

a. A cognitive appraisal of oneself
b. A feeling of wholeness
c. Determined completely by one's environment
d. Un-defined

96. In the Self-Concept Theory of Hattie, internal harmony among opinions, values, and attitudes is called:

a. Self-complexity
b. Self-verification
c. Self-consistency
d. Self-regulation

97. Self-concept is:

a. Subject to confirmation from others
b. Culturally bound

c. Multi-faceted
d. All of the above

98. Purposes of self-disclosure include:

a. Exploring oneself
b. Locating oneself in relation to others
c. Social control
d. All of the above

99. The General Adaptation Syndrome, as identified by Hans Selye, has the following stages:

a. Surprise, alertness, reaction
b. Inflexibility, adaptation, engulfment
c. Alarm, resistance, exhaustion
d. Openness, closedness, paranoia

100. In the structural approach to role theory, roles are considered:

a. Subject to change depending on immediate circumstances
b. Fixed positions with certain expectations and demands
c. Responses to a number of things in the environment
d. Synonymous with job descriptions

101. Role taking refers to:

a. Socialization into a role
b. The process of moving into a role that was previously held by another person
c. The process of imagining oneself in the place of another
d. Being taken by surprise by the expectations of a certain role

ANSWERS

1. a
2. c
3. d
4. d
5. d
6. b
7. d
8. c
9. b
10. a
11. c
12. d
13. a
14. d
15. a
16. d
17. a
18. b
19. a
20. a
21. b
22. c
23. b
24. b
25. d
26. a
27. c
28. d
29. c
30. b
31. a
32. c
33. d
34. c
35. d
36. d
37. b
38. b
39. d
40. b
41. d
42. d
43. c
44. c
45. c
46. b
47. d
48. a
49. d
50. b
51. c
52. d
53. b
54. d
55. c
56. c
57. d
58. d
59. d
60. c
61. b
62. d
63. b
64. c
65. b
66. d
67. a
68. a
69. a
70. b
71. b
72. d
73. c
74. c
75. b
76. c
77. c
78. a
79. c
80. c
81. b
82. d
83. b
84. a
85. a
86. c
87. d
88. b
89. c
90. a
91. a
92. c
93. a
94. c
95. a
96. c
97. d
98. d
99. c
100. b
101. c

Bibliography

Adler, A. (1983). *The practice and theory of individual psychology.* Totowa, NJ: Helix Books.

Archer, R. L. (1987). Commentary: Self-disclosure, a very useful behavior. In V. J. Derlega & J. H. Berg (Eds.), *Self-Disclosure: Theory, Research and Therapy* (pp. 329–341). NY: Plenum Press.

Aguilera, D. (1990). *Crisis intervention: Theory and methodology* (6th ed.). St. Louis: C. V. Mosby.

Bandler, R., & Grinder, J. (1975). *The structure of magic I.* Palo Alto: Science and Behavior Books.

Bandler, R., & Grinder, J. (1976). *The structure of magic II.* Palo Alto: Science and Behavior Books.

Berne, E. (1961). *Transactional analysis in psychotherapy.* NY: Ballantine.

Berne, E. (1964). *Games people play.* New York: Grove press.

Bowen, M. (1971). Family therapy and family group therapy. In H. Kaplan & B. Sadok (Eds.), *Comprehensive group psychotherapy* (pp. 384–421). Baltimore: Williams & Wilkins.

Bowen, M. (1978). *Family therapy in clinical practice.* NY: Jason Aronson.

Carter, B., & McGoldrick, M. (1988). *The changing family life cycle: A framework for family therapy.* New York: Garden Press.

Clements, I. W., & Buchanan, D. M. (1982). *Family therapy: A nursing perspective.* NY: John Wiley & Sons.

Dollard, J., & Miller, N. E. (1950). *Personality and psychotherapy: An analysis in terms of learning, thinking and culture.* NY: McGraw-Hill.

Drapela, V. J. (1987). *A review of personality theories.* Springfield, IL: Charles C. Thomas.

Ellis, A. (1977). The basic clinical theory of rational-emotive therapy. In A. Ellis & R. Grieger (Eds.), *Handbook of rational-emotive therapy* (pp. 3–34). NY: Springer.

Erikson, E. (1963). *Childhood and society* (2nd ed.). NY: W.W. Norton & Co. Inc.

Falco, S. M., & Lobo, M. L. (1990). Martha E. Rogers. In J. George: *Nursing theories: The base for professional practice.* Norwalk, CT: Appleton & Lange.

Fawcett, J. (1984). *Analysis and evaluation of conceptual models of nursing.* Philadelphia: F. A. Davis.

Foster, P. C., & Janssens, N. P. (1990). Dorothea E. Orem. In J. George (Ed.), *Nursing theories: The base for professional nursing practice.* Norwalk, CT: Appleton & Lange.

Galbreath, J. G. (1990). Sister Callista Roy. In J. George (Ed.), *Nursing theories: The base for professional nursing practice.* Norwalk, CT: Appleton & Lange.

George, J. B. (Ed.) (1990). *Nursing theories: The base for professional nursing practice* (3rd ed.). Norwalk, CT: Appleton & Lange.

Gilligan, C. (1982). *In a different voice.* Cambridge, MA: Harvard University Press.

Glasser, W. (1975). *Reality therapy: A new approach to psychiatry.* NY: Harper & Rowe.

Haley, J. (1987). *Problem-solving therapy,* (2nd. ed.). San Francisco: Jossey Bass Publishers.

Hardy M. E., & Conway, M. E. (1988). *Role theory: Perspectives for health professionals* (2nd ed.). Norwalk, CT: Appleton & Lange.

Hardy, R. E. (1991). *Gestalt psychotherapy: Concepts and demonstrations in stress, relationships, hypnosis and addiction.* Springfield, IL: Charles C. Thomas.

Hattie, J. (1991). *Self-concept.* Hillsdale, NJ: Lawrence Erlbaum Associates.

Helm, P. (1991). Family therapy. In G. W. Stuart & S. J. Sundeen (Eds.), *Principles and practice of psychiatric nursing* (pp. 827–851). St. Louis: Mosby.

Horney, K. (1945). *Our inner conflicts: A constructive theory of neurosis.* NY: W. W. Norton & Company.

Kerr, M., & Bowen, M. (1988). *Family evaluation: An approach based on Bowen's Theory.* NY: W. W. Norton.

Kohlberg, L. (1984). *The psychology of moral development.* San Francisco: Harper & Row.

Leininger, M (1991). *Culture care diversity and universality: A theory of nursing.* NY: National League for Nursing Press.

Madanes, Cloe (1981). *Strategic family therapy.* San Francisco: Jossey Bass Publishers.

Maslow, A. H. (1987). *Motivation and personality* (2nd. ed.). NY: Harper & Row.

Meleis, A. I. (1985). *Theoretical nursing: Development and progress.* Philadelphia: J. B. Lippincott.

Minuchin, S., & Nichols, M. (1993). *Family healing.* NY: The Free Press.

Moreno, J. L. (1946). *Psychodrama: Volume I.* Boston, MA: Beacon Press.

Perls, F. S., Hefferline, R. F., & Goodman, P. (1977). *Gestalt therapy.* NY: Bantam Books.

Piaget, J. (1967). *The child's conception of the world.* London: Routledge & Kegan Paul Ltd.

Polit, D. F., & Hungler, B. P. (1991). *Nursing research principles and methods.* Philadelphia: J. B. Lippincott.

Pulaski, M. A. (1971). *Understanding Piaget.* NY: Harper & Row.

Riehl, J. P., & Roy, S. C. (1980). *Conceptual models for nursing practice* (2nd ed.). NY: Appleton-Century Crofts.

Rogers, C. (1961). *On becoming a person.* Boston: Houghton Mifflin.

Rogers, M. (1983). *The theoretical basis of nursing.* Philadelphia: F. A. Davis.

Satir, V. (1967). *Conjoint family therapy.* (rev. ed.). NY: Science and Behavior Books.

Schultz, D. (1987) *Theories of personality.* Monterey, CA: Brooks/Cole.

Scroggs, J. R. (1985). *Key ideas in personality theory.* NY: West Publishing Company.

Skinner, B. F. (1974). *About behaviorism.* NY: Alfred A. Knopf.

Stuart, G. W., & Sundeen, S. J. (1991). *Principles and practice of psychiatric nursing.* St. Louis: C. V. Mosby.

Sullivan, H. S. (1953). *The interpersonal theory of psychiatry* NY: W. W. Norton.

Van Servellen, G. M. (1984). *Group and family therapy.* St. Louis: C. V. Mosby.

Von Bertalanffy, L. V. (1934). *Modern theories of development: An introduction to theoretical biology.* London: Oxford University Press.

Wilson, H. S., & Kneisl, C. R. (1992). *Psychiatric nursing* (4th ed.). Menlo Park, CA: Addison-Wesley.

Yalom, I. D. (1983). *Inpatient group psychotherapy.* NY: Basic Books.

Yalom, I. D. (1985). *Theory and practice of group psychotherapy* (3rd ed.). NY: Basic Books.

Zuckerman, M. (1991). *Psychobiology of personality.* NY: Cambridge University Press.

Mental Disorders Due to Substance Abuse

Therese K. Killeen

Psychoactive Substance Use Disorders

- Definition
  1. A primary, chronic disease with genetic, psychosocial, and environmental factors influencing its development and manifestations
  2. Progressive and fatal
  3. Characterized by the following continuous or periodic behavior:
     a. Impaired control over substance use
     b. Preoccupation with the drug
     c. Use of the drug despite adverse consequences
     d. Distortions in thinking, most notably denial (ASAM/NCAdd Committee, 1990)
  4. Recent Epidemiologic Catchment Area (ECA) statistics show that among the general population there is a 13.7% lifetime prevalence of alcohol abuse and/or dependence. Lifetime prevalence of drug abuse and/or dependence is 6.17%.
- Signs and Symptoms
  1. Criteria established by the Diagnostic and Statistical Manual of Mental Disorders (APA, 1993) for psychoactive substance **dependence** include the occurrence of at least three of the following in the same 12-month period:
     a. Use of amounts greater than intended
     b. Attempts at control
     c. Excessive time spent in obtaining, using, recovering
     d. Use despite social obligations or hazards
     e. Use despite recurrent problems
     f. Presence of *tolerance*—needing increasing amounts of substance to produce desired effect or markedly diminished effect with continued use of same amount of substance
     g. Presence of withdrawal or use to avoid or relieve *withdrawal symptoms*—a pathophysiological state of disquilibrium brought on by an abrupt discontinuation, or rapid decrease in, dosage of a psychoactive substance
  2. Criteria for psychoactive substance abuse (PSA) include:

a. Recurrent use resulting in a failure to fulfill major role obligations
b. Continued use despite having persistent or recurrent social or interpersonal problems caused or exacerbated by the effects of the substance
c. Recurrent use in hazardous situations
d. Recurrent substance-related legal problems

3. Psychoactive substances with abuse potential include: alcohol, sedative/hypnotics, amphetamines, cocaine, cannabis, hallucinogens, narcotics, phencyclidine, inhalants, caffeine, nicotine

- Differential Diagnoses

1. DSM-IV Disorders with similar symptoms/presentations
   a. Mood/Depressive Disorders
   b. Anxiety
   c. Psychotic Disorders
   d. Personality Disorders
   e. Impulse Control Disorders
   f. Adjustment Disorders
   g. Sleep Disorders
   h. Sexual Dysfunction Disorders
   i. Amnesia, Dementia, and Delirium Disorders
2. Substance use from other DSM-IV (APA, 1993) disorders
   a. Symptoms developed during or within a month of significant substance intoxication or withdrawal
3. Evidence that symptoms are better accounted for by a disorder that is not substance induced include:
   a. Symptoms precede onset of the substance abuse/dependence.
   b. Symptoms persist for a substantial period of time after the cessation of acute withdrawal or severe intoxication.
   c. Symptoms persist for a substantial period in excess of what would be expected given the character, duration, or amount of the substance used.

   d. Other evidence suggests the existence of an independent non-substance induced disorder (history of recurrent non-substance-related episodes).

4. Common laboratory values associated with PSA
   a. Gamma-Glutamyltransferase (GGT), Aspartate aminotransferase (AST), Mean Corpuscular Volume (MCV) commonly increased in alcoholism
   b. Blood Alcohol Concentration (BAC)—increased with alcohol ingestion—predictor of tolerance
      (1) BAC > 100 mg/ml on routine clinical exam
      (2) BAC > 150 mg/ml without evidence of gross neurological impairment
      (3) BAC > 300 mg/ml recorded at any time
   c. Urine drug screening (UDS) detects presence of drug in the urine. Diagnostic limitations include:
      (1) Short "window" of detection of metabolites
      (2) Intermittent use patterns of abusers
      (3) Issues of civil liberties

5. Assessing alcohol and drug involvement
   a. Drug and/or drink of choice
   b. Other types of substances used
   c. Minutes/hours since last use of substances
   d. Past history of and response to withdrawal
   e. Amount, duration frequency, and route of administration
   f. Pattern of use (episodic vs. continuous)
   g. Family history of alcohol and/or drug abuse
   h. History of delirium tremens, seizures, falls, blackouts, or injury to self or others
   i. Use interferes with job, relationships, or other areas of functioning
   j. Expected and experienced effects of substance on mood and behavior

k. Context of substance use (solitary vs. social consumption)

l. Access and availability of substances

6. Medical complications associated with PSA

   a. Hepatic complications—alcoholic fatty liver, alcoholic hepatitis, alcoholic cirrhosis

   b. Gastrointestinal complications—esophagitis, gastritis, pancreatitis associated with alcohol

   c. Cardiovascular complications—cardiomyopathy, hypertension, arrhythmias associated with alcohol and cocaine

   d. Neurological complications

      (1) Stroke, seizures associated with alcohol and cocaine

      (2) Polyneuropathy, alcoholic dementia, Wernicke-Korsakoff Syndrome (thiamine deficiency) associated with alcohol

   e. Nutritional complications—vitamin and iron deficiency, malnutrition associated with alcohol

   f. Pulmonary damage associated with smoking crack and cannabis

   g. Infectious disease complications—increased chance of hepatitis, HIV, sexually transmitted diseases mostly related to high risk behaviors associated with PSA

   h. Obstetrical complications—premature labor and delivery, spontaneous abortion, abruptio placenta associated with cocaine

   i. Teratogenic complications

      (1) Low birth weight, prematurity, small head circumference, anomalies associated with cocaine, cannabis, nicotine

      (2) Neonatal withdrawal most commonly associated with narcotics and sedative hypnotics

      (3) Fetal alcohol syndrome (FAS) characterized by:

         (a) Growth retardation

         (b) Central nervous involvement—developmental delay, neurological or intellectual impairment

(c) Facial dysmorphology

7. Behavioral indicators associated with substance use disorders
    a. Deterioration of personal appearance
    b. Decreased productivity
    c. Isolation and secretive behavior
    d. Difficulty in personal relationships
    e. Mood fluctuations
    f. Difficulty in meeting deadlines
    g. Elaborate excuses for behavior
    h. Decreased motivation and energy

- Mental Status Variations
    1. Acute alcohol, sedative/hypnotic intoxication
        a. Disinhibition and increased confidence
        b. Slurred speech
        c. Impaired insight, judgment and memory
        d. Decreased concentration
        e. Altered motor skills and sensory perception
        f. Mood swings
    2. Acute cocaine (stimulant) intoxication
        a. Euphoria
        b. Grandiosity
        c. Psychomotor agitation
        d. Hypervigilance
        e. Impaired judgment
        f. Elevated blood pressure, tachycardia
        g. Visual/tactile hallucinations
    3. Marijuana intoxication
        a. Excitement and dissociation of ideas
        b. Distortions of time and space

c. Diminished attention span and memory
d. Deterioration of motor skills
e. Increased appetite
f. Dry mouth
g. Tachycardia

4. Acute hallucinogen intoxication—"tripping"
   a. Anxiety and feeling of loss of control
   b. Paranoid ideation/suspiciousness
   c. Delusions and hallucinations
   d. Confusion and delirium
   e. Distortion of time, place, distance
   f. Impaired judgment
5. Acute narcotic intoxication
   a. Euphoria and sense of well being
   b. Analgesia, sedation, and somnolence
   c. Lethargy and apathy
   d. Pupillary constriction
   e. Decreased respirations and hypotension
6. Alcohol withdrawal syndrome—usually appears 6 hours after a substantial fall in BAC, peaks at about 24 to 36 hours and subsides after 48 hours
   a. Tremulousness
   b. Malaise
   c. Anorexia, nausea, vomiting
   d. Hyperreflexia
   e. Tachycardia, increased blood pressure
   f. Irritability
   g. Insomnia
   h. Diaphoresis

i. Perceptual distortions

j. Possible seizures

7. Delirium tremens—5% incidence—most severe manifestation of alcohol withdrawal—onset between 72 to 96 hours after cessation of drinking
   a. Gross tremors and agitation
   b. Disorientation
   c. Confusion
   d. Hallucinations
   e. Hyperpyrexia
   f. Increased psychomotor and autonomic nervous system activity
8. Cocaine withdrawal—24 hours after cessation or reduction in use
   a. Fatigue
   b. Depression
   c. Insomnia/hypersomnia
   d. Psychomotor agitation
   e. Intense cravings or desire to use
9. Narcotic withdrawal—onset depends on drug's half life and chronicity of use, peaks between 36 to 72 hours, subsides by 5 to 8 days
   a. Anorexia
   b. Stomach cramps and diarrhea
   c. Lacrimation and rhinorrhea
   d. Muscle aches
   e. Mild elevations in temperature, respiratory rate, pulse and blood pressure
   f. Profuse sweating
   g. Insomnia
   h. Irritability and restlessness
10. Dual diagnosis—concomitant existence of a substance abuse and psychiatric disorder.

Results of the most recent Epidemiologic Catchment Area (ECA) data show that 29% of the US population with current psychiatric diagnosis had a lifetime history of alcohol or drug abuse/dependence. Approximately 20–40% of substance abusers also meet DSM-III-R criteria for a psychiatric disorder (Robins & Ruger, 1990). Psychopathology can be both a cause and consequence of alcohol and drug use.

a. Ross and colleagues (1988) cited the most common lifetime psychiatric disorders in substance abusers as follows:
   (1) Antisocial personality disorder—47%
   (2) Phobias—26%
   (3) Psychosexual dysfunction—24%
   (4) Major depression—20%
   (5) Dysthymia—9%
b. The psychiatric disorders that have the highest lifetime rate of substance abuse (Reiger, 1990) are as follows:
   (1) Antisocial personality disorder—84%
   (2) Schizophrenia—47%
   (3) Bipolar disorders—61%
   (4) Panic disorder—25%

- Nursing Diagnosis—see Table 1.

Table 1

Multidimensional Assessment

Medical Problem Areas	Nursing Diagnosis
I. Intoxication/ withdrawal	Comfort, alteration in; Injury, potential for; Violence, potential for
II. Biochemical conditions/complications	Tissue integrity, impaired; Nutrition, Alteration in; Sleep pattern disturbance; Infection, potential for
III. Emotional/behavioral conditions/complications	Anxiety; Coping, ineffective individual; Thought processes, altered; Sensory-perceptual alterations; Self-esteem disturbance;

		Social interaction, impaired; Impaired communication; Personal identity disturbance;
IV.	Treatment acceptance/resistance	Denial, ineffective; Fear; Knowledge deficit; Non-compliance;
V.	Relapse potential	Adjustment, impaired; Decisional conflict; Diversional activity, altered; Role performance, altered; Spiritual distress;
VI.	Recovery environment	Coping, ineffective family; Home maintenance, altered

- Genetic/Biochemical Origins and Biochemical Approaches

  1. Etiology

     a. Dopamine D2 receptor gene found in alcoholics

     b. Family studies

        (1) Children of alcoholics are three to four times more likely to experience alcohol problems.

        (2) Adoptees are more likely to have alcoholism if a biological parent had alcoholism despite being raised by non-alcoholic parents.

        (3) There is more concordance of alcoholism in identical twins despite their being raised separately.

     c. EEG changes—markedly reduced P3 wave amplitude in response to visual stimuli in abstinent sons of alcoholic; this was also found in abstinent, formerly severe chronic alcoholics.

     d. Sensitivity to alcohol—Family history positives are less sensitive to both positive and negative effects of alcohol. Women suffer medical consequences of alcoholism 10 to 14 years sooner than men.

     e. Neurocognitive differences

        (1) Increase in cognitive deficits (visual, perceptual, and memory) in abstinent sons of alcoholic fathers compared to sons without any alcoholic relatives

     f. Hormonal differences

(1) Alcohol usually increases prolactin levels. However, after alcohol administration, sons of alcoholics had significantly lower prolactin levels than did sons of nonalcoholics.

2. Pharmacotherapy interventions

a. Agents to treat withdrawal

(1) Alcohol

(a) Benzodiazepines—high abuse potential; side effects—oversedation, disinhibition, mild to moderate central nervous system depressant when ingested with alcohol

(b) Carbamazepine (tegretol)— anticonvulsant, no abuse potential, ''antikindling'' effect (kindling occurs when repeated subthreshold stimulation to the brain raises the seizure threshold). Inadequately treated withdrawals could have cumulative kindling effect, thereby producing future withdrawals of increased severity.

(2) Opiates

(a) Clonidine—alpha adrenergic agonist, decreases autonomic symptoms; side effects—sedation, hypotension

(b) Flexeril—muscle relaxant; side effects—dizziness, lightheadedness, dry mouth, drowsiness, nausea and vomiting

(c) Buprenorphine—partial narcotic agonist

b. Agents to decrease craving

(1) Alcohol

(a) Naltrexone—narcotic antagonist, non-addicting, may block the euphoric effects of alcohol; side effects—increased liver enzymes, gastro-intestinal irritation, lightheadedness, drowsiness, slight increase in blood pressure

(2) Cocaine

(a) Bromocriptine, amantadine pergolide—dopamine

agonist, more effective in the acute phase of recovery; side effects—dizziness, lightheadedness, headache, nausea

(b) Carbamazepine (tegretol)—may reverse the cocaine-induced ''kindling'' and the cocaine-receptor sensitivity that results from chronic cocaine use; side effects—initial sedation, hepatotoxicity, platelet dysfunction, thrombocytopenia, hand tremor, ataxia at high doses

c. Maintenance agents

(1) Opiates

(a) Methadone—synthetic narcotic, decreases risky behavior associated with opiate use, longer duration of action, not a treatment modality in itself, usual dose 40 to 120 mg

(b) Buprenorphine—partial agonist, at increasing doses acts as an antagonist

d. Agents to decrease consumption

(1) Alcohol

(a) Disulfiram (antabuse)—aversion therapy, interferes with the metabolism of alcohol, producing unpleasant side effects when mixed with alcohol. These symptoms include facial flushing, heart palpitations, increased heart rate, dyspnea, nausea, vomiting, decreased blood pressure. Patients should be instructed to avoid over-the-counter cough medicines, aftershave lotions, vinegar, mouthwashes, non-alcoholic beer (contains small amount of alcohol), and foods cooked with alcohol while taking this drug and for 14 days after drug has been discontinued.

(2) Opiates

(a) Naltrexone—blocks euphoric effects

e. Agents to treat protracted abstinence—continued unpleasant state of low grade withdrawal—includes sleep disruption, anhedonia, anergia, irritability, nervousness, restlessness, conditioned cravings

(1) 5HT reuptake inhibitors—fluoxatine, sertraline, citalopram

(2) Tricyclic antidepressant—imipramine, desipramine

- Intrapersonal Origins/Psychotherapeutic Interventions

1. Psychological theory

a. Substance use as an adaptive attempt by the user to cope with, or compensate for, particular psychological deficits such as dysregulation of affect, poor object relations, and impaired judgment and self care.

b. Khantzian (1985) believes people are drawn to substances in an attempt to self medicate emotional distress (rage, aggression, depression, anxiety, low self esteem).

c. Use of immature, rigid defense mechanisms, such as denial, dependency, regression, projection, and displacement often characterize this population. Other theories recognize that the psychological dysfunctions seen in substance abusers are more the consequence of the drug use and drug seeking behavior than the cause. Interventions tied to psychological theory include:

(1) Allow expression of honest feelings and reinforce efforts to cope in appropriate ways.

(2) Help patient explore, accept, and own both positive and negative aspects of self.

(3) Help patient identify aspects of self that he/she would like to change.

(4) Help patient regain a feeling of empowerment by pointing out the choices he/she has available.

(5) Help patient recognize and focus on strengths and accomplishments.

2. Social learning theory—basis for cognitive-behavioral/relapse prevention therapy

a. Views addiction as a result of interacting factors:

(1) Personal experience and past learning

(2) Situational antecedents

(3) Biological make-up

(4) Cognitive processes

(5) Reinforcement contingencies

b. Marlatt (1984) believes the lack of coping skills or positive outcome expectations increase the possibility of a relapse (return to dysfunctional pattern of abuse).

c. Goals of relapse prevention are:

(1) Identify high risk situations, people, places and things.

(2) Identify negative emotions—boredom, loneliness, depression, anxiety, guilt, self-depreciation.

(3) Monitor thinking and increase awareness.

(4) Plan in advance successful avoidance and coping strategies.

(5) Use slips, lapses, and relapses for future planning, not as treatment failures.

- Family Dynamics/Family Therapy

1. Substance abuse is the central theme around which family life is organized. Family rituals and routines, interactional patterns, and problem solving abilities are altered (Steinglass, P., Bennett, L., Wolin, S. & Reiss, D., 1987).

2. Substance abuse as a symptom of underlying family system dysfunction (Bowen, 1978). Families are undifferentiated. Members cannot act independently of the whole. Family system is highly stressed and fails to meet members' basic nurturing needs. There is suppression and denial of emotional expression. Communication is indirect, inconsistent, and conflictual. Boundaries are weak and constantly changing.

Families accommodate to the addiction, thus ''enabling'' i.e., making it easier for the addict to continue using.

3. Co-dependency—condition afflicting the significant other which affects the whole personality and all relationships, that arises in part

from living with chemical dependency; often synonymous with adult children of alcoholics (ACOA). Characteristics include:

a. Low self esteem and loss of identity

b. Seeking of external sources of fulfillment

c. Need for approval from others

d. Fear of abandonment

e. Inability to express anger

f. Possible behavior that is controlling, rigid, perfectionistic, and overresponsible

g. Tendency to rescue others at the expense of their own needs

4. Strategies in family therapy

   a. Assess the family system—level of denial, level of education and insight—use genogram.

   b. Look for strengths to reinforce.

   c. Discourage blaming of members.

   d. Educate family about chemical dependency and refer to AL-ANON / AL-ATEEN for support.

   e. Assist with the process of emotional separation and reactiveness to the substance abuse behavior.

   f. Model effective communication and attitudes.

   g. Support/reinforce healthy change.

- Group Approaches (used more frequently in substance abuse treatment)—advantages include:

  1. Peer support and confrontation

  2. Reflection on family of origin issues

  3. A place to practice newly learned interpersonal skills

  4. Specific groups include:

     a. Psychoeducational groups—didactic lectures and discussions on such topics as the disease concept of addiction, the addictive cycle, biopsychosocial consequences of substance abuse, dual diagnosis, relapse prevention, communication skills, assertiveness, and relaxation

b. Self-help groups

(1) Grounded in the conception that substance abuse is a medical and spiritual disease, the belief is that there is an internal causation for chemical dependency beyond the individual's control.

(2) Groups offer support and mutual sharing and are open to all who share the common goal of recovery from a variety of substances and conditions.

(3) The twelve steps provide the roadmap one must follow to reach recovery.

(a) Admit powerlessness and unmanageability of life.

(b) Need greater power to restore sanity.

(c) Turn life and will over to God.

(d) Take a moral inventory.

(e) Admit nature of wrongs.

(f) Be ready to have God remove character defects.

(g) Ask God to remove shortcomings.

(h) Make a list of people harmed and willingness to make amends.

(i) Make amends.

(j) Continue personal inventory.

(k) Improve conscious contact with God.

(i) Carry message of spiritual awakening to other alcoholics.

4. Critics of the twelve steps believe this approach is not appropriate for everyone and complain about the reference to God. Proponents endorse a broader, more spiritual versus religious definition of God or Higher Power.

- Milieu Interventions—based on staff providing a safe, corrective environment that enhances the development of more adaptive coping skills and interpersonal behaviors

1. Biological/physical supportive measures—detoxification occurs in

the early phase of recovery and involves safely tapering off substance of abuse, thereby minimizing the physical discomfort associated with withdrawal.

a. Monitor for signs and symptoms of withdrawal—use Clinical Instrument for Withdrawal from Alcohol (CIWA) to measure both subjective and objective symptoms of withdrawal from alcohol, benzodiazepines, sedative/hypnotics. This enables the nurse to dose more accurately the amount of detoxification medication that is administered.
b. Use safety and fall precautions.
c. Use seizure precautions.
d. Maintain nutritional and hydration needs.
e. Decrease stimuli in the environment—quiet, dimly lit atmosphere.
f. Convey acceptance and reassurance.
g. Reorient when indicated.

2. Psychosocial supportive measures during rehabilitative phase of recovery
   a. Formulate treatment goals and expected outcomes with patient.
   b. Role model self-acceptance, assertiveness, and responsibility.
   c. Maintain consistency in care—requires a high degree of communication among staff.
   d. Confront in an empathic, respectable manner, always focusing on the dysfunctional behavior and not the individual.
   e. Identify and work through countertransference issues.
   f. Provide structure—use daily activity schedule.
   g. Use self disclosure only when appropriate and in the context of therapy.
   h. Use behavioral contracts with contingencies.
      (1) Reinforce compliance and achievement.
      (2) Issue consequences for noncompliance.
   i. Use on the spot conflict management.

j. Assist with task assignments and homework.
k. Use rehearsal and role playing of newly learned skills.

3. Clinical nurse specialist interventions
   a. Theory-based psychotherapy—individual, group, family
   b. Evaluation, treatment recommendation, and appropriate referral
   c. Consultant as an expert in the field of chemical dependency
   d. Staff support and management functions
   e. Interventions with the client presenting with complex problems
   f. Staff education and supervision
   g. Preventative functions—community awareness and education
   h. Research functions—participate and/or initiate protocols that may improve future interventions and care of the substance abusing population
   i. Professional development—committee memberships, publications, presentations, learning opportunities

- Community Resources
  1. Self-help support group meetings
     a. Alcoholic Anonymous (AA)
     b. Narcotic Anonymous (NA)
     c. Cocaine Anonymous (CA)
     d. Secular Organizations for Sobriety (SOS)—geared more toward individuals with agnostic view of spirituality
     e. AL-ANON, NAR-ANON and ALATEEN—Family/significant others and teenagers living with or involved with a substance abuser
     f. Adult Children of Alcoholics (ACOA)
  2. Prevention groups—special interest groups developed for community awareness and education, public policy making, introducing and changing legislation related to alcohol and substance use
     a. Drug Abuse Readiness Education (DARE)
     b. Mothers Against Drunk Drivers (MADD)

c. ''Just say no'' campaign

d. ''Hugs not drugs'' campaign

- Interventions with the Impaired Nurse—Cahill (1992) and colleagues estimate 7% of registered nurses abuse substances.

1. Use team approach, nonpunitive attitude, 2 to 10 professional associates of impaired colleague who share a nonjudgmental attitude (to include one recovering peer and one with experience in chemical dependency if posssible).

2. Present documented evidence, always prefacing testimony with positive remarks.

3. Give impaired nurse a chance to respond.

4. State available options and allow an opportunity for voluntary entry into treatment.

   a. Diversion programs—facilitate re-entry into practice without licensure sanctions

   b. Regulatory legal action—nurse reported to the state board for suspected chemical dependency is dealt with under the Nurse Practice Act and the Administrative Procedure Act.

   c. Criminal legal action—nurse who diverts a control substance from a facility or obtains a controlled substance by fraud is in violation of the Controlled Substance Act.

5. Make arrangements to monitor progress.

Questions
Select the best answer

1. Ms. P presents to the community substance abuse center for an evaluation. She states that she does not have a substance, abuse problem but agreed to the evaluation at her husbands insistence. The appropriate initial statement would be:
   a. Do you drink often?
   b. Your husband is concerned about your drinking?
   c. What makes you think that you do not have a drinking problem?
   d. How much do you drink?

2. A useful tool that can be helpful in assessing the severity of withdrawal from alcohol is:
   a. Inventory of drinking situations
   b. Comprehensive drinker profile
   c. Michigan alcohol screening tool
   d. Clinical instrument for withdrawal from alcohol

3. Mr. C, a 40-year-old male with a diagnosis of alcohol dependence, is admitted to the inpatient unit for detoxification. Nursing supportive measures during this time would include all but the following:
   a. Monitor vital signs
   b. Provide quiet, dimly lit atmosphere
   c. Confront denial
   d. Encourage fluids by mouth

4. Mr. C completes detoxification and rehabilitation and is discharged on Antabuse (disulfiram) 250 mg to be taken every morning. He should be warned to avoid all of the following substances except:
   a. Mouthwash
   b. Cough elixirs
   c. Non-alcoholic beer
   d. antidepressant medication

5. When assessing whether or not a patient has a problem with alcohol or drugs, which criteria is the best indicator:
   a. How much a person uses
   b. How often a person uses
   c. The level of interference with physical, emotional, and social functioning

d. Positive laboratory findings

6. All of the following are signs of delirium tremens except:

   a. Confusion
   b. Visual hallucinations
   c. Seizures
   d. Stroke

7. Ms. D is admitted to the emergency room with suicidal ideations. Urine drug screen reveals the presence of cocaine in the urine. When questioned with this finding Ms. D denies any use of cocaine. The most appropriate nursing response would be:

   a. "This test is very accurate, Ms. D you must not be telling the truth."
   b. "You are depressed because you have used cocaine."
   c. "Were you in a room with other people who were smoking crack!"
   d. "Have you ever used drugs in the past?"

8. Important questions in assessing for potential withdrawal from alcohol would include all but:

   a. When was your last drink and how much did you drink?
   b. What family or relationship problems has your alcohol use caused for you?
   c. During the last month, what is the longest period of time that you have gone without any alcohol?
   d. Do you experience any physical discomfort when you go without alcohol for a few hours or a few days?

9. The prevalence of substance abuse in the psychiatric population is about:

   a. 35%
   b. 50%
   c. 15%
   d. 75%

10. Laboratory values that are often altered by alcoholism include all but:

    a. Aspartate aminotransferase (AST)
    b. Gamma-Glutamyltransferase (GGT)
    c. Mean corpuscular value (MCV)
    d. White blood cell count (WBC)

11. Genetic studies in alcoholism support which of the following statements:

    a. Alcoholism is mostly influenced by environmental factors.
    b. Sons of alcoholics are four times more likely to have problems with alcohol or drugs.
    c. There is no definitive research that links alcoholism to genetic etiology.
    d. If both parents have alcoholism there is a 75% chance that each child will have an alcohol or drug problem.

12. Mr. F is participating in a six-week intensive outpatient substance abuse treatment program for his crack/cocaine addiction. During the third week of treatment he tests positive for cocaine in his urine. The most appropriate intervention would be to:

    a. Refer to inpatient treatment
    b. Dismiss from the Intensive outpatient program
    c. Meet with the patient individually to discuss the slip/relapse
    d. Confront the patient in group

13. Common alcohol-related medical complications include all but:

    a. Arteriosclerosis
    b. Cardiomyopathy
    c. Cirrhosis of the liver
    d. Gastritis

14. Which statement most accurately describes gender differences in alcoholism:

    a. There are no gender differences with regard to epidemiology, etiology, and treatment implications.
    b. Alcoholism is a disease that mostly afflicts men.
    c. Women experience fewer problems with alcohol.
    d. Women experience the medical consequences of alcoholism 10 to 14 years earlier than men.

15. Nurse K is a nurse counselor working for a university. Ms. G is a 22-year-old sophomore that has been referred to Nurse K for an evaluation because of her declining grades and poor class attendance. What would be the most appropriate line of questioning for Ms. K to pursue?

    a. Your advisor tells me that you are doing poorly in school?
    b. Have you been spending more time partying than concentrating on your schoolwork?

c. Can you tell me what has been happening around you that may be affecting your school work?
d. Are you using any drugs?

16. Ms. G continues to smoke marijuana and her school problems are getting worse. Your best intervention would be to:

a. Call her parents and inform them of her drug use
b. Tell her she will be expelled if she does not quit using drugs
c. Refer to substance treatment and monitor compliance and progress
d. Do not intervene, as patient probably needs to suffer the consequences of her use

17. Serious medical complications associated with cocaine abuse include all but:

a. Kidney failure
b. Seizures
c. Stroke
d. Cardiac Arrhythmias

18. Sedative/hypnotics are cross-addicted with:

a. Alcohol
b. Opiates
c. Stimulants
d. Hallucinogens

19. Mr. L is a 50-year-old male with a history of chronic back pain from a car injury that occurred 5 years ago. He has been taking Darvocet-N 100 over the past several years and reports taking up to 15 tablets a day. His medical doctor no longer feels comfortable giving Mr. L prescriptions for pain and refers him to substance abuse treatment. Mr. L is admitted to the inpatient unit for narcotic detoxification. He is very fearful that he will be denied pain medication and left to suffer. The most appropriate nursing intervention would be:

a. Reassure Mr. L that his pain will be managed while his narcotic is being slowly tapered.
b. Explain to Mr. L that he is addicted to narcotics and must not use them anymore.
c. Explain to Mr. L that his pain threshold has been lowered due to his narcotic abuse and he will not need pain medication.
d. Tell Mr. L that he will have tylenol and aspirin available for pain management.

20. Withdrawal from opiates include all but the following:
    a. Muscle cramps
    b. Tachycardia
    c. Sedation
    d. Diarrhea

21. Based on the information, an appropriate nursing diagnosis for Mr. L would include all of the following but:
    a. Injury, potential for
    b. Comfort, alteration in
    c. Self care deficit
    d. Knowledge deficit

22. The benefit of methadone substitution over heroin use is that it:
    a. Serves as an anticraving agent
    b. Diminishes risky behavior associated with heroin use
    c. Is effective as a detoxification agent
    d. Can be stopped abruptly without any withdrawal

23. A person who allows the addiction to continue by taking over the responsibilities of the addict is said to be:
    a. Caring
    b. Supportive
    c. Controlling
    d. Enabling

24. Beneficial components of group psychotherapy with the substance abusing patient include all of the following except:
    a. Self disclosure
    b. Peer confrontation
    c. Guidance from group leader
    d. Group nurturance

25. The limitations of urine drug testing for substances of abuse include all but:
    a. Often produces false positives
    b. ''Short'' window of detection of metabolites
    c. Intermittent abuse patterns of abusers

d. Issues of civil liberties

26. Fetal alcohol syndrome requires the presence of all of the following characteristics except:

 a. Heart defects
 b. Facial dysmorphology
 c. Growth retardation
 d. Central nervous system dysfunction

27. The CNS leads a multi-family group. Ms.T is a 40-year-old housewife who is very angry at her husband because he recently spent the couple's entire savings on cocaine. Ms.T feels very frustrated with her husband's addiction and would like to learn to support him in his recovery. The CNS's best suggestion would for Ms.T:

 a. To leave her husband
 b. To take charge of the family finances
 c. Not to get involved in her husband's recovery
 d. To attend AL-ANON meetings to explore how significant others cope with their loved one's addiction

28. From a family systems perspective Chemical dependency can be viewed as:

 a. A lack of the family's ability to problem solve
 b. Lack of communication
 c. Lack of family organization and interactional patterns
 d. A symptom of underlying family dysfunction

29. Ms. R is a 50-year-old woman married to an alcoholic. During individual counseling Ms. R states that her husband's drinking interferes with their social activities. His behavior when drinking embarrasses and humiliates her. An appropriate response would be to advise Ms. R to:

 a. Stop going to activities
 b. Continue to go to activities without focusing on her husband's drinking, letting him take responsibility for the consequences of his drinking behavior
 c. Encourage Ms. R to keep a watchful eye on her husband, frequently reminding him how much he has had to drink
 d. Make sure she is available at activities so that she can drive her husband safely home

30. Appropriate goals for the milieu management of a residential substance abuse program would include all of the following except:

    a. To maintain a restricted environment
    b. To maintain the safety of the patient
    c. To provide consistent, structured care
    d. To support the patient's recovery effort

31. Ms. G is a 67-year-old female with a long history of alcoholism. She currently has cirrhosis of the liver. In order to be put on a list to receive a liver transplant, she must complete an inpatient substance abuse program. Additionally, she must sustain 6 months of abstinence. On admission Ms. G states that the only reason she is here is to receive a new liver. An appropriate initial response would be:

    a. How did you get cirrhosis of the liver?
    b. You sound angry about having to participate in substance abuse treatment.
    c. Treatment requires having insight into your alcoholism.
    d. You are concerned about your liver disease?

32. An evaluation criterion for Ms.G's plan of care would be:

    a. Understand the reasons for her drinking
    b. Verbalize her dependence on alcohol
    c. Recognize situations which put her at high risk for drinking
    d. Discuss her alcoholism openly in group

33. An example of a violation of the Controlled Substance Act would be:

    a. Driving under the influence of alcohol
    b. Drinking or using drugs at work
    c. Possession of an illegal substance outside of work
    d. Diverting a controlled substance from a facility

Answers

1. b
2. d
3. c
4. d
5. c
6. d
7. d
8. b
9. a
10. d
11. b
12. c
13. a
14. d
15. c
16. c
17. a
18. a
19. a
20. c
21. c
22. b
23. d
24. c
25. a
26. a
27. d
28. d
29. b
30. a
31. d
32. b
33. d

Bibliography

American Psychiatric Association (1993). Substance-related disorders. In APA (4th ed.), *Diagnostic and statistical manual of mental disorders,* DSM-IV Draft criteria. Washington, DC: APA.

American Society of Addiction Medicine/National Council on Addictions Committee (ASAM/NCAdd Committiee, 1990).

Bowen, M. (1978). *Family therapy in clinical practice.* New York: Jason Aronson.

Cahill, J., Cassidy, K., Daly, S., Deutisch, D., Hodgson, B., Hodgson, J., Johnson, P. & McMahon, E. (1992). *Nurses handbook of law and ethics.* Springhouse, PA: Springhouse Corporation.

Frances, R. J., & Miller, S. I. (1991). *Clinical textbook of addictive disorders.* NY: Guilford Press.

Kaufman, E., (1992). A current approach to psychodynamic psychotherapy of substance—dependent individuals. In D. Greenfield (Ed.), *Treating diverse disorders with psychotherapy.* San Francisco: Jossey-Bass.

Kaufman, E., & McNaul, J. (1992). Recent developments in understanding and treating drug abuse and dependence. *Hospital and Community Psychiatry. 43*(3), 223–236.

Khantzian, E. J. (1985). The self medication hypothesis of addictive disorders: Focus on heroin and cocaine dependence. *American Journal of Psychiatry, 142*(11), 1259–1264.

Marlatt, G. A., & George, W. H. (1984). Relapse prevention: Introduction and overview of the model. *British Journal of Addiction, 79*(3), 261–273.

Miller, N. (Ed.). (1991). *Comprehensive handbook of drug and alcohol addiction.* NY: Marcel Decker.

Naegle, M. A. (1992, 1993). *Substance abuse education in nursing (Vol. I,II,III).* NY: National League for Nursing.

Reiger, D. A., Farmer, M. E., Rae, D. S., Locke, B. Z., Keith, S. J., Judd, L. L., & Goodwin, F. K. (1990). Comorbidity of mental disorders with alcohol and other drug abuse: Results from the Epidemiologic Catchment Area Study. *Journal of American Medical association. 246*(19), 2511–2518.

Robins, R. N., & Ruger, D. A. (1990). *Psychiatric disorders in America.* NY: Free Press.

Ross, H. E., Glaser, F. B., & Germanson, T. (1988). The prevalence of psychiatric disorders in patients with alcohol and other drug problems. *Archives of General Psychiatry.* 48, 43–51.

Steinglass, P., Bennett, L., Wolin, S., & Reiss, D. (1987). *The alcholic family.* NY: Basic Books.

Straussner, S. L. (1993). *Clinical work with substance abusing clients.* NY: Guilford Press.

Wallace, B. (1992). *The chemically dependent: Phases of treatment and recovery.* NY: Brunner/Mazel.

Weddington, W. W. (1992). Use of pharmacologic agents in the treatment of addiction. *Psychiatric Annals, 22*(8), 425–429.

Anxiety and Stress-Related Disorders

Karma Castleberry

Anxiety Disorders

Generalized Anxiety Disorder (GAD)

- Definition: Unrealistic or excessive worry accompanied by symptoms of motor tension, autonomic arousal, and vigilance
- Signs and Symptoms
  1. Motor tension—shaky, muscle tension, fatigability
  2. Autonomic arousal—shortness of breath, tachycardia, dry mouth, dizziness, nausea, diarrhea, dysphagia
  3. Vigilance—insomnia, feels ''keyed up''
  4. Not limited to discrete periods or discrete stimuli
  5. Often accompanied by depression or another anxiety disorder
  6. Considerable impairment in quality of life (Massion, Warshaw, & Keller, 1993)
  7. Levels of anxiety
     a. Mild—slight physical arousal, sharp perceptions, ability to learn well
     b. Moderate—physical symptoms apparent, narrowing of perceptual field
     c. Severe—physical symptoms problematic, difficulty concentrating, very apprehensive
     d. Panic—terror, little ability to concentrate, difficulty breathing, palpitations, fear of dying
- Differential Diagnoses
  1. Physical disorders such as hyperthyroidism and mitral valve prolapse
  2. Caffeine or stimulant abuse
  3. Withdrawal from alcohol or sedatives
  4. Panic or Obsessive Compulsive Disorders
  5. Anxiety disorder due to a general medical condition (APA, 1994)
- Mental Status Variations

1. Appearance—sweating, cold, clammy hands, exaggerated startle response, flushing, or chills
2. Psychomotor Activity—restless, trembling, twitching
3. Mood—irritable, anxious, apprehensive
4. Concentration—difficult to concentrate
5. Insight—impaired; clients often seek treatment for physical symptoms and do not associate physical and emotional responses with anxiety.

- Nursing Diagnoses
  1. Anxiety
  2. Coping, ineffective individual
  3. Family process, altered
  4. Fear
  5. Powerlessness
  6. Parenting, altered, high risk for
  7. Knowledge deficit
  8. Role performance, altered
  9. Sleep pattern disturbance
- Genetic/Biological Origins
  1. Some evidence of genetic link (25% first-degree relatives) (Kaplan & Sadock, 1991)
  2. Persons with GAD have increased sympathetic tone, greater response, and slower adaptation to stress (Kaplan & Sadock, 1991).
  3. Gamma aminobutyric acid (GABA), which is a principle inhibitory CNS neurotransmitter, may have diminished activity.
  4. Possible genetic link between alcoholism and anxiety disorders (Haack & Alim, 1991)
- Biochemical Approaches
  1. CNS effects of anti-anxiety agents linked to GABA-chloride channel receptor complex (Zorumski & Isenberg, 1991)

2. Benzodiazepines increase the affinity of binding sites for GABA, resulting in a greater influx of chlorine ions into the neuron.

3. Barbiturates bind to chloride channels, leaving channel open so that chloride flows 4 to 5 times longer (Zorumski & Isenberg, 1991).

4. Both benzodiazepines and barbiturates thus allow neurons to become hyperpolarized and, therefore, more inhibited than by the usual action of GABA alone.

The following table outlines anti-anxiety medications.

Table 1

Commonly Used Medications for Anxiety Disorders

Generic Name	Trade Name	Dosage (mg/day)
Benzodiazepines		
Alprazolam	Xanax	0.5–6
Chlordiazepoxide	Librium	5–100
Clonazepam	Klonopin	1.5–10
Clorazepate	Tranxene	7.5–60
Diazepam	Valium	2–60
Lorazepam	Ativan *	2–6
Oxazepam	Serax *	30–120
Temazepam	Restoril *	15–30
Triazolam	Halcion *	0.125–0.5
Barbiturates		
Butabarbital	Butisol	45–120
Propanediols		
Meprobromate	Equanil	400–1600
Azaspirodecanediones		
Buspirone	BuSpar	15–25

* short acting

5. Special Nursing Concerns
   a. Can cause physical and psychological addiction
      (1) Adhere to prescribed dosage.
      (2) Withdrawal begins 12 to 48 hours after last dose, lasts for 12 to 48 hours, with some symptoms persisting for weeks.
      (3) Reduce drug gradually to prevent seizures.
   b. Benzodiazepines with long half lives (1 to 8 days)
      (1) Cumulative effects

(2) Possible compensatory hyperexcitable state upon withdrawal

c. Monitor for blood dyscrasias: CBC with differential, sore throat, fever.

d. Monitor for liver dysfunction: nausea, upper abdominal pain, jaundice, fever, rash, liver function studies.

e. May increase depression: monitor, assess for suicide potential

f. Alcohol potentiates depressant effects.

(1) Behavioral dyscontrol, sedation, and psychomotor effects (Watsky & Salzman, 1991)

(2) Do not use alcohol.

g. May produce sedation that impairs ability to handle machinery or autos

h. Teach client to monitor side effects of medication.

- Intrapersonal

1. Origins

a. Psychodynamic—Anxiety results from unconscious conflict or emergence of unacceptable drives (often related to dependent, sexual, or aggressive content).

(1) Anxiety serves as a signal that repression of drive or conflict is not working.

(2) If repression doesn't contain drives, then other defense mechanisms employed (conversion, displacement, regression).

b. Behavioral—Anxiety is a conditioned response to a specific stimulus, or a learned, internal response (perhaps from imitating parental anxiety responses or reinforced by others).

c. Cognitive—Anxiety results from faulty or dysfunctional thoughts about events.

(1) Overestimate danger

(2) Underestimate ability to cope

2. Psychotherapeutic interventions.

a. Psychodynamic

(1) Long-term, insight-oriented therapy

(2) Focus on resolution of conflicts underlying anxiety

b. Behavioral

(1) Relaxation training—Progressive Muscle Relaxation (PMR) or Autogenic Training Techniques (Lichstein, 1988)

(2) Breathing techniques

(3) Biofeedback

(4) Identification of physical responses that trigger anxiety

c. Cognitive

(1) Identify and challenge dysfunctional thoughts (self-statements) that trigger anxiety.

(2) Replace with positive coping statements.

(3) Evaluate accurately presence of danger.

(4) Encourage use of log (diaries) and homework for subsequent analysis of relationship between thoughts and feeling of anxiety.

d. Therapeutic touch (Heidt, 1991)

- Family Dynamics/Family Therapy

1. Children of parents with GAD are likely to see the world as dangerous and themselves as vulnerable.

   a. May be excessively protected

   b. May be excessively dependent

2. Family member with GAD may exhibit altered role performance and require other family members to assume greater or inappropriate responsibility (Barloon, 1993).

3. Family member with GAD may become family's "weak one," or the scapegoat.

4. Family treatment emphasizes the following:

   a. Knowledge of GAD and treatment

   b. Cognitive restructuring for all family members to challenge and correct collective assumptions about danger and coping

   c. Promotion of differentiation, especially in children
   d. Re-establishment of healthy role performance

- Group Approaches
  1. Therapy—Group therapy offers opportunities for feedback, realistic self-appraisal, and support when changing behavior patterns.
     a. Insight-oriented to resolve unconscious conflicts
     b. Psychoeducational approaches to increase understanding of nature of GAD and learn coping strategies
     c. Cognitive group therapy to challenge and correct dysfunctional cognitions
     d. Assertiveness Training

- Milieu Interventions
  1. Create a safe, supportive environment.
  2. Use goal-oriented contract to focus treatment.
  3. Use diary/logs to record manifestation of anxiety (thoughts, emotions, physiological responses), the situation, course of events, efficacy of intervention.
  4. Teach role of dysfunctional cognitions (danger and inability to cope) in creating/maintaining anxiety.
  5. Teach analysis of negative self-statements and replace with rational, positive statements and receive feedback from other clients.
  6. Teach relaxation techniques, monitor practice of relaxation techniques, and assist to implement when experiencing anxiety.
     a. Breathing techniques
     b. Progressive muscle relaxation
     c. Autogenic training
  7. Assist to develop alternative means of coping such as exercising, taking warm baths, or talking to staff and other clients.
  8. Promote activities that increase self-confidence through progressively more difficult challenges.
  9. Plan leisure activities to deal with "free time."
  10. Encourage resumption of family, work, and social roles.

11. Refer to partial hospitalization program or outpatient services (Waddell & Demi, 1993).

- Community Resources
  1. GAD often treated by primary care providers such as family doctors and nurse practitioners
     a. CNS may provide consultation, individual, group, and family therapy.
     b. Work collaboratively.
  2. Provide support groups or parenting classes for persons with anxiety disorders.
  3. Teach how to access general community resources to enhance support base.

Phobias

- Definition: Persistent, excessive, irrational fear of a particular object or situation that actually poses no threat
- Signs and Symptoms
  1. Specific Phobias
     a. Fear of animals (snakes, spiders, dogs)
     b. Claustrophobia
     c. Fear of air travel
     d. Realizes fear is irrational, usually little impairment
  2. Social Phobia—fear of being exposed to scrutiny, humiliated, or embarrassed by others
     a. Specific fears—choking on food in restaurant, trembling when writing
     b. General fears—saying foolish things
     c. Realizes irrationality, usually mild impairment
  3. Agoraphobia—fear of being in a place or situation from which there might be difficult or embarrassing escape, or in which, should symptoms become very embarrassing or incapacitating, there might be no help available (Kaplan & Sadock, 1991)—such as:

a. Fears heart attack, depersonalization, loss of bladder control, etc.

b. Limits travel, crowds, or being outside the home alone to avoid symptom development

c. Mild (some avoidance or tolerance of anxiety) to severe (housebound or unable to leave the house unaccompanied)

- Differential Diagnoses
  1. Panic Disorder with Agoraphobia
  2. Avoidant Personality Disorder
  3. Obsessive Compulsive Disorder
  4. Post-traumatic Stress Disorder
  5. Schizophrenia (with delusions)
- Mental Status Variations
  1. Appearance and Behavior—normal unless faced with feared stimulus, then exhibits symptoms of severe anxiety
  2. Mood—commonly depressed, often related to degree of impairment
  3. Thought—persistent, irrational fear of object or situation
- Nursing Diagnoses
  1. Anxiety
  2. Coping, ineffective individual
  3. Family process, altered
  4. Fear
  5. Knowledge deficit
  6. Powerlessness
  7. Role performance, altered
  8. Self-esteem
  9. Social interaction, impaired
- Genetic/Biological Origins
  1. Biological inability to habituate to certain situation

2. Possible genetic component with higher concordance in first-degree relatives

- Biochemical Approaches
  1. Anti-anxiety agents in combination with behavioral approaches
  2. Anti-anxiety agents if behavioral approaches ineffective
  3. Antidepressants for clients with depressive features
     a. MAOIs in particular for social phobias
     b. Imipramine for panic disorders with agoraphobia (Mavissakalian & Perel, 1992)
  4. Beta-adrenergic antagonists which block the sympathetic response (e.g., propranolol) are helpful in situational anxiety such as stage fright (Glod, 1991)
- Intrapersonal
  1. Origins
     a. Psychodynamic—Phobia is an outward manifestation of inner, unresolved childhood conflicts.
        (1) Anxiety is displaced (when repression fails) upon an object or situation that symbolizes the conflict.
        (2) Conflicts are often sexual (oedipal) or related to separation anxiety.
     b. Behavioral
        (1) Classical conditioned response - Phobia develops when anxiety occurs as one is confronted with a naturally frightening stimulus and becomes paired with a neutral stimulus.
        (2) Operant theories—Person learns to avoid a stimulus for anxiety, and the reduction in anxiety reinforces the behavior.
  2. Psychotherapeutic interventions
     a. Psychodynamic—Insight-oriented therapy to resolve childhood conflicts, understand secondary gain, and to find healthy ways to deal with anxiety
     b. Behavior Therapy (most effective treatment)

(1) Systematic Desensitization

(a) Design, with client, list of anxiety-provoking stimuli related to the object/situation from the least to most frightening

(b) Teach PMR to induce deep relaxation.

(c) Induce/maintain relaxed state, while client imagines each anxiety-provoking stimulus.

(d) When desensitized to one stimulus, move up the scale, until relaxation can be maintained throughout entire list of stimuli

(e) Apply technique in vivo.

(2) Flooding—intensive exposure to stimulus in vivo or through imagery until fear can no longer be felt

(3) Neurolinguistic Programming

- Family Dynamics/Family Therapy

1. When role performance (work, family, social contacts) is impaired, family dynamics are altered, and other members assume additional responsibilities.
2. Children of phobic mothers are encouraged to be overly dependent and solicitous to mother's needs (Barloon, 1993).
3. Children sense fears of outside world or objects.
4. Family therapy for role restructuring, support of therapy and change, and reduction of secondary gain of all members

- Group Approaches

1. Therapy

a. Psychodynamic insight-oriented group therapy

b. Psychoeducational group—focus on understanding phobic disorders and learning relaxation techniques

c. Social skills training—modeling, rehearsing, coaching to improve communication

d. Supportive therapy to provide reality-testing and feedback within a group of others seeking to make similar changes

(1) May provide "here and now" experience in facing phobic social situations

2. Self-help groups (affiliated with Phobia Society of America, Rockville, MD) may be present in some communities.

- Milieu Interventions (Unlikely to be hospitalized unless severely impaired)
  1. Provide safe, supportive environment, free of ridicule for phobia.
  2. Goal-oriented contract for treatment.
  3. Employ anxiety-reducing techniques (PMR, breathing, etc.) to decrease general arousal.
  4. Conduct systematic desensitization (imagined or in vivo).
  5. Engage in activities that increase feelings of power and self-esteem.
  6. Reinforce what is learned in individual, group and family sessions.
  7. Referral to outpatient support groups.
- Community Resources
  1. Outpatient therapy
  2. Support groups

Panic Disorders

- Definition: Recurrent, unexpected, intense periods of extreme apprehension and terror without clear precipitant
- Signs and Symptoms
  1. Begins with rapidly increasing symptoms of fear and doom, palpitations, tachycardia, dyspnea, sweating, hyperventilation
  2. Lasts 30 to 60 minutes; may include symptoms of depersonalization, derealization, paresthesia, fainting, dizziness, choking, nausea, chest pain, flushes or chills
     a. First attacks often in phobogenic situation
     b. Subsequent attacks are spontaneous (uncued, unexpected) (Ballenger & Fryer, 1993; Faravelli, Pallanti, Biondi, Paterniti, & Scarpato, 1992)
  3. Clients usually try to seek help, focusing on cardiac or respiratory symptoms.

   a. Believe to be dying
   b. Often seen in emergency room
   c. Fear going "crazy"
4. May be accompanied by agoraphobia, fearing panic attacks will occur in setting without help
5. Between episodes, anticipatory anxiety, vigilant for onset of another attack
6. Ranges from mild (one attack per month or limited number of symptoms), to severe (8 panic attacks per month)
7. Often accompanied by depression

- Differential Diagnoses
  1. Note whether panic disorder is or is not accompanied by agoraphobia.
  2. Physical disorders such as mitral valve prolapse, hyperthyroidism, hypoglycemia, or pheochromocytoma
  3. Withdrawal from psychoactive substances
  4. Caffeine or stimulant abuse
  5. Alcohol abuse
  6. GAD, PTSD
  7. Somatization Disorder
- Mental Status Variations
  1. Appearance—anxious, perspiring, choking, difficulty breathing
  2. Behavior—trembling, hyperventilation
  3. Mood—may be depressed (including suicidal)
  4. Speech—stammering, difficulty speaking
  5. Thought—ruminating, preoccupation with fear of death or doom
  6. Memory—impaired
  7. Concentration—decreased, confusion
  8. Orientation—confused

- Nursing Diagnoses
  1. Anxiety
  2. Coping, ineffective individual
  3. Family processes, altered
  4. Fear
  5. Hopelessness
  6. Knowledge deficit
  7. Parenting, altered
  8. Powerlessness
  9. Role performance, altered
  10. Self-esteem, chronic low
  11. Social isolation
  12. Violence, high risk for, self-directed
- Genetic/Biological Origins
  1. First-degree relatives of clients with panic disorders affected (20%) and higher concordance rate with monozygotic twins (Katon, 1989)
  2. Mitral value prolapse present in about half of all persons with panic disorders (cardiac and respiratory symptoms similar in both disorders)
  3. Increased sympathetic responsiveness; sensitivity to CO_2 and lactate; alterations in blood flow and metabolic activity in brain (Kaplan & Sadock, 1991)
- Biochemical Approaches
  1. Antidepressants, especially imipramine, desipramine, and some MAOIs
     a. Increase therapeutic dose slowly to decrease adverse effects such as orthostatic hypotension.
     b. Decrease in panic attacks by 2 to 4 weeks
     c. Teach about dietary restriction with MAOIs.
     d. Remain on drug 6 to 12 months after symptom relief, then taper off slowly.

2. Benzodiazepines, especially clonazepam
3. Serotonin-reuptake inhibitors (sertraline, paroxetine) currently being investigated for treatment.

- Intrapersonal

1. Origins
   a. Psychodynamic—Panic occurs when defenses against anxiety (repression, displacement, and avoidance) are ineffective.
      (1) Symbolic nature often related to abandonment and separation anxiety
      (2) Traumatic separations in childhood may increase vulnerability by producing autonomic nervous system stimulation (Free, Winget, & Whitman, 1993; Shear, Cooper, Klerman, Busch, & Shapire, 1993).
   b. Behavioral
      (1) Parental behavior modeling or classical conditioning.
      (2) Demonstration of cognitions of exaggerated vulnerability, inability to cope, and general negative views of self. Catastrophic interpretations of anxiety symptoms which provide more arousal and symptoms
      (3) Stressful life events—Persons with panic disorders report greater frequency of life events that pose danger and threat (Katon, 1989).
2. Psychotherapeutic interventions
   a. Psychodynamic—insight-oriented therapy to focus on origin of anxiety, symbolism, secondary gain, and resolution of early conflicts
   b. Behavioral—most effective (Clum, 1990)
      (1) Psychoeducation regarding origin and maintenance of panic attacks
      (2) Desensitization—real or imagined phobic situation
      (3) Cognitive restructuring to decrease self-statements that promote anxiety and to increase positive, coping statements (Beck, Sokol, Clark, Berchick, & Wright, 1992)

(4) Reinforcement of mastery

(5) Relaxation techniques—breathing, PMR, and imagery

- Family Dynamics/Family Therapy
  1. Clients with agoraphobia may always require family members to stay close by
     a. Marital discord
     b. Dependent upon children
  2. Altered role performance (work, family, social situations) increases responsibility of other family members.
  3. Family education about origin, nature, and treatment of disorder
  4. Family therapy to restructure communication and roles to support change
- Group
  1. Therapy
     a. Insight-oriented
     b. Cognitive therapy
     c. Support groups
  2. Self-Help
     a. Community self-help groups
- Milieu
  1. Provide safe, supportive environment.
  2. Establish goal-oriented treatment contract.
  3. Assist client to employ relaxation and cognitive techniques when panic attack first begins.
  4. Label experience as a "panic attack" and anxiety.
  5. Promote socialization with peers.
  6. Engage in activities that promote self-esteem.
  7. Assist client's use of cognitive strategies to decrease anticipatory anxiety associated with possible future panic attacks.
  8. Reinforce learning from individual, groups, and family sessions.

9. Refer to outpatient therapy.

- Community Resources
    1. Outpatient therapy
    2. Support groups

Obsessive Compulsive Disorder (OCD)

- Definition: Recurrent persistent obsessions and/or compulsions that interfere with functional abilities, occupation, social activities, and interpersonal activities
- Signs and Symptoms
    1. Obsession—unwanted, repeated and uncontrollable thoughts, images or impulses
        a. Unable to break thought cycle through distraction in conversation or other tasks
        b. Common themes of losing things, blasphemy, fears of disease, contamination, sexual behavior, or aggression (Simoni, 1991)
        c. Increased anxiety if resisted
    2. Compulsions—repeated, unwanted patterns of behavior that are often responses to obsessions
        a. Involve excessive cleaning, washing, checking, counting, or repeating
        b. Increased anxiety and dread if compulsions are resisted
    3. Intervention usually not sought until basic needs are not met or when physical and/or emotional exhaustion occurs of either client or significant other
        a. Most present with both obsessions and compulsions
- Differential Diagnoses
    1. Obsessive Compulsive Personality Disorder
    2. Major depression with obsessive thoughts
    3. Hypochondriasis
    4. Tourette's Syndrome
    5. Temporal lobe epilepsy

6. Schizophrenia

- Mental Status Variations
    1. Appearance—special dress pattern, abraded hands
    2. Behavior—ordering and arranging environment of examiner, touching, licking, spitting, repeating rituals
    3. Mood—depressed, anxious
    4. Thought—intrusive sounds, words, music, sexual images or impulses; thoughts of doom, concerns with germs, dirt, etc.
    5. Insight—understands obsessions and compulsions are irrational
- Nursing Diagnoses
    1. Anxiety
    2. Coping, ineffective individual
    3. Family process, altered
    4. Injury, high risk for
    5. Powerlessness
    6. Role performance, altered
    7. Social interaction, impaired
    8. Thought process, altered
- Genetic/Biological Origins
    1. Abnormal activity in basal ganglia which may be repository for latent behavior patterns found in both OCD and other neurologically caused movement disorders such as tics, epilepsy, and Sydenham's Chorea (Griest, Rapaport, & Rasmussen, 1990)
        a. Vigilance and grooming behavior in primitive humans may have been of evolutionary advantage.
        b. OCD behavior is remarkably similar regardless of cultures, ethnicity, or age.
    2. OCD symptoms decrease with selective serotonin re-uptake inhibitors (SSRIs) and increase with serotonin antagonists.
    3. Some evidence of increased prevalence of disorder in first-degree relatives

- Biochemical Approaches
  1. Clomipramine (antidepressant)
     a. 250 mgm/day ceiling dose because of lowered seizure threshold
     b. Side effects—orthostatic hypertension; anticholingengic effects (dry mouth, constipation, urinary retention, tachycardia) weight gain, ejaculatory failure, impotence, drowsiness
     c. Patient teaching—take at bedtime to minimize side effects; management of side effects; avoidance of alcohol; care in operating machinery or driving; OCD symptom relief in 6 to 12 weeks (Greist et al., 1990; Whitley, 1991)
     d. Discontinue gradually under supervision
  2. Paroxetine and sertraline currently investigated for treatment of OCD
- Intrapersonal
  1. Origins
     a. Psychodynamic—Unacceptable thoughts and impulses are isolated, but threaten to break through into consciousness so that compulsive acts are performed to undo the possible consequences, should the unacceptable become conscious.
        (1) May arise during anal stage since much OCD involves cleanliness or aggressive preoccupation
        (2) Note both ambivalence and magical thinking.
     b. Behavioral
        (1) Obsessions as conditioned stimulus to anxiety
        (2) Compulsions arise when a behavior reduces the anxiety associated with the obsessions.
  2. Psychotherapeutic interventions
     a. Insight-oriented, psychodynamic therapy to develop acceptable expression of thoughts and impulses
     b. Supportive therapy
     c. Behavioral therapies have greatest effectiveness.

(1) Combine with pharmacotherapy.

(2) Employ gradual extinction of rituals by exposure to anxiety-producing situations, and increase in the time before engaging in compulsive act (response delay).

(3) Reduce obsessive thoughts by thought-stopping (such as snapping a rubber band on the wrist when obsessive thought appears).

(4) Reduce obsessive thoughts through semantic satiation (write a few words of the obsession and then rewrite or say aloud many times until fear no longer evoked).

d. Therapeutic touch (Hill & Oliver, 1993)

- Family Dynamics/Family Therapy

1. Family members may constantly reassure the client which reinforces the obsession.

2. Family may assist patient to avoid situations which trigger OCD which worsens the fear cycle.

3. Family therapy:

a. Emphasize remaining neutral (not reinforcement through reassurance).

b. Avoid reasoning with client (increases anxiety).

c. Avoid ridicule.

d. Assist with response delay (Greist et al., 1990).

- Group Approaches

1. Supportive group therapy

2. Self-help groups in community are often affiliates of Obsessive Compulsive Foundation Inc. (New Haven, CT)

- Milieu Interventions

1. Provide safe, supportive environment, free from ridicule.

2. Establish goal-oriented treatment plan and daily structure.

a. Initially, do not interfere with rituals.

b. Plan daily schedule to allow time for rituals.

c. Gradually reduce amount of time spent on rituals in collaboration with treatment team.

3. Assist with self-care if needed.
4. Reinforce what is learned from individual, group, and family session.
5. Assist to implement thought-stopping or response delay as designed by the primary therapist.
6. Promote activities that reduce anxiety such as physical activity, and vary sufficiently in order not to produce a substitute ritual.
7. Promote clear and direct verbal communication of feeling.
8. Engage in developing plan for use of leisure time, involving social interaction and hobbies that are less anxiety producing.
9. Refer to outpatient therapy.

- Community Resources
  1. OCD Foundation

Post-traumatic Stress Disorder (PTSD)

- Definition: A response to severe emotional or physical trauma characterized by (1) intrusive re-experiencing of the trauma, (2) emotional numbing, and (3) increased arousal (Davidson & Foa, 1991)
- Signs and Symptoms
  1. Stressors may include war experiences, assault, rape, serious accidents, abuse, and natural catastrophes (Glod, 1993; Kline, Sydnor-Greenberg, Davis, Pincus, & Frances, 1993).
  2. Common trauma experience—overwhelming fear, loss of control, helplessness, and fear of being annihilated (Herman, 1992)
     a. Person witnesses or experiences events that involve actual or threatened death or severe physical harm.
     b. Reacts with fear, helplessness, or horror (APA, 1994)
  3. Recurrent intrusive thoughts of trauma in dreams, thoughts, flashbacks, or events similar to stressor
  4. Numbing or constriction (avoidance)
     a. Avoidance of thoughts/feeling/recollections about trauma

   b. Avoidance of persons/situations which provoke memory of original trauma
   c. Psychogenic amnesia, dissociation
   d. Marked diminished interest in significant activities, persons, or the future
5. Increased arousal—sleep disturbances, temper outbursts, hypervigilance and difficulty concentrating, exaggerated startle response (APA, 1994)
6. Response may be delayed weeks to many years.
7. Standard definition of PTSD (DSM) tends better to fit survivors of circumscribed events and fails to address symptoms and personality manifestation resulting from prolonged, repeated trauma (Herman, 1992).

- Differential Diagnoses
  1. Factitious Disorder
  2. Borderline Personality Disorder (Gunderson & Sabo, 1993)
  3. Schizophrenia
  4. Depression
  5. Panic Disorder
  6. Generalized Anxiety Disorder
  7. Acute Stress Disorder (APA, 1994)
     a. Similar origin and presentation as PTSD, but occurs within 4 weeks of traumatic event
     b. Symptoms last from 2 days to 4 weeks.
- Mental Status Variations
  1. Behavior—vigilant, restless
  2. Mood—anxious, depressed, blunted affect, guilty
  3. Perceptual Experiences—flashbacks, derealization, dissociation
  4. Thought—preoccupation with trauma
  5. Memory—impaired
  6. Concentration—impaired

- Nursing Diagnoses
    1. Post trauma response
    2. Grieving, dysfunctional
    3. Self mutilation, high risk for
    4. Spiritual distress
    5. Violence, high risk for, self-directed or directed at others
- Genetic/Biological Origins
    1. Increased baseline sympathetic arousal may predispose; after trauma, baseline elevated
    2. Trauma response includes the following:
        a. Immediate, excessive arousal, especially cardiovascular and neuromuscular systems
        b. Arousal of sympathetic system that leads to difficulty in distinguishing perceptual cues
        c. Original hyperarousal easily evoked after trauma by variety of cues
        d. Autonomic arousal becomes neurologically entrained (Mejo, 1990).
    3. Regulation of endogenous opioids altered
        a. When stressor subsides, opioids may decrease.
        b. Withdrawal symptoms similar to PTSD
        c. May be ''addicted'' to trauma
- Biochemical Approaches
    1. Antidepressants—tricyclic antidepressants (TCAs) and monoamine oxidase inhibitors (MAOIs)
    2. Propranolol
    3. Carbamazepine
    4. Avoid MAOIs/benzodiazepines if abusing drugs/alcohol
- Intrapersonal
    1. Origins

a. Psychodynamic view—trauma reactivates previous, unresolved childhood conflicts.

   (1) Regression, repression, denial and undoing defense mechanisms

   (2) Secondary gain when dependency needs met

b. Cognitive—brain attempts to process through alternate blocking and acknowledging the event until a new mental scheme which incorporates the trauma is devised (Herman, 1992; Karl, 1989).

c. Personal resilience—persons who construct meaning of the event, connections with others, who actively attempt to cope, and who have strong internal locus of control withstand trauma with fewer symptoms (Herman, 1992).

d. Some evidence that those who dissociate at time of trauma have higher risk for PTSD (Bremner, Southwick, Brett, Fontana, Rosenheck, & Charney, 1992; Bremner, Steinberg, Southwick, Johnson, & Charney, 1993)

2. Psychotherapeutic Interventions (all aimed at empowerment and reconnection with others)

   a. Psychoeducation regarding the recovery process (tailor to particular traumas)

   b. Expressive therapies (art, dance, music) translate visual and sensorimotor memories, especially those not encoded in cognitive systems, into meaningful symbols and verbal representations to be integrated (Bowers, 1992).

   c. Purpose of individual therapy to:

      (1) Connect present distress (relationships, work, physical health, mood) to trauma.

      (2) Cease minimizing the trauma.

      (3) Construct new, caring relationship with self.

      (4) Set boundaries on relationships with others.

      (5) Confront abusive family-of-origin—mixed results (few admit abuse and usually blame victim).

   d. Herman's (1992) three-stage model for recovery

(1) Safety

(a) Name the problem.

(b) Restore control.

(c) Establish safe environment.

(2) Remembrance and mourning

(a) Reconstruct the story, including meaning of the event.

(b) Transform traumatic memories.

(c) Mourn traumatic loss.

(3) Reconnection

(a) Learn to fight.

(b) Reconcile with oneself.

(c) Reconnect with others.

(d) Find survivor mission.

(e) Resolve trauma.

(f) Hypnosis (McCann & Pearlman, 1990)

(g) Systematic desensitization

(h) Cognitive therapy (usually integrated)

- Family Dynamics/Therapy

1. Family roles altered as PTSD symptoms experienced
2. Some children develop affective symptoms, become rescuers or disengage from parent who has PTSD.
3. Family may expect quicker recovery than what is possible.
4. Family can help clarify events, listen, and connect distortions (Mejo, 1990).
5. Abusive families-of-origin may deny, punish, and attempt to enforce conspiracy of silence.
6. Family Therapy

   a. Support victim in recovery.

   b. Meet needs of all family members.

c. Maintain awareness of how trauma affects views of self, family, and world.

d. Develop shared frame of reference for trauma.

e. Central issues of blame, responsibility, and trust (McCann & Pearlman, 1990)

- Group (Group experiences with survivors of similar traumas helpful, length variable.)

1. Adult Survivors of Childhood Sexual Abuse

a. Long-term group therapy, usually outpatient

b. Goals

(1) Reduce isolation, shame, guilt, and sense of deviance.

(2) Restructure family-induced behaviors.

(3) Develop new, more realistic patterns of interaction.

c. Group serves as surrogate family (Kreidler, 1991).

(1) Victims often blamed by family for disclosing or overreacting

(2) Group serves as training ground for new behaviors

(a) Analyze effect of family's messages and beliefs on view of self and world.

(b) Learn and practice assertive behaviors.

(c) Do not reinforce helplessness or powerlessness.

(3) Support and validate strengths/worth.

(4) Handle successfully displaced hostility, regression, dissociation, extreme, anxiety or depression, self destructive behaviors (Kreidler & Hassan, 1992; Urbancic, 1989).

(5) 12-step groups

(6) Short-term stress management

(7) Trauma—focused groups

2. Combat trauma groups

a. Often long term

b. Goals

(1) Share experiences.
(2) Work through problems in social adaptation.
(3) Manage aggression towards other.
(4) Make sense of trauma in life.

- Milieu Interventions
  1. Create a safe environment, including a trusting relationship with staff and no harm contract.
  2. Educate client about recovery process.
  3. Assist client to employ stress management techniques (relaxation techniques, exercise, cognitive strategies).
     a. Reduce general arousal.
     b. Employ techniques when anxiety increases or with intrusive memories.
  4. Support client's ability to gain control over memories.
     a. To retrieve during therapy
     b. To set aside
  5. Teach client to manage physiological symptoms of PTSD, including sleep disorders.
  6. Listen to client's story, respecting ability to disclose and to stop remembering.
  7. Engage in activities that promote self-esteem.
  8. Assist in making plans to use leisure time.
  9. Encourage social interaction.
  10. Address spiritual issues.
  11. Develop system of social support in community.
  12. Assist to devise realistic plans for future, including therapy, occupation, and relationships.
- Community Resources
  1. Twelve-step programs
  2. Community outreach program

3. National Organization for Victim Assistance (Washington, D.C.)—a clearinghouse for all victim assistance

Somatoform Disorders

Conversion Disorder

- Definition: Loss or change in physical functioning not explained by any known pathophysiological disorder
- Signs and Symptoms
  1. Temporally related to psychological factors
  2. Symptom fulfills a need or deals with a conflict
  3. Symptom not under voluntary control
  4. Examples—paralysis, blindness, mutism, paresthesias, pseudocyesis, vomiting
- Differential Diagnosis
  1. Rule out medical disorders, especially neurological diseases.
  2. Schizophrenia
  3. Depression
  4. Somatization disorder
  5. Hypochondriasis
- Mental Status Variations
  1. Mood—La belle indifference, inappropriate for physical symptoms
  2. Perceptual disturbances—may be blind, but does not bump into objects; stocking or glove anesthesia
  3. Insight—unaware of relationship between psychological conflict and appearance of symptoms
- Nursing Diagnoses
  1. Anxiety
  2. Communication, impaired verbal
  3. Coping, ineffective individual
  4. Family process, altered

5. Knowledge deficit
6. Role performance, altered
7. Possible—sensory-perceptual alterations, physical mobility, impaired

- Genetic/Biological Origins
  1. CNS arousal disturbance which may diminish awareness of bodily sensations
  2. Subtle impairments in verbal communication, memory, alteration, suggestibility noted in neuropsychological testing
  3. More than half diagnosed with neurological disorder in 3—4 years after Conversion Disorder
- Biochemical Approaches (None indicated)
- Intrapersonal
  1. Origins
     a. Conversion of anxiety into physical symptom
        (1) Conflict usually sexual or aggressive
        (2) Symptom allows both disguising impulse and partially expressing
        (3) Symptoms have symbolic relationship to conflict
        (4) Communicates special needs
     b. Conversion symptoms reinforced by family or society, plus secondary gain
     c. Symptoms replace verbal language
  2. Psychotherapeutic interventions
     a. Psychodynamic insight-oriented psychotherapy to explore conflicts
     b. Focus therapy on stress and coping.
     c. Hypnosis to uncover traumatic events
     d. Brief, solution-focused psychotherapy
- Family Dynamics/Family Therapy
  1. Family rules negate direct expression of conflict.

2. Illness may be family-accepted means to avoid taking action.
3. Family may encourage secondary gain.
4. Therapy to improve verbal communication, conflict resolution, and restructuring of family interactional patterns

- Group Approaches
  1. Emphasis on coping with stress
  2. Assertiveness training
- Milieu Interventions
  1. Minimize sick role behavior.
  2. Encourage verbal expression of needs and conflicts.
  3. Assist staff and patients to reinforce verbalization and functional behavior, and ignore impairments reducing secondary gain.
  4. Help client understand relationships between conflict, symptoms, and gain.
  5. Teach new coping skills to decrease anxiety.

Hypochondriasis

- Definition: Preoccupation with and unrealistic interpretation of physical symptoms and sensations as a serious disease
- Signs and Symptoms
  1. Preoccupation with health state in spite of medical reassurance
  2. Not of delusional quality (can admit possibility of exaggeration)
  3. May be organ-system related or related to a particular bodily function
  4. Experience anguish over physical state
  5. Tend to see multiple practitioners
- Differential Diagnoses
  1. Medical disorders with multiple organ system involvement (AIDS, endocrine disorders, MS, SLE, some neoplasms)
  2. Generalized Anxiety Disorder
  3. Panic Disorder

4. Conversion and Somatization Disorders

- Mental Status Variations
  1. Appearance—apprehensive, anguished
  2. Mood—depressed, anxious
  3. Thought—preoccupied with seriousness of physical symptoms
  4. Insight—impaired
- Nursing Diagnoses
  1. Anxiety
  2. Coping, ineffective individual
  3. Fear
  4. Self esteem disturbance
  5. Social interaction, impaired
  6. Role performance, altered
- Genetic/Biological Origins
  1. Some evidence of increased prevalence in twins
  2. Physiological lower threshold tolerance for discomfort
- Biochemical Approaches
  1. Medication only for coexistent anxiety or depression
  2. Avoid reinforcing through medication
- Intrapersonal
  1. Origins
     a. Repression of aggressive and hostile impulses with displacement into somatic complaints
        (1) Anger originates in past losses
        (2) Displacement solicits help (which later is rejected)
     b. Cognitive schema focusing on bodily sensations—tendency to amplify and misinterpret symptoms of emotional arousal and to think in concrete rather than emotional terms
     c. Sick role offers respite from responsibilities of life

   d. May begin with physical illnesses in childhood or following a severe medical problem as an adult
   e. Atonement for real or imagined wrong doings (Ford, Katon, & Lipkin, 1993)
2. Psychotherapeutic interventions
   a. Usually resistant to psychiatric treatment unless occurs in medical setting
   b. Focus on stress reduction and coping
   c. Avoid reinforcements of sick role as a solution to life problems

- Family Dynamics/Therapy
  1. Family may reinforce sick role behavior.
  2. Family conflict over client distress and medical treatment
  3. Family roles may be altered.
  4. Family may have low ability to deal directly with stressful situations or obligations
- Group Psychotherapy
  1. Social support
  2. Social interaction
- Milieu Interventions
  1. Often treated on medical unit
  2. Teach rational interpretation of bodily sensations.
  3. Assist to identify relationship between physical symptoms and stress.
  4. Teach techniques to cope with anxiety including talking, exercise, and relaxation techniques.
  5. Meet physical needs, but avoid reinforcing.
  6. Encourage social interaction and constructive use of leisure time.
  7. Teach problem-solving techniques for personal difficulties.
  8. Refer to outpatient therapy.

Somatization Disorder

- Definition: A chronic relapsing syndrome of multiple somatic symptoms for which there is no medical explanation
- Signs and Symptoms
    1. Symptoms include gastrointestinal, pain, cardiopulmonary, conversion, sexual, and female reproductive.
    2. History of several years' duration, beginning before age 30
    3. High utilization of health services: physician visits, excessive surgery, psychiatric services, multiple medications
    4. Associated with changes in life style due to illness
    5. Typically, new symptoms arise during times of emotional distress.
    6. Chaotic social lives
    7. Often accompanied by depression and anxiety (Katon, Lin, VonKorff, Russo, Lipscomb, & Bush, 1991; Simon & VonKorff, 1991)
    8. Existence of primary gain (keep conflicts out of awareness) and secondary gain (benefits of illness)
- Differential Diagnoses
    1. Medical illnesses, especially those with fluctuating presentation such as multiple sclerosis and systematic lupus erythematosus
    2. Anxiety
    3. Depression
    4. Hypochondriasis
- Mental Status Variations
    1. Appearance—may be dressed in exhibitionistic manner
    2. Behavior—seductive, coy
    3. Mood—present as depressed, anxious, with cavalier attitude about symptoms
    4. Thought—medical history disorganized, vague, with dramatic, exaggerated description of symptoms
    5. Insight—none, believes physically ill

- Nursing Diagnoses
  1. Communication, impaired verbal
  2. Coping, ineffective individual
  3. Family processes, altered
  4. Social interaction, impaired
  5. Knowledge deficit
- Genetic/Biological Origins
  1. Inconclusive—dominant hemisphere dysfunction, abnormal cortical function, EEG abnormalities
  2. Possible common genetic background with Antisocial Personality Disorder
  3. Increased risk of Somatization Disorder in first-degree relatives
- Biochemical Approaches
  1. No specific biochemical treatment
  2. If presents with prominent anxiety or depression, may treat with antidepressants or antianxiety agents, but clients tend to misuse
- Intrapersonal
  1. Origins
     a. Substitute somatic symptoms for repressed impulses
     b. Somatization as social communication
        (1) To control or maintain relationships
        (2) Gain disability or divert attention
     c. Somatization as emotional communication
        (1) Symptoms express emotional state
        (2) Coping with environmental stress
     d. Somatic disorders associated with childhood abuse (Glod, 1993)
  2. Psychotherapeutic interventions
     a. Requires close collaboration of medical and mental health practitioners managing chronic condition

(1) Establish trusting relationship with one medical care provider.

(2) Schedule regular visits at frequent intervals, decrease frequency over time.

(3) Provide physical examination of pertinent organ system, but avoid diagnostic procedures, tests, and surgeries

(4) Emphasize interest in patient and symptoms and will continue to follow (Smith, 1990).

(5) Avoid suggestion that symptoms do not exist or are unsubstantiated.

(6) Treat anxiety or depression if present.

(7) Encourage continued employment or rehabilitation if necessary.

b. Solution-focused, brief therapy approaches

- Family Dynamics/Family Therapy

1. Children taught to somatize, rather than to deal with issues verbally
2. Readjust roles to accommodate symptoms and illness behavior.
3. Use somatization as means to mediate relationships.
4. Female clients often choose alcoholics or men with antisocial personality disorders as partners (Smith, 1990).
5. Family therapy aimed at clear, congruent communication, role restructuring, and increasing self-esteem of family members

- Group Approaches

1. Time-limited group therapy with emphasis on improving socialization skills and ability to cope
2. Group therapy with emphasis on how to cope with multiple medical problems

- Milieu Interventions

1. Monitor and assess client's physical status.
2. Attend to physical needs in supportive, but non-reinforcing way.
3. Reinforce verbal expression of needs and feelings.

4. Assist other staff and patients to understand that physical complaints are experienced as "real" (Ford et al., 1993).
5. Help client realize connection between psychological stress and onset of somatic symptoms.
6. Teach new coping skills including use of social relationships and other techniques to decrease anxiety.
7. Maintain consistent approach by all personnel.
8. Support self-care abilities and appropriate role performance, including occupational.

Pain Disorder

- Definition: Severe prolonged pain for which there is no organic basis for the pain and/or the intensity
- Signs and Symptoms
  1. Various manifestations-low back pain, headache, or chronic pelvic pain
  2. Preoccupation with pain
  3. Often follows physical trauma
  4. Analgesics usually do not help
  5. Frequent visits to physicians for relief
  6. Usually refuses to consider psychological origins
  7. Depression usually present
  8. Difficulties in diagnosing because of diverse definitions of pain (King & Strain, 1992)
- Differential Diagnoses
  1. Organic disorders
  2. Depression
  3. Hypochondriasis
  4. Conversion Disorder
- Mental Status Variations
  1. Appearance—antalgic position, diaphoretic, tense

2. Behavior—restless
3. Mood—depressed
4. Thought—preoccupied with pain
5. Concentration—impaired
6. Insight—unaware of psychological factors

- Nursing Diagnoses
  1. Coping, ineffective individual
  2. Family process, altered
  3. Hopelessness
  4. Knowledge deficit
  5. Pain, chronic
  6. Physical mobility, impaired
  7. Role performance, altered
  8. Self-esteem disturbance
  9. Social interaction, impaired
- Genetic/Biological Origins
  1. Greater prevalence in first-degree relatives
  2. Greater incidence of alcoholism and depression in families
  3. Endorphin deficiency
  4. Lower serotonin levels in CNS
- Biochemical Approaches
  1. Analgesics and anxiety agents unhelpful and ineffective; possibility of addiction
  2. Antidepressants, especially amitriptyline, imipramine, and doxepin; anafranil, sertraline
  3. Biofeedback training
  4. Transcutaneous nerve stimulation
  5. Exercise programs/physical therapy
  6. Acupuncture

- Intrapersonal
    1. Origins
        a. Punishment for guilt
        b. Pain behaviors may be reinforced by attentiveness or avoidance of unwanted responsibilities.
        c. Control of others
        d. Stabilization of marriage/family relationships
    2. Psychotherapeutic interventions
        a. Rehabilitate client to usual social/occupational roles.
        b. Discuss psychological causes and secondary gain common to all pain.
        c. Cognitive restructuring
        d. Relaxation techniques
        e. Supportive psychotherapy
- Family Dynamics/Therapy
    1. Family as a whole may be stabilized by pain experience.
    2. Teach family members how to respond to client's pain.
    3. Discuss secondary gain and power in sick role behavior.
    4. Restructure roles, communication patterns, and responsibilities.
    5. Deal with issues of individual and family self-esteem.
- Group
    1. Pain support groups
    2. Exercise groups
    3. Psychoeducational (pain management) groups
    4. Assertiveness training
- Milieu Intervention
    1. Help client apply relaxation and cognitive techniques for pain relief and tension reduction.
    2. Encourage social interaction and participation in activities.

3. Teach about stress—pain-relaxation relationships
4. Encourage verbal, rather than somatic, communications.
5. Avoid reinforcing pain behaviors.
6. Encourage self-care in ADLs.
7. Help client to find ways of assisting others.
8. Design plan for use of leisure.
9. Refer for rehabilitation, pain management, or vocational training.

- Community Resources
  1. Pain management clinics

Factitious Disorder

Factitious Disorder

- Definition: Physical or psychological symptoms intentionally produced or feigned (APA, 1994)
- Signs and Symptoms
  1. Desires role of patient
  2. Compulsive quality
  3. May travel from hospital to hospital, seeking admission for different illnesses under different names
  4. Extremely convincing in presentation of physical or psychological symptoms
     a. With physical presentation of symptoms, may be called "Munchausen" syndrome
     b. Children are presented as the ill one by a parent, but rarely
- Differential Diagnoses
  1. True physical disorder
  2. Somatoform Disorder
  3. Personality Disorders
  4. Schizophrenia
  5. Malingering

- Mental Status Variations
  1. Variance depends upon symptoms produced
  2. Thoughts—conflicts and discrepancies in content
  3. Information not corroborated by significant other
- Nursing Diagnoses
  1. Communication, impaired
  2. Coping, ineffective individual
  3. Role performance, altered
- Genetic/Biological Origins—none identified
- Biochemical Approaches—none
- Intrapersonal
  1. Origins
     a. Found caretakers or hospital as caring with previous illnesses and seek continuance
     b. History of parental deprivation
     c. Those who seek surgery or painful treatment may seek punishment.
     d. Identify with relatives with genuine illnesses.
     e. Defenses employed: Repression, identification, identification with aggressor, and symbolization (Kaplan & Sadock, 1991)
  2. Psychotherapeutic intervention
     a. Early recognition and referral for factitious disorder to avoid unnecessary treatment
     b. Avoid setting client up as adversary.
     c. Usually avoidance of meaningful therapy
- Family Dynamics/Family Therapy
  1. Psychoeducation about disorder
  2. Assist family not to enable client, but to support therapy.
- Group Approaches—none

- Milieu Interventions
  1. Create a safe environment.
  2. Assist caregivers to understand nature of disorder.
  3. Avoid reinforcing gain from illness.
  4. Assist to find means to meet needs for nurturance.

Dissociative Disorders

Dissociative Amnesia

- Definition: Dissociative disorder in which person is suddenly unable to recall memories
- Signs and Symptoms
  1. Not ordinary forgetfulness
  2. Can recall other information, learn, and function coherently
  3. Most common during wars and natural disasters
  4. Amnesia
     a. Localized—short time period
     b. Generalized—for whole lifetime of experiences
     c. Selective—amnesia for some, but not all events
     d. Continuous—forgets successive events as they occur, but alert at the time
  5. Primary and secondary gain
  6. Terminates abruptly
- Differential Diagnoses
  1. Medical conditions: neoplasms, infections, epilepsy post concussion
  2. Wernicke-Korsakoff syndrome
  3. ECT
  4. Drug-induced (LSD, steroids, benzodiazepines, barbiturates)
  5. Transient global amnesia usually caused by TIAs
- Mental Status Variations

1. Mood—often depressed
2. Memory—impaired
3. Orientation—variable
4. Insight—impaired

- Nursing Diagnoses
  1. Anxiety
  2. Coping, ineffective individual
  3. Thought processes, altered
  4. Powerlessness
- Genetic/Biological Origins
  1. Origins—no definitive explanations
- Biochemical Approaches
  1. Thiopental and sodium amytal interviews to recover memories
- Intrapersonal
  1. Origins
     a. Psychoanalytic: Expressed or fantasized forbidden wish
        (1) Usually sexual or aggressive
        (2) Cannot deal with, so uses repression and denial
     b. Emotional trauma (Saxe, van der Kolk, Berkowitz, Chinman, Hall, Lieberg, & Schwartz, 1993)
        (1) Strong emotional response
        (2) Psychological conflict
  2. Psychotherapeutic intervention
     a. Psychotherapy to deal with emotional responses to trauma
     b. Psychotherapy aimed at resolution of unacceptable impulses or behavior
     c. Hypnosis to uncover memories
     d. Stress management
- Family Dynamics/Family Therapy

1. If natural disaster affected all family members, reconstruct collective memory.
2. All family members affected by client's distress
   a. Family education to understand condition of individual client
   b. Family therapy to help family members make sense of trauma and/or impulse expression

- Group Approaches
  1. If traumatic event, may benefit from support group of survivors
  2. Group psychotherapy usually not indicated
- Milieu Intervention
  1. Treated primarily on outpatient basis or in general hospital
  2. Create safe environment.
  3. Mutually develop contract for care.
  4. Provide opportunities to talk about traumatic event and its meaning.
  5. Teach coping strategies to deal with anxiety actively (rather than dissociation).
  6. Assist in devising realistic future plans.

Dissociative Fugue

- Definition: Dissociative disorder characterized by physically traveling from usual environment, inability to recall important aspects of identity and the assumption of a new identity
- Signs and Symptoms
  1. Old and new identities do not alternate.
  2. New identity incomplete
  3. Unaware of having forgotten
  4. Lasts hours to days; rarely months
- Differential Diagnosis
  1. Organic mental disorders such as temporal lobe epilepsy
  2. Psychogenic Amnesia
  3. Malingering

- Mental Status Variations
  1. Memory—amnesia for identity and important aspects of life
  2. Insight—unaware of memory impairment
- Nursing Diagnoses
  1. Anxiety
  2. Coping, ineffective individual
  3. Personal identity disturbance
  4. Thought processes, altered
- Genetic/Biological Origins
  1. Origins: No definitive explanation
  2. Heavy alcohol abuse may predispose, but may be primarily psychological effect.
- Biochemical Approaches
  1. Amobarbital or Thiopental interviews to uncover identity
- Intrapersonal
  1. Origins
     a. Response of withdrawal (by dissociation) to psychological stressors: war, family, marital, and occupational (Saxe et al., 1993)
  2. Psychotherapeutic interventions
     a. Hypnosis to uncover memories/identity
     b. Psychotherapy
        (a) Uncover identity and memories
        (b) Deal with sources of stress more effectively
     c. Couples therapy if marital situation a source of stress
     d. Stress management
- Family Dynamics/Therapy
  1. Family of origin or current family setting may be source of conflict.
     a. Family rules may prohibit overt expression of distress.

b. All family members affected by behavior and loss (for some period of time) of family member.

2. Psychoeducation to understand client's condition
3. If family dynamics are source of stress, family therapy to improve communication, problem-solve, and deal with crisis

- Group Approaches

    a. If trauma victim (war, natural disaster), support groups

- Milieu Interventions
    1. Treat primarily on outpatient basis.
    2. Create safe environment.
    3. Help to reconstruct memories and identity.
    4. Assist to create meaning of fugue episode.
    5. Teach coping skills to deal with anxiety.
    6. Refer for therapy or other continued assistance in managing stressors.
- Community Resources
    1. Support groups for managing specific stressors

Depersonalization Disorders

- Definition: Dissociative disorder in which client experiences recurrent alterations in perception of self
- Signs and Symptoms
    1. Described as "detached from reality," "dreamlike," or detached from one's body
    2. Self feels strange, unreal
    3. Able to function during the experience
    4. Client distressed about depersonalization experience
    5. May be episodic or chronic
- Differential Diagnoses
    1. Organic Disorder—neurological, metabolic
    2. Schizophrenias

3. Anxiety
4. Obsessive Compulsive Disorder (OCD)
5. Psychoactive Substance Abuse

- Mental Status Variations
  1. Mood—anxious, depressed
  2. Perception—feelings of detachment from self and/or environment, feeling of physical change in body
  3. Insight—impaired
- Nursing Diagnoses
  1. Anxiety
  2. Coping, ineffective individual
  3. Personal identity disturbance
  4. Sensory—perceptual alterations
- Genetic/Biological Origins
  1. Organic disease—neoplasms, epilepsy, and metabolic disorders
  2. Sensory deprivation
  3. Drug-induced-psychoactive drugs, especially hallucinogens, cannabis
- Biochemical Approaches
  1. Anxiety agents (if anxiety a component)
  2. Treatment of underlying organic disorder
- Intrapersonal
  1. Origin
     a. Internal conflict
     b. Disturbance in ego functioning
     c. Severe emotional distress (Saxe et al., 1993)
  2. Psychotherapeutic Interventions
     a. Insight—oriented psychotherapy
     b. Stress management

c. Deal with past traumas, if present

- Family Dynamics/Family Therapy
  1. Family may exhibit poor coping mechanisms to deal with internal family conflict or outside stressors
     a. Family myths of strength may prohibit admission of family pain
     b. Family rules may prohibit verbal expression of feelings
  2. Psychoeducation about disorder
  3. Family therapy if family dynamics are stressors or influence coping with anxiety
- Group Approaches
  1. Support groups for specific stressors (parenting, occupational)
  2. Stress management group
- Milieu Interventions (rarely treated inpatient)
  1. Create safe environment.
  2. Educate about disorder.
  3. Assist client to examine relationship between anxiety and depersonalization.
  4. Teach stress management and problem-solving techniques.
  5. Plan for use of leisure time.

Dissociative Identity Disorder or Multiple Personality Disorder (MPD)

- Definition: Dissociative disorder in which person has two or more separate, distinct personalities (alters), each with relatively enduring pattern of perceiving, relating to, and thinking about, self and environment
- Signs and Symptoms
  1. At least 2 personalities dominant, recurrent (APA, 1993)
  2. Core personality usually unaware of alters when first seeks treatment
  3. Personalities may represent different ages, genders, races. Most have at least one child alter.
  4. Personalities with different influence and power over one another

5. Communicate with one another through executive alter or through inner dialogue (Curtin, 1993)
6. Amnesic symptoms for childhood experiences, or ''lose time'' when alternate personality present for period of time
7. Sleep disturbances, self mutilation, substance abuse, headaches
8. Physiological responses (including allergies) vary in different alters
9. Issue of therapists ''creating'' memories and alters (North, Ryall, Ricci, & Wetzel, 1993)
    a. Verbal/nonverbal behavior of therapist may create false memories in suggestible client.
    b. Public as well as some health care providers doubt validity of the diagnosis.

- Differential Diagnoses
    1. Psychogenic fugues
    2. Psychogenic Amnesia
    3. Schizophrenia
    4. Borderline Personality Disorder
- Mental Status Variations
    1. Appearances—dress style, grooming, mannerisms may vary from session to session; marked changes in nonverbal behavior, handedness within sessions; blinking, eye roll, twitches with switching
    2. Speech—marked changes within brief period of time (style, accent, vocabulary)
    3. Mood—depressed, anxious; switches rapidly within sessions
    4. Thought processes—loose association with rapid switches
    5. Perceptual—hallucinations (auditory/visual)—voices usually experienced within patient's head
    6. Memory—some long-term memory deficits
    7. Judgment—erratic, depending upon age, personality
    8. Insight—initially not aware of alters

- Nursing Diagnoses
  1. Anxiety
  2. Coping, ineffective individual
  3. Personal identity disturbance
  4. Self-mutilation, high risk for
  5. Violence, high risk for, directed at self and/or others
- Genetic/Biological Origins
  1. Higher incidence in first-degree relatives
  2. Possible psychobiological ability to dissociate or to be hypnotized
  3. Self mutilation possibly biologically entrained (Winchell & Stanley, 1991)
- Biochemical Approaches
  1. Generally do not respond to psychotropic medications
  2. Antidepressants, antianxiety agents, or antipsychotics may provide symptomatic relief or help control behavior (Putnam & Lowenstein, 1993)
  3. No specific medication to treat MPD
- Intrapersonal
  1. Origins
     a. Prolonged and severe physical, emotional , or sexual abuse as a child
     b. Dissociation helps child cope by creating new personalities to experience and deal with various aspects of time periods of the trauma.
     c. Alters serve various purposes (protection, expression of anger, organizer)
  2. Psychotherapeutic interventions
     a. Individual therapy stages (Putnam, 1989)
        (1) Making diagnosis
        (2) Initial interventions

(a) Meet personalities
(b) Take history
(c) Develop working relationship with system

(3) Initial stabilization
(a) Contract with alters
(b) Contract with entire system
(c) Stabilize uncontrollable behaviors

(4) Acceptance of diagnosis
(a) Some alters do not accept presence of others
(b) Issue throughout treatment

(5) Development of communication and cooperation
(a) Internal communication
(b) Establish cooperation toward common goals
(c) Development of internal decision-making process
(d) Facilitation of switching

(6) Metabolism of the trauma
(a) Major treatment task
(b) Uncover trauma
(c) Abreaction

(7) Resolution and integration
(a) Some elect integration
(b) Others remain multiples

(8) Development of postresolution coping skills
(a) Learn new coping skills
(b) Take on tasks previously split
(c) Deal with reactive depression

b. Hypnosis uniformly endorsed (Putnam & Lowenstein, 1993)

- Family Dynamics/Family Therapy
  1. Family of origin characteristics (Braun, 1986)

   a. United front to community, but internal, severe conflict
   b. Socially isolated
   c. One caretaker with severe pathology; one abuses, one labels
   d. Contradictory messages to child, inconsistent expectations
   e. Rigid religious/mystical beliefs
   f. Secrecy and denial

2. Family therapy with family of origin. Adjunct to primary individual therapy
   b. Complicated by severe family pathology and secrecy
   c. Occasionally include selected family members
   d. Abusers not included in therapy (Braun, 1986)

3. Family therapy with partners and children
   a. Marital therapy helpful adjunct
   b. Help family members avoid promoting dissociation.
   c. Help to deal with hostile personalities.
   d. Understand process of therapy and integration.
   e. Evaluate children and treat for abuse (if present).
   f. Confirm children's experience with parental behavior and label as illness.

- Milieu Interventions
  1. Hospitalize when self-harm or danger toward others.
     a. Support during abreaction.
     b. Provide structure and safety.
     c. Create mutually designed contract so that treatment goals understood by alters.
     d. Establish primary nurse for each shift.
  2. Maintain consistent, accurate understanding of MPD and client by all staff members to avoid splitting.
  3. Provide safe, consistent environment.

4. No-harm contract—homicide, suicide, self-mutilation (Winchel & Stanley, 1991)
5. Teach techniques to provide:
    a. Anxiety reduction
    b. Personal, emotional safety
    c. Control of switching
    d. Avoidance of self-mutilation, based upon particular meaning of the behavior (Favazza & Rosenthal, 1993)
6. Educate about nature of disorder, existence and function of personalities, course of therapy, and integration.
7. Assist staff and clients to treat alters as they present.
8. Help other clients understand MPD client's behavior, attention from the staff, and their own reactions.
    a. Include in-ward non-therapy activities, but exclude from general group sessions.

Adjustment Disorders

Adjustment Disorders

- Definition: Maladaptive or pathological response to a psychosocial stressor (Strain, Hammer, Huertas, Lam, & Fulop, 1993)
- Signs and Symptoms
    1. Sources of stressors—events, such as job loss, acute or chronic illness, divorce, or specific developmental milestones (beginning school, getting married, etc.)
        a. The more numerous or more disturbing the stressors, the greater effect on adjustment (Schatzberg, 1990).
        b. Previous history of adjustment disorder puts person at more risk.
    2. Distress experienced is in excess to what is expected.
    3. Significant impairment in social, occupational, or school functioning (APA, 1993)
    4. Occurs within 3 months of stressor's onset

a. Symptoms may be delayed.

b. Disorder may continue with prolonged stressor or inability to adapt.

5. Commonly diagnosed in medical settings (Schatzberg, 1990)

6. Manifestations vary:

   a. Depressed mood

      (1) Sadness

      (2) Tearfulness

      (3) Hopelessness

   b. Anxiety

      (1) Palpitations

      (2) Agitation

      (3) Jitteriness

   c. Conduct disturbances

      (1) Violate rights of others

      (2) Violate social norms

   d. Combinations of the above

7. Physical complaints such as headache or backache are more common in the elderly

- Differential Diagnoses

  1. Generalized Anxiety Disorder
  2. Depression
  3. Somatization Disorder
  4. Post-traumatic Stress Disorder
  5. Uncomplicated bereavement
  6. Conduct Disorder

- Mental Status Variations

  1. Varies considerably, depending upon manifestation
  2. Appearance—visibly distressed

3. Psychomotor Activity—restless, agitated
4. Mood—Anxious, Depressed
5. Concentration—Impaired
6. Thought—Preoccupation with stressors or physical symptoms
7. Insight—May attribute symptoms to onset of stressor

- Nursing Diagnoses
  1. Coping, ineffective individual
  2. Family process, altered
  3. Parenting, altered, high risk for
  4. Role performance, altered
  5. Adjustment, impaired
  6. Grieving, dysfunctional
  7. Post-trauma response
- Genetic/Biological Origins
  1. Psychological insult produces aberration of autonomic regulation and emotional lability Popkin, Callies, Colon, & Stiebel, 1990).
  2. Note early responsiveness of REM (rapid eye movement) sleep waves to emotional turmoil (Cartwright & Wood, 1991).
     (1) Decreased delta sleep initially
     (2) Continues if stress unresolved
  3. Physical changes associated with aging, particularly sleep deprivation, may contribute to symptoms (Turnbull, 1989).
  4. Possible constitutional predisposition
- Biochemical Approaches
  1. Anti-depressive or anti-anxiety agents on a short-term basis (Horowitz, Stinson, & Field, 1991)
  2. Limited use of hypnotics to aid sleep
  3. Tendency for overprescription of sedatives and tranquilizers in early phase of coping with stressor (Cartwright & Wood, 1991)

a. Benzodiazepines which decrease delta sleep may compound problems of insomnia.

b. Beta-blockers decrease anxiety but little effect on depressive component.

4. Teach client to avoid alcohol, caffeine, nicotine, and street drugs (Horowitz, et al., 1991).

5. Therapeutic touch (Heidt, 1991)

- Intrapersonal

1. Origins

a. Psychoanalytic view: early parent-child relationship shapes ability to respond to stressors in later life (Kaplan & Sadock, 1991)

b. Cognitive/Behavioral (Strain et al., 1993)

(1) Cognitive coping styles reflect personal attitude and meaning of the event.

(2) Field independent persons use isolation and intellectualization.

(3) Field dependent persons use repression and denial.

2. Psychotherapeutic interventions

a. Crisis intervention/brief therapies

(1) Clarify meaning of the event.

(2) Engage social support.

(3) Create active interventions to ameliorate the stressor.

b. Process memories/associations elicited by the stressor.

(1) Dose-by-dose approach to difficult topics (Horowitz, Stinson, & Field, 1991)

(2) Teach techniques to keep emotions at tolerable level.

c. Cognitive/Behavioral (Turnbull, 1989)

(1) Desensitization

(2) Flooding

(3) Stress management techniques

(a) Autogenic Training/PMR

(b) Hypnosis

(c) Meditation

(4) Assertiveness Training

(5) Cognitive re-structuring

d. Interpersonal support and reassurance

- Family Dynamics/Family Therapy

1. Family members affected by client's response to stressors, or may have experienced the stressors themselves

2. Family therapy

a. Clarify meaning of the event.

b. Support effective coping techniques of individuals and entire family system.

c. Decrease secondary gain system-wide.

d. Facilitate decision-making and reality-testing.

e. Educate about the course of adapting to a stressor.

- Group Approaches

1. Short-term group psychotherapy with problem-solving, supportive focus

2. Self-help groups developed to deal with particular stressors (e.g., divorce, death, stroke, diabetes)

a. Common bond

b. Experience in adjusting

c. Chance to share coping techniques

d. Source of continuing support

e. Pragmatic in nature

- Milieu Interventions (Inpatient or home setting)

1. Protect from excessive stimulation.

2. Provide structure in activities, environment, and safety.

3. Teach about adjustment process.

4. Support biological functioning (eating, sleeping, etc.).
5. Emphasize trust in the future, social support, and self-efficacy (Horowitz et al., 1991).
6. Focus on active recollection, re-telling story while differentiating between reality and fantasy (group and/or family helpful).
7. Reinforce increased communication with others.
8. Reduce external demands to allow for work on stressors.
9. Reinforce conscious control over ruminations or recollections.
10. Deal with recurrent stressors, shame over vulnerability, anger, and sadness (Horowitz et al., 1991).

- Community
  1. Refer to community self-help groups.
  2. Refer to community resources to deal with specific stressors.
  3. Mobilize neighbors, churches, and other naturally occurring groups to lend help.

Questions
Select the best answer

Generalist Level

1. Ms. Smith, who has panic attacks, comes to where you are sitting and says "it's happening again. I can't breathe. I know I'm going to die." She is breathing with difficulty. She has been attending a group to learn more about panic attacks and how to avert them. Your best response is:

   a. "Let me take your blood pressure."
   b. "You know what to do—start your exercises."
   c. "You're experiencing anxiety; that's what you are feeling."
   d. "Tell me what's been going on."

2. Persons with recurrent panic disorders usually present with:

   a. High level of general anxiety
   b. Cardiac/respiratory symptoms of distress
   c. La belle indifference
   d. Clear precipitants

3. A priority nursing diagnosis for Sandra, an agoraphobic, who will not leave her house without her husband accompanying her is:

   a. Post trauma response
   b. Parenting, altered
   c. Fear
   d. Denial, ineffective

4. Mr. Lee has a generalized anxiety disorder. You will be teaching him some relaxation techniques. When is the best time for him to learn?

   a. When he is only mildly anxious
   b. Immediately after feeling severe distress
   c. In the middle of a time of moderate distress
   d. After taking an anti-anxiety agent

5. Jim, who suffers from severe flashbacks of war experiences, and has just been admitted, sits on the lounge, apart from other clients. Your best response is:

   a. Let him remain apart until he's ready to disclose.
   b. Introduce him to two other veterans on the unit with similar problems.
   c. Suggest that he work on a crossword puzzle until dinner.

d. Observe him for flashbacks.

6. Symptoms of autonomic arousal in the PTSD client include:
   a. Hypersomnia
   b. Tachycardia
   c. Alexithymia
   d. Hypotonic musculature

7. Which mental status variations would you expect for a client diagnosed as having PTSD?
   a. Thought: Delusion of Grandeur
   b. Perceptual: Derealization
   c. Memory: Impaired recent memory
   d. Mood: Inappropriate, silly

8. Physiological monitoring of clients using benzodiazepines includes:
   a. CBC with differential
   b. Kidney function studies
   c. Blood pressure
   d. Serum benzodiazepine levels

9. Jerry, a miner, was injured a year ago and hasn't been able to return to work because of severe low back pain. His neurologist could find no organic reason for his continuing pain. Which of the following psychiatric diagnosis best fits Jerry's clinical picture?
   a. Factitious disorder
   b. Hypochondriasis
   c. Pain disorder
   d. Conversion disorder

10. Nursing diagnoses for Jerry might include all but:
    a. Role performance, altered
    b. Pain, chronic
    c. Post trauma response
    d. Family processes, altered

11. An explanation for Jerry's continued pain in spite of his neurologist's findings is:

a. Secondary gain
b. High endorphin levels
c. High serotonin levels
d. Repression of unacceptable impulses

12. Treatment of Jerry's chronic pain is likely to include all but which of the following?

a. Exercise program
b. Biofeedback-assisted relaxation
c. Pain support group
d. Anti-anxiety agents

13. John has been preparing for running a marathon for over a year. "It's my 40th birthday present to myself" he explains. The morning of the race, his wife finds him still in bed, his legs paralyzed. John tells her that he guesses he can't race after all. What mental status variations might you expect?

a. Mood: Depressed, anxious
b. Mood: La belle indifference
c. Mood: Blunted affect
d. Mood: Relieved

14. The symptoms of a conversion disorder may be related to:

a. Heightened autonomic arousal
b. Displacement of aggression
c. Mid-life crisis
d. Symbolic relationship with conflict

15. Mae has an intense argument with her 15-year-old daughter who visits her daily in the hospital where Mae is being treated for hypochondriasis. Mae sends her daughter home and asks the nurse for medication for her stomach. "I wonder if she'll regret this when I'm dead of stomach cancer?" she states. Your best reply is:

a. "Let's talk about what just happened."
b. "This antacid will help."
c. "Teenagers just go through those phases."
d. "Mae, there is *no* sign of stomach cancer. You're not about to die."

16. A client with a conversion disorder hospitalized in a psychiatric facility will require which approach by nursing staff:

a. Anticipate and meet self-care needs of client
b. Encourage attendance at expressive therapies
c. Reinforce verbal expression of needs
d. Remind the client that his difficulties are not real

17. When an MPD client is hospitalized for serious self-inflicted cuts, the no-harm contract should include:

a. Ward privileges gained for no self-harm
b. Clear alternatives to follow when feeling the urge to cut
c. Provision of antipsychotics for increased agitation
d. Discharge from the hospital if there is self harm

18. Which is true about the resolution of MPD?

a. Clients must integrate alters
b. All traumatic incidents must be remembered
c. Many clients experience a reactive depression
d. Some alters always exist, although hidden

19. Given the diagnosis of depersonalization disorder, which nursing diagnosis is most likely to result from assessment?

a. Powerlessness
b. Grieving, dysfunctional
c. Personal identify disturbance
d. Depersonalization alteration

20. Treatment of dissociative amnesia includes all modalities *except:*

a. Hypnosis
b. Stress management
c. Anti-anxiety agents
d. Psychotherapy

21. Mrs. Peters who has experienced a traumatic automobile accident in which three persons were burned to death, tells you that she just wants to "put it behind her." She refuses to talk about the accident or attend activities, and says, "I just want my nerve pills." Your best response is:

a. "Nerve pills are highly addictive. You need to learn to relax."
b. "I can see why you'd like to put it behind you. It must have been very scary."
c. "You are right. It's important to carry on and not dwell on the past."

d. "I hope you'll talk to your doctor about this."

22. Mrs. Peters asks why she has to go to art therapy this morning. "I'm no artist. My hobby is gardening. I'd rather go gardening. I'd rather just stay here and watch a little television." Which is your best response?

 a. "Art therapy is one way to express yourself. You don't have to be an artist—just be willing to try the activity."
 b. "Art therapy may give you an idea about undiscovered talents. You just might be a great artist inside."
 c. "Art therapy is good, but I'll see if we can't schedule you for the green house activity instead."
 d. "I'll stay here and talk with you while you watch TV."

23. Mrs. Peters finally decides to participate in art therapy. She returns to the unit red-eyed and clutching a paper covered with heavy red scrawls. She stops and shows it to you. The best response would be:

 a. "That's really good. That red must be the fire."
 b. "Let's put this up for the other patients to see."
 c. "This is very strong—tell me about it."
 d. "If art therapy was too troubling, I do have some medication for you."

24. Mary has been diagnosed as having a depersonalization disorder. Which experience might she relate during your initial nursing assessment?

 a. "This feeling is so weird—I feel just 'unreal.' "
 b. "I haven't been able to take care of the kids; I just sit around."
 c. "It's no big deal."
 d. "I have dreams that I just can't get out of."

Advanced Practice Level

1. Chris, a successful music major, is preparing for his recital next week. He has experienced severe stage fright in the past and once, refused to perform at all. Which of the following biochemical approaches is most likely to be employed in conjunction with behavioral therapy for his difficulty?

   a. Mono-amine oxidase inhibitor
   b. Tricyclic antidepressant
   c. Beta-adrenergic antagonist
   d. Antiparkinsoniam agent

2. Your client, Fred, attends a men's group for adult survivors of childhood sexual abuse. Some men in the group are currently confronting their families, but Fred is unsure of his course of action. Your best response is:

   a. "Most families welcome the honesty as difficult as it is for everyone."
   b. "You've been learning to be assertive. This is probably the next step."
   c. "If you don't confront your father now, you'll always feel powerless."
   d. "That's a difficult decision. What would you like to have happen with your family?"

3. A Vietnam veteran who served at a field hospital late in the war becomes symptomatic of PTSD after a long period of what seemed excellent adjustment. Her husband and children have joined her in your office to talk about what's happening. They ask if she has PTSD. What is your best response?

   a. Yes, she has PTSD, but we are going to let "bygones" be "bygones" and work on other things in therapy.
   b. "I think there is a different problem. PTSD occurs much sooner."
   c. "She has symptoms of PTSD which are difficult not just for her, but for all of you."
   d. The problem is rooted in the past, family can do nothing now.

4. Family therapy for the PTSD client and her family will meet all but one of the following goals:

   a. Develop a shared frame of reference for the trauma
   b. Support the victim in recovery
   c. Reduce secondary gain by limiting trauma talk to therapy sessions only
   d. Address issues of trust, responsibility, and blame

5. Now, three weeks after the hurricane, Charley cannot remember anything about

his 36- hour ordeal, trapped under debris from his house until he was finally rescued. This is best described as:

a. Dissociative amnesia, localized
b. Dissociative amnesia, generalized
c. Dissociative amnesia, continuous
d. Dissociative amnesia, selective

6. A community support group for flood victims asks you, the CNS, to talk about symptoms of PTSD. The group has been meeting since the disaster six months ago. One woman asks why she continues to have periodic, recurrent dreams and thoughts about the flood. Which is your best reply?

a. "Your mind is attempting to work through what happened, a little bit at a time."
b. "You are probably thinking too much. Try to stop these thoughts."
c. "You could be guilty about surviving."
d. "At this time, you have a serious problem. Have you seen your doctor?"

7. One hypothesis why PTSD clients may continue to engage in dangerous activities and have recurrent interpersonal difficulties is related to:

a. serotonin excesses
b. autonomic entrainment
c. endogenous opioid withdrawal
d. dysregulation of GABA

8. Leonard has recently avoided going out to eat with his family at restaurants. He claims the food is better at home, and that other people may watch him eat and critique his table manners. The most appropriate psychiatric diagnosis is:

a. Schizophrenia with delusions
b. Agoraphobia
c. Avoidant Personality Disorder
d. Social Phobia

9. The client presenting with a somatization disorder typically:

a. Exaggerates the seriousness of minor symptoms into major health problems
b. Refuses medication, preferring to "work it out alone"
c. Has a chaotic social life
d. Understands the stress-physical symptoms relationship

10. Joan, who obsessively thinks about her children dying in a house fire, is learning to use thought-stopping techniques. Such techniques include:

    a. Practicing progressive muscle relaxation
    b. Discussing with a staff member the likelihood of a house fire
    c. Snapping a rubber band on her wrist when the thought of fire occurs
    d. Reminding herself of the home fire alarm system

11. Anxiety-reducing techniques such as autogenic\training or progressive muscle relaxation are best employed by a person who fears flying on airplanes:

    a. When anxiety rises to intolerable levels
    b. When the plane takes off and lands
    c. Prior to feeling autonomic arousal
    d. Only in practice settings

12. The psychoanalytic explanation for a phobic disorder involves:

    a. Classical conditioned responses
    b. Reaction formation
    c. Displacement
    d. Avoidance

13. Group therapies for the treatment of agoraphobia include:

    a. Social skills training
    b. Medication education
    c. Art or movement therapies
    d. Gestalt approaches

14. Systematic desensitization includes all but which of the following?

    a. In vivo exposure
    b. Deep muscle relaxation
    c. Understanding why stimuli are anxiety provoking
    d. Cognitive coping self-statements

15. Peggy is hospitalized because of emotional exhaustion. Her husband reports that she has become increasingly preoccupied with cleaning the house over the past year. Always a meticulous housekeeper, she is now afraid that the house is contaminated by environmental toxins. She is up most of the night, trying to clean and decontaminate. When her husband attempts to have her rest, she becomes distraught. The most accurate psychiatric diagnosis is:

a. Obsessive compulsive disorder
b. Obsessive compulsive personality disorder
c. Schizophrenia, paranoid type
d. Major depression

16. Probable nursing diagnoses include all but:

a. Coping, ineffective individual
b. Anxiety
c. Role performance, altered
d. Home maintenance management, impaired

17. Clomipramine (Anafranil), 250 mgm every morning, is ordered for Peggy. After taking the medication for a week, she complains of being too sleepy to participate in morning activities. Which of the following actions might the CNS suggest?

a. Tell her the sleepiness will soon disappear
b. Recommend the medication be taken at bedtime
c. Request the medication be discontinued immediately
d. Reschedule her activities to late afternoon

18. The most effective treatment of panic disorders is:

a. Reworking previous traumatic separations
b. Family therapy
c. Cognitive restructuring
d. Provision of a stress-free environment

19. Persons prone to high levels of anxiety tend to have which dysfunctional thoughts?

a. Negative views about the self, world, and future
b. Overestimation of the support of others
c. Overestimation of danger
d. ''Black or white'' thinking

20. Mrs. Stevens has been taking Alprazolam (Xanax) 2.0 mgm/day for six months. She wants to become pregnant and, in preparation, goes off the medication. She currently experiences little anxiety. She has learned a variety of coping techniques in therapy. Your best response to her desire to discontinue the Xanax is:

a. ''Since you are doing so well, go ahead and stop taking your Xanax.''

b. ''You should remain on benzodiazepines for at least one year.''
c. ''Should you decide to discontinue Xanax, it's important to very slowly reduce the dose.''
d. ''You might want to try a shorter-acting medication like Oxazepam (Serax) as a substitute.''

21. Susan was admitted at 3 a.m. to the emergency department of a medical center, complaining of stomach pain which she believes is cancer. Although she admits to having eaten some ''real spicy food'' the evening before, she is insistent on having an upper and lower GI series immediately. She is anxious, despite her doctor's reassurance. Which is a likely psychiatric diagnosis?

    a. Conversion disorder
    b. Hypochondriasis
    c. Pain disorder
    d. Generalized anxiety disorder

22. A primary focus of treatment for Susan will be:

    a. Dietary instructions and antacids
    b. Stress management techniques
    c. Insight-focused psychotherapy
    d. Rehabilitation efforts

23. Upon questioning your client during the intake interview, she relates that she hears voices inside her head, as if in a conversation. Which psychiatric diagnosis best fits these experiences?

    a. Schizophrenia
    b. PTSD
    c. MPD
    d. Panic Disorder

24. Family therapy with partners and children of MPD clients is aimed at which of the following?

    a. Help children access child alters
    b. Help children deal with hostile alters
    c. Help children ignore inconsistent parental behavior
    d. Help children parent the child alters

25. The most efficacious approach for dealing with a client who has a somatization disorder is to:

a. Use antidepressants
b. Closely collaborate with the primary care provider
c. Confront the unreality of the symptoms
d. Provide brief, problem-focused therapy

Answers

Generalist Level

1. c	9. c	17. b
2. b	10. c	18. c
3. c	11. a	19. c
4. a	12. d	20. c
5. b	13. b	21. b
6. b	14. d	22. a
7. b	15. a	23. c
8. a	16. c	24. a

Advanced Practice Level

1. c	10. c	19. c
2. d	11. c	20. c
3. c	12. c	21. b
4. c	13. a	22. b
5. a	14. c	23. c
6. a	15. a	24. b
7. c	16. d	25. b
8. d	17. b	
9. c	18. c	

Bibliography

American Psychiatric Association. (1993). *Diagnostic and statistical manual of mental disorders* (4th ed.). Washington, DC: American Psychiatric Association.

Ballenger, J. C., & Fyer, A. J. (1993). Examining criteria for panic disorder. *Hospital and Community Psychiatry, 44*(3), 226–228.

Barloon, D. E. (1993). Effects on children of having lived with a parent who has an anxiety disorder. *Issues in Mental Health Nursing, 14,* 187–199.

Beck, A. T., Sokol, L., Clark, D. A., Berchick, R., & Wright, F. (1992). A crossover study of focused cognitive therapy for panic disorder. *American Journal of Psychiatry, 149*(6), 778–783.

Bowers, J. J. (1992). Therapy through art: Facilitating treatment of sexual abuse. *Journal of Psychosocial Nursing, 30*(6), 15–24.

Braun, B. G. (1986). Treatment of multiple personality disorder. Washington, DC: American Psychiatric Press.

Bremner, J. D., Southwick, S., Brett, E., Fontana, A., Rosenheck, R., & Charney, D. S. (1992). Dissociation and posttraumatic stress disorder in Vietnam combat veterans. *American Journal of Psychiatry, 149*(3), 328–332.

Bremner, J. D., Steinberg, M., Southwick, S. M., Johnson, D. R., & Charney, D. S., (1993). Use of the structural clinical interview for DSM-IV dissociative symptoms in posttraumatic stress disorder. *American Journal of Psychiatry, 150*(7), 1011–1014.

Cartwright, R., & Wood, E. (1991). Adjustment disorders of sleep: The sleep effects of a major stressful event and its resolution. *Psychiatry Research, 39,* 199–209.

Clum, G. A. (1990). Coping with panic. Pacific Grove, CA: Brooks/Cole.

Curtin, S. L. (1993). Recognizing multiple personality disorder. *Journal of Psychosocial Nursing, 31*(2), 29–33.

Davidson, J. R., & Foa, E. B. (1991). Refining criteria for posttraumatic stress disorder. *Hospital and Community Psychiatry, 42*(3), 259–261.

Davis, M., Eshelman, E. R., & McKay, M. (1988). *The relaxation and stress reduction workbook.* (3rd ed.). Oakland, CA: New Harbinger.

Draucker, C. B. (1992). The healing process of female adult incest survivors: Constructing a personal residence. *Image, 24*(1), 4–8.

Faravelli, C., Pallanti, S., Biondi, F., Paterniti, S., & Scarpato, M. A. (1992). Onset of panic disorder. *American Journal of Psychiatry, 149*(6), 827–828.

Favazza, A. R., & Rosenthal, R. J. (1993). Diagnostic issues in self-mutilation. *Hospital and Community Psychiatry, 44*(2), 134–140.

Ford, C. V., Katon, W. J., & Lipkin, M. (1993). Managing somatization and hypochondriasis. *Patient Care, 27*(2), 31–34.

Free, N. K., Winget, C. N., & Whitman, R. M. (1993). Separation anxiety in panic disorder. *American Journal of Psychiatry, 150*(4), 595–599.

Glod, C. A. (1993). Long-term consequences of childhood physical and sexual abuse. *Archives of Psychiatric Nursing, 7*(3), 163–173.

Glod, C. A. (1991). Psychopharmacology and clinical practice. *Nursing Clinics of North America, 26*(2), 1991.

Greist, J. H., Rappaport, J. L., & Rasmussen, S. A. (1990). Spotting the obsessive compulsive. *Patient Care, 24*(9), 47–73.

Gunderson, J. G., & Sabo, A. N. (1993). The phenomenological and conceptual interface between borderline personality disorder and PTSD. *American Journal of Psychiatry, 150*(1), 19–27.

Haack, M. R., & Alim, T. N. (1991). Anxiety and the adult child of an alcoholic: A comorbid problem. *Community Health, 13*(4), 49–60.

Heidt, P. R. (1991). Helping patients to rest: clinical studies in therapeutic touch. *Holistic Nursing Practice, 5*(4), 57–66.

Herman, J. (1992). *Trauma and recovery.* NY: Basic Books.

Hill, L., & Oliver, N. (1993). Therapeutic touch and theory-based mental health nursing. *Journal of Psychosocial Nursing, 31*(2), 19–22, 27.

Horowitz, M., Stinson, C., & Field, N. (1991). Natural disasters and stress response syndromes. *Psychiatric Annals, 21*(9), 556–562.

Kaplan, H., & Sadock, B. (1991). *Synopsis of Psychiatry.* (6th ed.). Baltimore: Williams & Wilkins.

Karl, G. T. (1989). Survival skills for psychic trauma. *Journal of Psychosocial Nursing, 27*(4) 15–19.

Katon, W. J. (1989). *Panic disorder in the medical setting* (DHHS Publication No. ADM 89-1629). Washington, D.C.: U.S. Government Printing Office.

Katon, W. J., Lin, E., VonKorff, M., Russo, J., Lipscomb, P., & Bush, T. (1991). Somatization: A spectrum of severity. *American Journal of Psychiatry, 148*(1), 34–40.

King, S. A., & Strain, J. J. (1992). Revising the category of somatoform pain disorder. *Hospital and Community Psychiatry, 43*(3), 217–219.

Kline, M., Sydnor-Greenberg, N., Davis, W. W., Pincus, H. A., & Frances, A. J. (1993). Using field trips to evaluate proposal changes in DSM diagnostic criteria. *Hospital and Community Psychiatry, 44*(7), 621–623.

Kluft, R. P. (1991). Clinical manifestation of multiple personality disorder. *Psychiatric Clinics of North America, 14,* 605–629.

Kreidler, M. C. (1991). Breaking the incest cycle: The group as surrogate family. *Journal of Psychosocial Nursing, 29*(4), 28–32.

Kreidler, M. C. & Hassan, M. (1992). Use of an interactional model with survivors of incest. *Issues in Mental Health Nursing, 13,* 149–158.

Lichstein, K. L. (1988). *Clinical relaxation strategies.* New York: Wiley.

Lowenstein, R. J. (1991). An office mental status examination for complex chronic dissociative symptoms and multiple personality disorder. *Psychiatric Clinics of North America, 14,* 567–604.

Massion, A. O., Warshaw, M. G., & Keller, M. B. (1993). Quality of life and psychiatric morbidity in panic disorder and generalized anxiety disorder. *American Journal of Psychiatry, 150*(4), 600–607.

Mavissakalian, M. & Perel, J. M. (1992). Protective effects of imipramine maintenance treatment in panic disorders with agoraphobia. *American Journal of Psychiatry, 149*(8), 1992.

McCann, I., & Pearlman, L. (1990). *Psychological trauma and the adult survivor.* New York: Brunner/Mazel.

McKay, M., Davis, M., & Fanning, P. (1981). *Thoughts and feelings: The art of cognitive stress intervention.* Oakland, CA: New Harbinger.

Mejo, S. L. (1990). Posttraumatic stress disorder: an overview of three etiological variables, and psychopharacologic treatment. *Nurse Practitioner, 15*(8), 41–45.

North, C. S., Ryall, J. M., Ricci, D. A., & Wetzel, R. D. (1993). *Multiple personalities, multiple disorders.* NY: Oxford University Press.

Pollock, D. (1992). Structured ambiguity and the definition of psychiatric illness: Adjustment disorder among medical inpatients. *Social Science & Medicine, 35*(1), 25–35.

Popkin, M., Callies A., Colon, E., & Stiebel, V. (1990). Adjustment disorders in medically ill inpatients referred for consultation in a university hospital. *Psychosomatics, 31*(4), 410–414.

Putnam, F. W. (1989). *Diagnosis & treatment of multiple personality disorder.* New York: Guilford.

Putnam, F. W. & Loewenstein, R. J. (1993). Treatment of multiple personality disorder: a survey of current practices. *American Journal of Psychiatry, 150*(7), 1048–1052.

Saxe, G. N., van der Kolk, B. A., Berkowitz, R., Chinman, G., Hall, K., Lieberg, G., & Schwartz, J. (1993). Dissociative disorders in psychiatric inpatients. *American Journal of Psychiatry, 150*(7), 1037–1042.

Schatzberg, A. (1990). Anxiety and adjustment disorder: A treatment approach. *Journal of Clinical Psychiatry, 51:*(11 supp), 20–24.

Shear, M. K., Cooper, A. M., Klerman, G. L., Busch, F. N., & Shapiro, T. (1993). A psychodynamic model of panic disorder. *American Journal of Psychiatry, 150*(6), 859–866.

Simon, G. E., & VonKorff, M. (1991). Somatization and psychiatric disorder in the NIMH epidemiologic catchment area study. *American Journal of Psychiatry, 148*(11), 1494–1500.

Simoni, P. S. (1991). Obsessive-compulsive disorder: The effect of research on nursing care. *Journal of Psychosocial Nursing, 29*(4), 19–23.

Smith, G. (1990). *Somatization disorder in the medical setting* (DHHS Publication No. ADM 90-1631). Washington, DC: U.S. Government Printing Office.

Spratto, G. R., & Woods, A. L. (1993). *RN's nurses drug reference.* Albany, NY: Delmar.

Strain, J., Hammer, J., Huertas, D., Lam, H. T., & Fulop, G. (1993). The problem of coping as a reason for psychiatric consultation. *General Hospital Psychiatry, 15*(1), 1–8.

Turnbull, J (1989). Anxiety and physical illness in the elderly. *Journal of Clinical Psychiatry, 50*(11, suppl), 40–45.

Urbancic, J. C. (1989). Resolving incest experiences through impatient group therapy. *Journal of Psychosocial Nursing, 27*(9), 5–10.

Waddell, K. L. & Demi, A. S. (1993). Effectiveness of intensive partial hospitalization program for treatment of anxiety disorders. *Archives of Psychiatric Nursing, 12*(1), 2–10.

Watsky, E. J., & Salzman, C. (1991). Psychotropic drug interactions. *Hospital and Community Psychiatry, 42*(3), 247–256.

Whitley, G. G. (1991). Ritualistic behavior: Breaking the cycle. *Journal of Psychosocial Nursing, 29*(10), 31–35.

Winchel, R. M. & Stanley, M. (1991). Self-injurious behavior: A review of the behavior and biology of self-mutilation. American *Journal of Psychiatry, 148*(3), 306–317.

Zorumski, C. F. & Isenberg, K. (1991). Insights into the structure and function of GABA-benzodiazepine receptors: Ion channels and psychiatry. *American Journal of Psychiatry, 148*(2), 162–173.

Schizophrenia and other Psychotic Disorders

Mary Fultz Spencer

Schizophrenia

- Definition: "A mental disorder with essential features of characteristic psychotic symptoms during the active phase of the illness, functioning below highest level previously achieved, failure in social development, and a duration of at least six months" (Wilson and Kneisl, 1992).
- Signs and Symptoms [DSM-IV Draft Criteria (APA, 1993)]
  1. Two of the following present a significant portion of time over a one-month period:
     a. Delusions
     b. Hallucinations
     c. Disorganized speech—derailment or incoherence
     d. Grossly disorganized or catatonic behavior
     e. Negative symptoms—affective flattening, alogia, or avolition
  2. Only one of the above symptoms are necessary in the presence of
     a. Bizarre delusions (i.e., involving a phenomenon that the person's culture would regard as totally implausible, e.g., thought broadcasting, being controlled by a dead person)
     b. Hallucinations of a voice with content having no apparent relation to depression or elation, or a voice keeping up a running commentary on the person's behavior or thoughts, or two or more voices conversing with each other.
  3. Social/occupational dysfunction
     a. In adults—work, interpersonal relations or self-care below level achieved before onset
     b. In children or adolescents—failure to achieve expected level of interpersonal, academic, or occupational achievement
  4. Continuous signs of the disturbance for at least six months including an active phase during which there were psychotic symptoms characteristic of schizophrenia and prodromal and residual phases including the following symptoms in DSM-III-R (APA, 1987)
     a. Withdrawal or social isolation
     b. Impairment in role functioning
     c. Odd behavior (e.g., talking to self in public)

d. Little attention to personal hygiene, bathing, manner of dress, overall self-care, and activities of daily living.

e. Odd speech characterized by circumstantiality, tangentiality, poverty of speech, or poverty of content of speech

f. Magical thinking including ideas of reference

g. Recurrent illusions or other perceptual experiences

h. A decrease in motivation, energy, or initiative

- Subtypes and Features (Townsend, 1988)

1. Paranoid Schizophrenia—characterized by extreme suspiciousness of others with hallucinations and delusions of a grandiose or persecutory nature
2. Catatonic Schizophrenia—features include stupor with waxy flexibility, mutism, posturing, or catatonic excitement characterized by extreme psychomotor agitation
3. Disorganized Schizophrenia—formerly known as Hebephrenic Schizophrenia, the individual may engage in inappropriate, silly behavior or may giggle inappropriately
4. Undifferentiated Schizophrenia—behavior is grossly disorganized and speech is incoherent with flat or grossly inappropriate affect; there may be delusions or hallucinations.
5. Residual Schizophrenia—absence of hallucinations and delusions; two or more residual symptoms are continued

- Differential Diagnosis

1. Bipolar affective disorder—clients who are in the manic phase and displaying psychotic features have been misdiagnosed as having schizophrenia.
2. Mood disorder with psychotic features
3. Organic illnesses—medical work-up is important to rule this out (Malone, 1990).
4. Substance abuse
5. Other disorders

a. Delusional disorders

b. Schizophreniform disorder

c. Schizoaffective disorder

d. Brief reactive psychosis

e. Induced psychotic disorder

Schizophreniform Disorder

- Definition/Signs and Symptoms
    1. Episode of symptoms of Schizophrenia which lasts at least one month but less than six months
    2. The more rapid the onset and the shorter the illness lasts the more likely the return to premorbid level of functioning
    3. Recurrence is unlikely.
- Differential Diagnosis
    1. Schizophrenia, schizoaffective and mood disorders
    2. Medical illness or result of substance abuse or medication.

Delusional Disorder

- Definition/Signs and Symptoms
    1. Non-bizarre delusions
    2. None of the folowing for more than a few hours
        a. Hallucinations
        b. Disorganized Speech
        c. Grossly disorganized or catatonic behavior
        d. Negative symptoms
    3. Functioning not markedly impaired except for the impact of the delusions
- Types of delusions (Townsend, 1988)
    1. Persecutory—clients believe others are after them or "out to get them"; they may feel they are being followed by the CIA or that others are poisoning their food.
    2. Jealous—the belief is held that one's sexual partner is unfaithful.

3. Erotomania—delusion is present that an individual in a higher status or position is in love with them.
4. Grandiose—the clients may believe that they have special knowledge or powers; they may believe that they are Jesus Christ or the President of the United States.
5. Somatic—belief that one's appearance is abnormal or there is a physical illness present

Unlike schizophrenia, the clients do not have an inappropriate or flat affect, they are able to attend to grooming and hygiene and can care for themselves. They do not isolate themselves.

- Elderly (Wilson & Kneisl, 1992)
  1. The mood may be manifested by anger, paranoia, and anxiety.
  2. Behaviors may include suspiciousness, aggression, and isolation.

Schizoaffective Disorder

- Definition: Major depressive episode or manic episode occurs concurrently with Schizophrenia symptoms
- Depression/Signs and Symptoms
  1. Depressed mood with sad affect
  2. Anhedonia with little social participation
  3. Decrease in energy or complaints of fatigue
  4. Decrease in appetite—sometimes an increase
  5. Insomnia or hypersomnia
  6. Feelings of guilt, worthlessness, hopelessness
  7. Decreased concentration or memory
  8. Crying spells
  9. Irritability
  10. Thoughts of death or suicide
- Mania/Signs and Symptoms
  1. Mood may be expansive, elevated, or irritable.

2. Need for sleep may be decreased.
3. Pressured speech
4. Racing thoughts with flight of ideas
5. Increase in energy
6. Sexual indiscretions
7. Spending sprees

Brief Psychotic Disorder

- Definition/Signs and Symptoms
    1. One of the following is present and not culturally sanctioned:
        a. Delusions
        b. Hallucinations
        c. Disorganized speech
        d. Grossly disorganized or catatonic behavior
    2. Onset is generally sudden with duration of symptoms of one month or less, but at least one day.
    3. Individual recovers to a normal level of functioning.
- Differential Diagnosis
    1. Schizophrenia—symptoms are similar due to hallucinations and delusions, but thought disorder is not as evident (Torrey, 1988).
    2. Drug-induced psychosis

Shared Psychotic Disorder (Folie a Deux)

- Definition (APA, 1993)
    1. A delusional system develops in the context of a close relationship with a person who already has a psychotic disorder with delusions.
    2. The delusion is similar in content to that of the person who already has the established delusion.
    3. The second person to develop delusions receives this diagnosis.
- Differential Diagnosis

1. Schizophrenia or another psychotic disorder
2. Substance abuse or a general medical illness

Psychotic Disorder (Secondary to General Medical Condition)

- Definition (APA, 1993): Delusions or hallucinations which
  1. Do not occur during the course of Delirium or Dementia
  2. Are not better accounted for by another mental disorder
  3. Are related to a medical condition as determined by
     a. History
     b. Physical Examination
     c. Laboratory Findings

Substance-Induced Psychotic Disorder

- Definition (APA, 1993): Delusions or hallucinations (these are not included if the client has insight that they are substance induced) which
  1. Develop during or within a month of significant substance intoxication
  2. Are in excess of what would be expected for the amount and type of substance abused
  3. Does not occur during the course of Delirium or Dementia
  4. Are not better accounted for by another psychotic disorder

Psychotic Disorder Not Otherwise Specified (APA, 1993)

- Postpartum psychosis which does not meet other DSM criteria
- Persistant auditory hallucinations in the absence of other features
- Psychosis where a more specific diagnosis is impossible;
- Mental Status Variations for Schizophrenia and Other Psychotic Disorders
  1. Appearance—often unkempt with clothing mismatched or in disarray; bathing, toileting, grooming, and dressing may be neglected.
  2. Speech—often disorganized, difficult to comprehend, or incoherent; Chesla in Wilson and Kneisl (1992, p.270) notes that there may be

poverty of speech or poverty of content of speech; may have concrete thinking or have difficulty with abstract concepts. For example, if the nurse were to ask the client, "What brings you to the hospital," he/she may reply, "an ambulance." Speech may also be rapid or pressured.

3. Motor activity—rocking movements or behaviors may be noted; important to distinguish rocking or restless motor movements from what may be extra-pyramidal symptoms of medications. Torrey (1988) notes that the individual may have increased or decreased blinking.
4. Mood—emotional ambivalence with difficulty with decision-making can occur; anxiety, aggression, or the tendency to withdraw; depressed or manic Schizoaffective Disorder.
5. Affect—flat or blunted in some cases; responses may be inappropriate or laughter may occur when a serious topic is discussed.
6. Thought content—delusions, hallucinations, neologisms, ideas of reference, paranoia, thought insertion, or thought broadcasting; assessing for suicidal and homicidal ideation is imperative. When assessing hallucinations, note if they are commanding the individual to harm others or inflict self-harm.
7. Thought processes—flight-of-ideas, looseness of associations, word salad, echolalia, or echopraxia; they may be disorganized with tangentiality or circumstantiality.
8. Judgment and insight—vary; some clients may not understand the need for medication or understand the illness.
9. Orientation/memory—varies with the disease process

- Nursing Diagnoses (See Table 1)
- Genetic/Biological Theories

1. Genetic theories of Schizophrenia (Torrey, 1988)
   a. Offspring of nonschizophrenic parents have a 1% chance of developing the disease.
   b. Offspring of one schizophrenic parent have a 13% chance.
   c. Offspring of two schizophrenic parents have a 46% chance.
   d. A twin of a dizygotic (non-identical) twin with schizophrenia has a 10%–15% chance of having schizophrenia.

Table 1

Possible Nursing Diagnosis for Clients with Schizophrenia and Other Psychotic Disorders

	Schizophrenia	*Delusional Disorder*	*Schizoaffective Disorder*	*Brief Psychotic Disorder*
Anxiety	X	X	X	X
Alteration in Nutrition	X		X	
Altered Thought Process	X	X	X	X
Diversional Activity Deficit	X		X	
Impaired Social Interaction	X			X
Impaired Verbal Communication	X	X		X
Post Trauma Response				X
Potential for Violence: Self-Directed or Directed at Others	X	X	X	
Self-Care Deficit	X	X	X	
Self-Esteem Disturbance	X		X	
Sensory Perceptual Alteration Auditory/Visual	X		X	X
Sleep Pattern Disturbance	X	X	X	X
Social Isolation	X	X	X	X

e. A twin of a monozygotic (identical) twin with schizophrenia has a 35%-50% chance of having schizophrenia.

f. Genetic inheritance is not the only cause since twins have identical genes.

g. A predisposition of some individuals to develop schizophrenia due to environmental influence may be inherited.

2. Biological origins

a. Dopamine Hypothesis—some cases of schizophrenia may be due to an excess of dopamine in key areas of the brain (Stuart and Sundeen, 1991); Dopaminergic agents (L-dopa and amphetamines) exacerbate psychotic behavior; Torrey (1988) cites the possibility of an excessive number of dopamine receptors found in the limbic system and basal ganglia.

b. Platelet Monoamine Oxidase (MAO) Theory—hypothesis is that individuals with schizophrenia have lower levels of MAO in the bloodstream; a decrease in levels of MAO would lead to increased levels of dopamine (Stuart and Sundeen, 1987).

c. Indolamine Hypothesis—possible defect in the metabolism of indolamine serotonin results in the production of hallucinogenic substances.

d. Brain Disease Hypothesis—CT scans indicate enlargement of lateral ventricles or third ventricles in the brain of some patients. Other abnormalities sometimes noted as atrophy of a portion of the cerebellum, abnormalities in brain density and brain asymmetry. Some MRI studies show a thickening of the corpus callosum. Schizophrenia may consist of several different diseases and the limbic system is the sight of pathology for some cases (Torrey, 1988).

e. Theory of two types of schizophrenia (Wilson and Kneisl, 1992).

(1) Type I—characterized by positive symptoms of schizophrenia: delusions, hallucinations, disorganized thinking. May be associated with increased dopamine receptors. Responds well to psychotropic medications.

(2) Type II—characterized by negative symptoms including withdrawal, flattening of affect, decreased motivation; does not respond as well to psychotropic medications.

f. Brief Psychotic Disorder—could possibly be due to a brief viral infection of the brain such as encephalitis (Torrey, 1988).

- Biochemical Interventions

1. Antipsychotic medications block dopamine receptors.
2. Used short term in Schizophreniform Disorder
3. Clients with Brief Psychotic Disorder usually recover whether or not they are treated with medication (Torrey, 1988)
4. Medications (See Table 2)
5. Dosages may vary widely among clients.
6. Fluphenazine (Prolixin) and haloperidol (Haldol) are available in intramuscular, injectable forms that are long-acting and released over two to three weeks (Wilson and Kneisl, 1992).

a. Reduces the need to take a pill each day.

b. Helps reduce ambivalence

Table 2

Medications

Classification	*Generic (Trade name)*	*Dosage Range*
Phenothiazines	Chlorpromazine (Thorazine)	100–1400mg
	Thioridazine (Mellaril)	200–800mg
	Mesoridazine (Serentil)	100–500mg
	Prochlorperazine (Compazine)	15–150mg
	Perphenazine (Trilafon)	8–64mg
	Trifluoperazine (Stelazine)	2–80mg
	Fluphenazine (Prolixin)	5–40mg
Thioxanthenes	Thiothixene (Navane)	6–60mg
Butyrophenones	Haloperidol (Haldol)	4–100mg
Dibenzoxazepines	Loxapine (Loxitane)	50–250mg
Dihydroindolones	Molindone (Moban)	20–225mg

7. Potential side effects of Antipsychotics

   a. Anticholinergic effects include constipation, dry mouth, blurred vision, urinary retention and hesitancy; Bethanechol is sometimes given for urinary retention; occurs due to the interference of nerve impulses by acetylcholine and epinephrine (Wilson and Kneisl, 1992).

   b. Extrapyramidal symptoms due to the medication's effects on the extrapyramidal tracts of the central nervous system. Symptoms include:

      (1) Pseudoparkinsonism—drooling, shuffling gait, rigidity, tremor, mask-like facies, pillrolling of the fingers and cogwheel rigidity; responds to anti-Parkinsonian medications.

(2) Akathisia—characterized by restlessness, pacing, the need to pace, or shifting from one foot to another; responds well to oral anti-Parkinsonian medications; ceases with discontinuation of the neuroleptic; generally occurs after weeks or months of treatment. Need to distinguish this from anxiety or agitation; i.e., if neuroleptic is increased, akathisia becomes worse.

(3) Dystonic reactions—involuntary muscular movements of neck, arms, legs, and face; includes torticollis and oculogyric crisis (rolling back of the eyes). Reversible with one of the antiparkinsonian agents; occurs early in treatment, sometimes after first dose; can be very frightening and painful for the client with sudden onset.

(4) Tardive Dyskinesia—characterized by difficulty swallowing, lip smacking, tongue protrusion, puckering, blinking, choreiform movements of the limbs and trunk; generally irreversible; usually occurs after a maintenance dose is discontinued or reduced; can try discontinuing medication and restarting another; all patients on long-term therapy are at risk.

c. Other Symptoms—include sedation, orthostatic hypotension, photosensitivity, decreased libido, weight gain, reduction of seizure threshold, amenorrhea; cholestatic jaundice is an allergic response to chlorpromazine; usually self-limiting. Agranulocytosis can also occur and may be noted when the patient gets an infection; it is a medical emergency.

d. Neuroleptic Malignant Syndrome—a medical emergency the symptoms of which include high fever, autonomic instability, tachycardia, increased pulse and respirations, muscle rigidity, elevated CPK, sweating, and hyperkalemia. It is believed to be caused by dopamine blockage in the hypothalamus (Wilson and Kneisel, 1992). This requires discontinuation of all drugs and maintenance of nutrition and hydration; ventilation may be required for respiratory failure as well as renal dialysis for renal failure. Bromocriptine or dantroline is sometimes given to decrease muscle contracting; it can occur at any time. Neuroleptics can be restarted with caution.

8. Clozaril (Clozapine)—one of the newest antipsychotic medications that has been proven beneficial in clients with schizophrenia who have had unsuccessful trials on other antipsychotics (Sandoz Pharmaceuticals, 1992)
   a. Causes fewer of the side effects common to other neuroleptics, such as restlessness and tremors
   b. Tardive dyskinesia does not occur.
   c. Effective in both ''positive'' and ''negative'' symptoms of schizophrenia
   d. Side effects—drowsiness, low blood pressure, headaches, irregular heartbeat, dizziness, fatigue, nausea and vomiting, constipation
   e. Caution—one or two people out of every 100 who are prescribed Clozaril will develop agranulocytosis; symptoms include any signs of infection including sore throat, flu-like symptoms, and fever; complete blood counts are assessed before the therapy and drawn weekly for the duration; if agranulocytosis occurs, the drug is not restarted.
9. Medications used to treat extrapyramidal symptoms:

   Trihexyphenidyl (Artane) 1–10mg/day

   Benzotrophine (Cogentin) .5–6mg/day

   Diphenhydramine (Benedryl) 50–200mg/day

   Amantadine (Symmetrel) 100–300mg/day

   Biperiden HCL (Akineton) 6–8mg/day

   (Sometimes are given prophylactically if likelihood of EPS is high, but not always.)
10. Medications used for Schizoaffective Disorder—in addition to neuroleptics, antidepressants, Lithium or Tegretol may be utilized, depending on the mood disorder.

- Intrapersonal Origins
  1. Chesla in Wilson and Kneisl (1992) outlines the interactional model for schizophrenia which delineates that biologic vulnerability along with environmental factors, social skills, and support of the individual are factors in the development of the illness.

2. Brief Psychotic Disorder generally appears after a significant psychosocial stressor, i.e.:
    a. Loss of a significant other
    b. Psychological trauma of combat
    c. Concentration camp victims
    d. Sensory deprivation situations (Torrey, 1988)

- Psychotherapeutic Intervention
    1. Communication—the client may communicate in symbols; listen actively for the theme.
    2. Hallucinations
        a. Observe for the client attending to internal stimuli.
        b. Note if the client talks or smiles to himself/herself.
        c. Encourage involvement in real conversations and/or structured activities.
        d. Administer medication as ordered and note response.
        e. Assess for the content of the hallucination; if the patient is having command hallucinations to harm self or others, provide for safety.
        f. Utilize judgment when providing for increased levels of observation as a client with command hallucinations may not be able to contract for safety.
        g. Chesla in Wilson and Kneisl (1992) notes that different disease processes are associated with various types of hallucinations.
            (1) Auditory and somatic hallucinations are associated with schizophrenia.
            (2) Olfactory and gustatory hallucinations are associated with seizure disorders.
            (3) Visual hallucinations may be noted with acute organic brain syndrome.
            (4) Tactile hallucinations are associated with acute alcohol withdrawal.

3. Delusions—delusional individuals may have delusions of grandeur, paranoia, or poverty. They may think they are a public figure or may believe they are being followed by the CIA.
   a. Do not argue with the client or deny the belief. This does not eliminate the delusion nor is trust gained by this approach.
   b. Focus on reality and talk about reality-oriented issues.
   c. Accept the client's need for the belief without actually reinforcing the belief.
   d. For the paranoid individual, it is helpful to assign the same staff member in a consistent way to build trust.
   e. If the client feels the food is poisoned, serve it in sealed containers.
   f. Administer medications and note response.
4. Withdrawn behavior
   a. Assist with food and fluid intake as well as hygiene.
   b. Townsend (1988) notes that an accepting attitude and "unconditional positive regard" (p.98) may decrease the sense of isolation.
   c. Gradually introduce the client into activities.
   d. Give positive reinforcement for participating.
   e. Allow time for being alone as well as provide structure.
5. Aggressive behavior
   a. Aggression against the self may be in the form of suicide or self-mutilation, particularly if there are command hallucinations present.
   b. Aggression towards others is also a possibility.
   c. Assess characteristics such as increased pacing, clenched fists, tense expression, irritability, agitation, threatening verbalizations (Townsend, 1988).
   d. Early intervention is important, keeping in mind the use of the least restrictive measures.
      (1) Decrease stimulation in the environment.
      (2) Administer prn medications and note response.

(3) Provide for a safe environment by removing dangerous objects.

(4) Encourage the client to spend quiet time in his/her room or in the quiet room.

(5) When approaching the client, do so from the side and not in a direct manner.

(6) A show of force may be necessary and is sometimes sufficient in redirecting the client and de-escalating a situation (Townsend, 1988).

(7) If redirection and medication as well as a decrease in stimulation are not effective, the client is at risk for hurting self or others; seclusion and restraint may be needed; these are not used as punishment. According to Fisher (Wilson and Kneisl, 1992), protocol includes:

   (a) Positioning the client to prevent aspiration.

   (b) Glasses, jewelry, shoes, or belts are removed to prevent injury to the self.

   (c) Constant observation is recommended due to the possibility of laryngeal spasms from neuroleptic medications.

   (d) Range-of-motion to the extremities should be performed every two hours and pulses, color, and temperature are to be assessed and documented. Blood clots and emboli may form if this is not done.

   (e) Nursing care includes hydration, nutrition, and elimination needs.

   (f) Documentation of the need for seclusion and/or restraint should be done by an RN. A flowsheet should be available to document the nursing care given as well as client response.

   (g) Assessment is ongoing and the patient may gradually be moved from 5-point restraints to 3-point and 2-point restraints; a client should *never* be left in only one restraint.

(h) The client is released from seclusion when behavior is under control and he/she is not in danger of hurting self or others.

6. In addition to interventions previously noted that are applicable to schizophrenia, the following may be utilized in Schizoaffective Disorder (Townsend, 1988)
   a. Potential for harm to self
      (1) Inquire about suicidal thoughts.
      (2) Create a safe environment by removing sharps and other harmful objects.
      (3) Encourage patient to contract for safety, noting that if command hallucinations are present, contracting may not be feasible.
   b. Social isolation
      (1) Spend time with patient.
      (2) Make brief, frequent contacts.
      (3) Gradually encourage participation in activities.
      (4) Encourage structure in the day.
   c. Alteration in nutrition
      (1) Encourage balanced diet with high fiber.
      (2) Intake, output, and caloric count when needed.
      (3) Daily weights.
      (4) Small, frequent meals may be better tolerated.
   d. Potential for injury
      (1) Decrease stimulation in the environment.
      (2) Encourage quiet time in room.
      (3) Promote safe environment—remove sharps, potentially harmful items.

- Family Dynamics/Family Therapy
  1. There is no proof that schizophrenia is caused byfamily interaction patterns. It is important that the family is involved in the care of the individual. The family is an integral part of the treatment plan and

has the best knowledge of the individual's illness and ability to function.

2. The illness affects the entire family system including careers, finances, schedules, and social life. Problems which recur most frequently are
   a. Failure to care for personal needs/hygiene
   b. Difficulty handling finances
   c. Withdrawal
   d. Odd personal habits
   e. Suicide threats
   f. Fears for the safety of client and family (Torrey, 1988)
3. Eliminating blame is important if family members blame each other; acceptance of the illness is the first step toward management of the illness; expectations for the client should be realistic (Torrey, 1988).
4. Anger may have to be addressed in family therapy.
5. Other questions to consider include
   a. The devotion of time to other family members
   b. Respite for the caregiver
   c. Home care versus a boarding home or halfway house
6. Family members require education and instruction; the discharged client may require reintegration within the family and role shifting may occur. The nurse should assess family attitudes toward the patient, the overall atmosphere in the family, and available emotional/social supports (Stuart and Sundeen, 1987)
7. Structure in the individual's day and a routine can provide some predictability. The family can provide responsibilities, simple chores and the like to enhance a sense of routine and accomplishment (Torrey, 1988; and Stuart and Sundeen, 1987).
8. Family members can be taught to recognize symptoms that may require a medication adjustment or hospitalization (Mason, 1988).

9. The family should encourage following the prescribed medication regimen, vocational rehabilitation (Mason, 1988).
10. Self-help groups such as the National Alliance for the Mentally Ill (NAMI), as well as Friends and Families of the Mentally Ill, can be beneficial.

- Group Approaches/Therapy and Self-help
  1. Traditional group therapy, insight-oriented groups or groups that are primarily interactional in nature are generally not helpful, since the individual has difficulty filtering stimuli (Torrey, 1988).
  2. Self-help groups may be more beneficial and focus on educational issues, support, and destigmatization of mental illness.
  3. Social skills training can occur in groups and would include introducing oneself, starting a conversation, and listening skills. Staff act as role models for the implementation of these skills (Chesla, 1992).
- Milieu Interventions
  1. A structured hospital environment provides therapeutic benefits for the individual (Garritson, 1992).
  2. Regular daily activities can provide a sense of predictability as well as a sense of accomplishment and reward.
  3. Treatment environment should emphasize involvement, organization and standards of safety; there should be established norms and rules (Stuart and Sundeen, 1987).
  4. Clients may feel safer if time is allowed for periods in their room.
  5. If the client feels threatened by milieu activities, encourage involvement with one other patient only (Chesla, 1992).
- Community Resources
  1. The Alliance for the Mentally Ill provides the family with support groups and educational programs.
  2. The local community mental health center is also a valuable resource; often, the client is followed on an outpatient basis through the mental health center and receives medication through this setting.
  3. Day treatment programs may be available.

4. Possibilities for placement include halfway houses or boarding homes depending on the client's abilities and skills.
5. Supplementary security income can provide a small, fixed income and may pay residential costs in a boarding home.

Questions
Select the best answer

1. Mr. Jones is a patient diagnosed with schizophrenia who is hospitalized on a psychiatric unit. You notice him standing motionless on one leg in the day area. This could most likely be an example of:

   a. Attention-seeking behavior
   b. Catatonic posturing
   c. A side-effect to neuroleptic medication.
   d. Catatonic stupor

2. During the initial assessment, the nurse inquires of Mr. Jones, "What brought you to the hospital?" Mr. Jones replies, "An ambulance." This is an example of:

   a. Deductive reasoning
   b. Abstract thinking
   c. Concrete thinking
   d. Poverty of content of speech

3. Mr. Jones is informed during his hospital stay that his brother has been diagnosed with cancer and will be undergoing surgery. Mr. Jones laughs upon hearing the news. Your understanding of this is:

   a. Mr. Jones is obviously not close to his brother.
   b. Mr. Jones possibly has a mood disorder.
   c. Mr. Jones is obviously anxious and upset by this news.
   d. Mr. Jones is displaying incongruence between the content of the communication and his emotions.

4. Mr. Jones comments that he hears voices of men telling him "bad things about myself. They say I should hurt myself." Your most appropriate initial response would be to:

   a. Reassure Mr. Jones of his safety and security by telling him the voices aren't real
   b. Provide for Mr. Jones' comfort and security by reminding him that he has never hurt himself in the past
   c. Assess the command hallucinations for potential destructiveness by asking specifically for the content.
   d. Tell him to ignore the voices and administer prn medications

5. You are working in the emergency room at the hospital when Mr. Brown comes in displaying hallucinations, delusions, and aggressive behavior. Possible Axis I diagnoses include:

   a. Bipolar Affective Disorder
   b. Schizoaffective Disorder
   c. Intermittant Explosive Disorder
   d. All of the above

6. The patient remarks repeatedly that he believes he is Jesus Christ and that he has come to save the world. This can best be described as:

   a. The defense of identification
   b. A delusion of grandeur
   c. An illusion
   d. An idea of reference

7. Mr. Brown continues to remark that the CIA is following him and that they are waiting outside the door to the emergency room. Your best response would be:

   a. "Mr. Brown, the CIA is not following you."
   b. "We've told the CIA to leave you alone."
   c. "I understand you feel that they are outside, but the CIA is not there and you're safe here."
   d. "Why do you think the CIA is out there?"

8. You notice during the assessment period that Mr. Brown is rocking back and forth on his feet and he appears to be restless. This could be an indication of:

   a. Extreme anxiety
   b. Extrapyramidal symptoms of medication
   c. Catatonic rigidity
   d. a & b

9. Ms. Smith recently admitted to an inpatient psychiatric facility. During the assessment she seems to be mimicking your body movements. This is an example of:

   a. Echopraxia
   b. Echolalia
   c. Mirroring the therapist
   d. Akathisia

10. Several hours after being admitted, Ms. Smith complained of feeling bugs crawling on her skin. This could be indicative of:

    a. Alcohol withdrawal
    b. A hallucination that is common among patients with schizophrenia.
    c. A side-effect to neuroleptic medications
    d. A seizure disorder

11. Ms. Smith displays paranoid behavior on the unit and becomes particularly suspicious. She comments that she suspects the food is being poisoned. A possible intervention would be to:

    a. Serve the food in sealed containers
    b. Serve small, frequent feeding
    c. Have Ms. Smith eat away from the other patients
    d. Have Ms. Smith prepare her own meals

12. Mr. Brown has been treated for the past several years with Prolixin. You notice that he is drooling, has a tremor, and there is a slight pillrolling of the fingers. This is the extrapyramidal symptom known as:

    a. Anticholinergic side effects
    b. Pseudoparkinsonism
    c. Tardive dyskinesia
    d. A dystonic reaction

13. Several days into the hospitalization, Mr. Brown complains of urinary retention, an anticholinergic side effect. Which of the following medications would be best to ease the urinary retention?

    a. Cogentin
    b. Artane
    c. Lasix
    d. Bethanechol

14. Mr. Brown has been on Cogentin along with the Haldol. You notice that in addition to the urinary retention, his face is flushed, and he has become disoriented. This is an example of:

    a. An exacerbation of the psychosis
    b. Anticholinergic side effect
    c. Early-onset dementia
    d. Brief reactive psychosis

15. Mr. Johnson is being treated with Haldol. He develops a fever of 102°, muscular rigidity, altered mental status, and diaphoresis. It is determined that he is suffering from neuroleptic malignant syndrome. Which laboratory findings are most likely to occur?

    a. An elevated Haldol level
    b. A decrease in the CPK level
    c. An increase in the CPK level
    d. A decrease in the white cell count

16. Possible complications from Neuroleptic malignant syndrome include the following:

    a. Marked dehydration, renal failure, and acute respiratory failure
    b. Liver failure
    c. Increased intracranial pressure
    d. Agranulocytosis

17. Nursing care for the client with NMS will include:

    a. The discontinuation of the Neuroleptic, maintenance of skin integrity and hydration, and the administration of Bromocriptine
    b. The gradual tapering of the Neuroleptic, the administration of Cogentin, and the maintenance of skin integrity and hydration
    c. The gradual tapering of the Neuroleptic, administration of Bromocriptine, and the maintenance of skin integrity and hydration
    d. The discontinuation of the Neuroleptic, maintenance of skin integrity and hydration, and the administration of Cogentin

18. Which of the following statements best describes characteristics about the onset and development of NMS?

    a. It is noted most commonly in male clients taking Haldol, so they are most at risk.
    b. The initial onset is insidious and is therefore difficult to detect.
    c. It develops only after months to years of treatment with Neuroleptic medications.
    d. The onset may be sudden and can occur after the first dose of the medication.

19. Which of the following is most likely true with regards to follow-up care for the individual who has experienced NMS?

a. Maintenance ECT may be used in lieu of medication to manage psychosis.
b. Neuroleptic medications are contraindicated.
c. Injectable forms of neuroleptics are contraindicated.
d. Neuroleptic medications may be restarted with caution.

20. Which best describes the action of antipsychotic medications?

a. They block dopamine receptors.
b. They decrease available amounts of serotonin and norepinephrine.
c. They enhance the availability of dopamine.
d. They block the re-uptake of dopamine to increase availability at receptor sites.

21. As a nurse employed at the community mental health center, you are a case manager for several clients taking Clozapine. The advantages of taking Clozapine include:

a. Follow-up is less frequent since tardive dyskinesia does not occur.
b. It is less likely to cause orthostasis.
c. Restlessness and tremors are less likely to occur.
d. It is more potent than phenothiazines.

22. Medication teaching about Clozaril *should include* which of the following:

a. Cautioning the client to report any signs of infection including sore throat, flu-like symptoms and fever
b. The importance of being compliant with having a complete blood count drawn at least monthly
c. Notifying the physician *immediately* about lip-smacking or vermiform movements of the tongue
d. Notifying the physician immediately at the onset of diarrhea and hand tremors

23. You are caring for a client who suffers from epilepsy and has been diagnosed recently as having schizophrenia. Teaching should include which of the following:

a. Antipsychotic medications should be used cautiously as they increase the seizure threshold.
b. Antipsychotic medications should be used cautiously as they decrease the seizure threshold.
c. Antipsychotic medications do not affect the seizure threshold.

d. Antipsychotic medications are contraindicated.

24. The following is indicative of a dystonic reaction:
    a. Oculogyric crisis and spasms of the back muscles
    b. Cogwheel rigidity and lip-smacking movements
    c. Shuffling gait and mask-like facies
    d. Urinary retention and leg stiffness

25. Nursing actions during a dystonic reaction may include:
    a. Turning the patient on his side
    b. Notifying the physician, administration of Cogentin and making sure respiratory support equipment is available
    c. Administration of IM physostigmine and bethanechol
    d. Decreasing stimulation in the environment as dystonia and agitation may appear similar

26. Which of the following statements about tardive dyskinesia is *most* accurate?
    a. Symptoms are generally reversible, particularly in the younger patient population.
    b. Symptoms may appear 1–10 days following administration of neuroleptic medication.
    c. It occurs most often in dehydrated patients.
    d. All patients on long-term neuroleptic therapy are at risk.

27. Your patient on neuroleptic medication complains of dizziness. Your *initial* intervention would be:
    a. Taking the patient's blood pressure sitting and standing
    b. Forcing fluids
    c. Prompt discontinuation of the medication and notifying the physician
    d. Instructing the patient to place his/her head between the knees

28. You are working with Mr. Green who has recently been prescribed Thorazine. He comes to the nurses stations and complains of blurred vision and constipation. Your most appropriate response would be:
    a. "I'll notify the physician right away as your dose is probably too high."
    b. "Those are possibly side effects of the medication and tolerance usually develops in several weeks. We can order a bulk diet for you."
    c. "I'll notify the physician right away and see if we can try a different medication."

d. Administer an anticholinergic medication.

29. A common hypothesis regarding the biological origin of schizophrenia is:

 a. The dopamine hypothesis which postulates that some cases of schizophrenia may be due to an excess of dopamine in the brain and/or an excessive number of dopamine receptors
 b. The disease is caused by enlarged lateral ventricles in the brain.
 c. The norepinephrine hypothesis which states that schizophrenia is due to an excess of this neurotransmitter which causes hallucinations
 d. All cases of schizophrenia are caused by viruses contracted in utero.

30. The most current family theory states:

 a. Research has indicated that schizophrenia is a direct result of dysfunctional family interaction.
 b. The individual with schizophrenia withdraws and hallucinates as a defense against a hostile family environment.
 c. There is no proof that schizophrenia is caused by family interaction patterns.
 d. An individual with schizophrenia is most likely to be the product of a cold, aloof mother and an absent, distant father.

31. Genetic studies of schizophrenia have indicated the following:

 a. A twin of a dizygotic twin with schizophrenia is just as likely as a monozygotic twin to have schizophrenia.
 b. A twin of a monozygotic (identical) twin with schizophrenia has a 75% chance or greater of having schizophrenia.
 c. A twin of a monozygotic (identical) twin with schizophrenia has a 35%–50% chance of having schizophrenia.
 d. Genetic inheritance is most likely the only cause of schizophrenia since family interactional patterns cannot be empirically studied.

32. Mr. Jones reports that he is hearing voices telling him to cut his wrists and he is highly agitated with complaints of fear and anxiety. The *most appropriate* intervention would be to:

 a. Administer medication and encourage Mr. Jones to contract for safety and to notify the nursing staff should the voices increase.
 b. Administer prn medication and encourage Mr. Jones to spend time in his room after checking for sharp objects and ensuring the environment is safe.

c. Administer prn medication, remove dangerous objects from the patient's environment, and place him on constant observation.
d. Administer prn medication and place him in closed door seclusion with safety checks every 15 minutes.

33. Ms.Williams who was admitted to the unit yesterday is withdrawn and keeps to herself on the unit. An appropriate intervention would be:

a. Encouraging Ms. Williams to attend all activities as prescribed in order to integrate into the milieu and feel a part of the group
b. Encouraging Ms. Williams to spend all day and early evening on the unit and locking the door to her room
c. Encouraging Ms. Williams to attend activities gradually with a supportive staff member
d. Electing Ms. Williams as the patient representative to increase her sense of confidence

34. Ms. Williams has not been eating and has difficulty bringing food to her mouth. The most appropriate intervention would be:

a. Place the spoon in the patient's hand, scoop food into it and say, "Eat a bite of this roast beef."
b. Place the patient on a liquid supplement only as this may be more easily tolerated.
c. Spoon feed the patient.
d. Allow the patient to eat in her room as she will be more comfortable away from the other patients.

35. Ms. Williams has difficulty trusting the staff members on the unit. Which of the following interventions is most likely to promote trust?

a. Using therapeutic touch in order to convey caring and concern for Ms. Williams
b. Encouraging the patient to engage in a one-to-one session for an hour on both morning and evening shifts
c. Assigning the same staff to work with Ms. Williams as often as possible
d. Encouraging Ms. Williams to play a game of cards with the other patients

36. Mr. Parker has been diagnosed with Paranoid Schizophrenia. You notice that he has been pacing, has a tense facial expression, and his fists are clenched. He tells you he is upset because he feels the other patients are after him. The most appropriate nursing intervention would be:

a. Convey your understanding of the need for the belief, but explain that the other patients do not wish to harm him.
b. Decrease stimulation in the environment.
c. Administer prn medication.
d. All of the above

37. Mr. Parker has escalated to the point where he is threatening others and he is having difficulty staying in his room. The decision is made to assist Mr. Parker by having him spend some time in the quiet room. Which of the following interventions will *most likely* promote safety?

a. Approach Mr. Parker with several other staff members in a quiet manner and escort him to the quiet room.
b. Approach Mr. Parker alone as he may feel more threatened with more than one staff member.
c. Place Mr. Parker in 4-point restraints and check on him every 15 minutes.
d. Force medicate him according to hospital policy.

38. Mr. Parker begins banging his head against the wall. It becomes necessary to place Mr. Parker in mechanical restraints in order that he not hurt himself. Nursing care should include the following:

a. Checking on Mr. Parker at least once an hour
b. Performing range-of-motion exercises every 2 hours and assessing circulation to the extremities
c. Removing all restraints if Mr. Parker becomes less agitated within 10 minutes
d. Gradually removing restraints until Mr. Parker has only one restraint remaining

39. The individual with schizophrenia may benefit from a group-oriented approach. Which of the following groups would be *most* appropriate?

a. A didactic as well as supportive group that provides social skills training
b. Insight-oriented
c. Cognitive-behavioral in order to assist with difficulties with self-care
d. Any of the above, depending on the individual patient

40. Mr. Williams who has been hospitalized for over a month due to exacerbation of schizophrenia will soon be discharged to his home where he will live with his parents and one younger brother. Which of the following recommendations will be most helpful to the family.

a. Provide Mr. Williams with a structured routine, including chores and other responsibilities.
b. Do not encourage spending time alone as this will increase a sense of isolation from the family.
c. Encourage Mr. Williams to take complete responsibility for medications and follow-up appointments.
d. Set goals for Mr. Williams as he may have difficulty doing this for himself.

Answers

1. b
2. c
3. d
4. c
5. d
6. b
7. c
8. d
9. a
10. a
11. a
12. b
13. d
14. b
15. c
16. a
17. a
18. d
19. d
20. a
21. c
22. a
23. b
24. a
25. b
26. d
27. a
28. b
29. a
30. c
31. c
32. c
33. c
34. a
35. c
36. d
37. a
38. b
39. a
40. a

Bibilography

American Psychiatric Association (1987). *Diagnostic and statistical manual of mental disorders* (3rd ed.), Washington, DC: APA.

Chesla, C. (1992). Applying the nursing process for clients with schizophrenia and other psychotic disorders. In H. S. Wilson & C. R. Kneisl (Eds.), *Psychiatric nursing* (pp. 258–284). Reading, MA: Addison-Wesley.

Garritson, S. H. (1992). Milieu therapy. In H. S. Wilson & C. R. Kneisl (Ed.), *Psychiatric nursing* (pp. 742–764). Reading, MA: Addison-Wesley.

Malone, J. A. (1990). Schizophrenia research update: Implications for Nursing. *Journal of Psychosocial Nursing. 28*(8), 4–9.

Papolos, D., & Papolos, J. (1992). *Overcoming depression.* New York: Harper Perennial.

Sandoz Pharmaceuticals (1992). *Understanding Clozaril® (Clozapine) therapy: A guide for patients and their families.* Sandoz Pharmaceuticals.

Stuart, G. W., & Sundeen, S. J. (1987). *Principles and practice of psychiatric nursing.* St. Louis: C. V. Mosby.

Stuart, G. W., & Sundeen, S. J. (1988). *Pocket guide to psychiatric nursing.* St. Louis: C. V. Mosby.

Torrey, E. F. (1988). *Surviving schizophrenia: A family manual.* New York: Harper & Row.

Townsend, M. C. (1988). *Nursing diagnoses in psychiatric nursing: A pocket guide for care plan construction.* Philadelphia: F. A. Davis.

Mood Disorders

Judith Haber

- Definition

    1. Mood disorders are characterized by a disturbance of mood (a prolonged emotion that colors the whole psychic life)

        a. Generally involves single or recurring depressive (unipolar) and/or manic (bipolar) episodes

        b. Also occurs as part of other non-mood conditions (eating, panic, obsessive-compulsive disorders)

        c. Occurs in drug or alcohol intoxication or withdrawal

        d. Occurs as consequences of non psychiatric medical conditions (cerebrovascular accident (CVA), dementia, diabetes, cancer, acquired immunodeficiency syndrome (AIDS), chronic fatigue syndrome (CFS), fibromyalgia, multiple sclerosis (MS) or as consequences of the use of selected prescription medications (See Table 1.)

Table 1

Medications Associated with Depression

Cardiovascular Drugs	*Hormones*
Alpha-Methyldopa	Oral Contraceptives
Reserpine	ACTH (corticotropin and glucocorticoids)
Propanolol	Anabolic steroids
Guanethidine	
Clonidine	*Psychotropics*
Thiazide diuretics	Benzodiazepines
Digitalis	Neuroleptics
Anticancer Agents	*Others*
Cycloserine	Cocaine (withdrawal)
	Amphetamines (withdrawal)
Anti-Inflammatory/Anti-Infective Agents	L-dopa
Non-steroidal anti-inflammatory agents	Cimetidine
Ethambutol	Rantidine
Sulfonamides	
Baclofen	
Metoclopramide	

- Prevalence

    1. Mood disorders 8–9% in general population; 24% in lst degree relatives; 10–15 million American people experience mood disorders at any given time.

2. First-degree relatives of persons with mood disorders have a higher rate of depression and mania than occurs in the general population.
3. Unipolar disorder (major depression) 7% in general population; first-degree relatives 18%; mean age of onset 20s to 30s
4. Bipolar disorder (manic-depressive illness) lifetime prevalence is 1–2%; 8% in first-degree relatives; represents 25–35% of mood disorders; mean age of onset is early 20s.
5. Recurrence rate—over 50% for unipolar and bipolar illness.
6. Suicide rate—1% in general population; people with a history of affective disorder—18%
7. Fifty percent of the annual suicides are associated with depression.
8. Fifteen percent of people with Bipolar I Disorder (BPI) untreated commit suicide.
9. Suicide occurs more frequently > 60; at risk are white single males.
10. Suicide rate is increasing in < 24 age cohort.

- Sex distribution
  1. Unipolar disorder females 2:1
  2. Bipolar disorder—equal male-female distribution; females have a higher depression to mania ratio.

Depressive Disorders

Major Depression (Unipolar, Endogenous)

- Definition: Depressed mood or loss of interest or pleasure in all or almost all activities, and associated symptoms for a period of at least 2 weeks, persisting and representing a change from previous functioning; can be mild, moderate or severe.
- Signs and Symptoms: Presence of at least 5 of the following (1–10) including presence of (1) or (2) (APA, 1993):
  1. Depressed mood most of day, nearly every day
  2. Diminished interest or pleasure in all, or almost all, activities

3. Significant weight loss or gain when not dieting (>5% of body weight in a month)
4. Insomnia or hypersomnia
    a. Initial insomnia/difficulty falling asleep (DFA)
    b. Middle insomnia (waking up during sleep and difficulty falling back to sleep)
    c. Terminal insomnia/early morning awakening (EMA)
5. Psychomotor retardation or agitation
    a. Slowed speech/pressured speech
    b. Slowed body movements/pacing, handwriting, inability to sit still, rubbing of hair, skin, clothing
    c. Decreased speech (poverty of thought)
    d. Muteness
6. Fatigue or loss of energy
7. Feelings of worthlessness or excessive or inappropriate guilt
8. Diminished ability to think or concentrate or indecisiveness
9. Recurrent thoughts of death
10. Psychotic features, such as hallucinations or delusions (focus on worthlessness and guilt)

- Differential Diagnosis
    1. Substance abuse
    3. Medications that may cause depressive symptomatology (See Table 1).
    4. Physical health problems that may cause or be associated with depressive symptoms.
    5. Non-mood psychiatric disorders
    6. Prior episodes of unipolar depression or bipolar disorder and/or suicide attempts
    7. Nodal events/stressful life events (postpartum, death of a spouse, job loss, geographic move, illness)

- Screening Instruments
  1. Patient Self-Report Questionnaires
     a. General Health Questionnaire (GHQ)
     b. Center for Epidemiological Studies—Depression Scale (CES-D)
     c. Beck Depression Inventory (BDI)
     d. Zung Self-Rating Depression Scale (ZSRDS)
  2. Clinician-Completed Rating Scales
     a. Hamilton Rating Scale for Depression (HRS-D)
     b. Montgomery-Asberg Depression Rating Scale (MADRS)
     c. Schedule for Affective Disorders and Schizophrenia (SADS)
     d. Inventory for Depressive-Symptomatology-Clinician Rated (IDS-C)
     e. Minnesota Multiphasic Personality Inventory (MMPI)
     f. Symptom 90 Checklist
- Laboratory tests—experimental
  1. Thyrotropin releasing hormone (TRH) stimulation test and cortico tropin-releasing hormone (CRH)—differentiate unipolar from bipolar disorders and mania from schizophrenia
  2. Dexamethasone suppression test (DMST)—dexamethasone is an exogenous steroid that suppresses blood levels of cortisol. Based on the premise that many depressed patients exhibit hyper-secretion of cortisol, a single (11 P.M.) dose of cortisol does not depress late afternoon cortisol levels. If the post dexamethasone cortisol level is ≥ 5 mg/ml, then it has escaped suppression, and support is added for a diagnosis of biological depression.
  3. Urinary MHPG—a major metabolite of norepinephrine (NE) is 3-methoxy -4-hyroxy-phenylglycol (MHPG); because this metabolite crosses the blood-brain barrier, its CNS activity can be estimated by measuring MHPG elimination in urine (peripheral MHPG is also secreted in urine). It is proposed that patients with low MHPG have less norepinephrine to metabolize and would respond to antidepressants that block norepinephrine reuptake; patients with normal or

high NE levels may have a serotonin deficient depression and may respond to drugs that block serotonin reuptake.

4. Sleep EEG (REM Latency Measurement)—Sleep EEGs indicate that depressed patients spend less time in the more refreshing slow-wave phases of sleep and have a shorter pre-REM phase (decreased REM latency) of 2–30 minutes versus 90 minutes.

Depression With Melancholic Features

- Definition: A severe form of major depressive episode occurring more commonly in older persons; believed to be particularly responsive to somatic therapy
- Signs and Symptoms: The presence of at least 4 of the following including presence of 1 or 2 below (APA, 1993):
    1. Loss of interest or pleasure in all, or almost all, activities
    2. Lack of reactivity to usually pleasurable stimuli
    3. Depression regularly worse in morning
    4. Early morning awakening (EMA)
    5. Psychomotor retardation or agitation
    6. Significant anorexia or weight loss
    7. Distinct quality of depressed mood
    8. Excessive or inappropriate guilt

Depression With Seasonal Pattern (Seasonal Affective Disorder)

- Definition: A temporal relationship between the onset of an episode of major depression or bipolar disorder, recurrent and a particular period of the year (APA, 1993)
- Signs and Symptoms
    1. Onset (i.e. regular appearance of depression begins in October to November) and remissions, or change from depression to mania or hypomania (i.e., depression disappears from mid-February to mid-April) occurs within a characteristic period of the year, and no non-seasonal episodes have occurred during that same period

2. At least 2 episodes of temporal mood disturbances in 2 consecutive years.
3. Seasonal episodes substantially outnumber any nonseasonal episodes that may have occurred over the individual's lifetime.

Dysthymic Disorder

- Definition: Chronic depressed mood for most of the day, for more days than not, as indicated by subjective account or observations made by others, for at least 2 years (APA, 1993)
- Signs and Symptoms: The presence while depressed of at least 3 of the following (1–14):
  1. Low self-esteem or self-confidence, or feelings of inadequacy
  2. Feelings of pessimism, despair, or hopelessness
  3. Generalized loss of interest or pleasure
  4. Social withdrawal
  5. Chronic fatigue or tiredness
  6. Feelings of guilt, brooding about the past
  7. Subjective feelings of irritability; or excessive anger
  8. Decreased activity, effectiveness, or productivity
  9. Difficulty in thinking reflected by poor concentration, poor memory or indecisiveness
  10. During the two year period of the disturbance, the person has not been without symptoms "1" & "2" for more than two months at a time.
  11. No major depressive episode during the first two years of the disturbance
  12. Has never had a manic or hypomanic episode
  13. Does not occur exclusively during the course of a chronic psychotic disorder
  14. Not due to the direct effects of a substance (i.e. drugs or abuse of medication) or a general medical condition (i.e. hypothyroidism)

Major Depression With Postpartum Onset

- Definition: Depressive episode, ranging from moderate to severe, following childbirth with or without psychotic features and/or manic episodes
- Signs and Symptoms
  1. Onset within 1 month following delivery; onset for non-psychotic postpartum depression is 2 weeks to 12 months following delivery—typically occurs within 6 months.
  2. Recurrence rate for psychotic postpartum depression at future deliveries is 33 to 51 percent.

Bipolar Disorders

A disorder of mood in which there is at least one or more manic or hypomanic episodes, usually with a history of one or more major depressive episodes (APA, 1993).

Bipolar I Disorder (BP I)

- Definition: Frank manic or hypomanic episdodes with or without major depressive episodes that occur in an alternating pattern separated by hours, weeks, months or years, interspersed with periods of euthymia (normal mood)
  1. Manic episode
     a. A distinct period during which the predominant mood is elevated, expansive, or irritable, causing marked impairment in occupational functioning, social activities, and relationships.
     b. Presence of at least 3 of the following (2–8) during the same period:
        (1) Elevated, expansive, or irritable mood lasting at least one week
        (2) Inflated self-esteem or grandiosity
        (3) Loquaciousness/pressure of speech
        (4) Flight of ideas/thoughts racing/looseness of associations
        (5) Distractibility
        (6) Increase in goal-directed activity ranging to frantic, disorganized activity

(7) Excessive involvement in pleasurable activities with harmful consequences (i.e., spending sprees, promiscuity, reckless business decisions and investments)

(8) Decreased need for sleep

c. Differential Diagnosis

(1) Hypomanic Episode

(2) Schizoaffective Disorder

2. Hypomanic Episode

a. A distinct period of sustained, elevated, expansive, or irritable mood, lasting throughout four days, that is clearly different from the nondepressed mood.

b. At least 3 of the following symptoms (1–7) have been present to a significant degree:

(1) Inflated self-esteem or grandiosity

(2) Decreased need for sleep

(3) More talkative or pressure to keep talking

(4) Flight of ideas/thoughts racing

(5) Distractibility

(6) Increase in goal directed activity

(7) Excessive involvement in pleasurable activities

c. Associated with:

(1) Unequivocal change in functioning

(2) Disturbance in mood and change in functioning are observable by others

(3) Episode not severe enough to cause marked impairment in social or occupational functioning, or to necessitate hospitalization

(4) No psychotic features

d. Differential Diagnosis—medication, substance abuse or general medical condition, (e.g., hyperthyroidism)

3. Depressive Episode
    a. Definition: Previously has had at least one manic episode, but currently in a major depressive episode
    b. Signs and Symptoms—see Major Depression

Bipolar II Disorder (BP II)

- Definition: Recurrent major depressive episodes with hypomania (APA, 1993)
- Signs and Symptoms
    1. One or more major depressive episodes
    2. At least one hypomanic episode
    3. Has never had a manic episode
    4. Mood symptoms not accounted for by Schizoaffective Disorder; not superimposed on Schizophrenia, Schizophrenoform Disorder, Delusional Disorder, or Psychotic Disorder NOS
    5. Not precipitated by somatic antidepressant treatment

Cyclothymic Disorder

- Definition: A chronic mood disturbance of at least 2 years duration involving numerous hypomanic episodes and periods of depressed mood or loss of interest or pleasure
- Signs and Symptoms
    1. Person not without a hypomanic or depressive episode for more than 2 months during a 2 year period
    2. Has not met criteria for a Major Depressive or Manic Episode
    3. For symptoms of depression, see Depressive Disorders
    4. For symptoms relating to hypomania, see Bipolar Disorders

Other Depression Related Phenomena Not Classified as Disorders (APA, 1993)

Bereavement/Grief (Uncomplicated)

- Definition: A depressive syndrome normally occurring in response to the death of a loved one or a significant loss.

- Signs and Symptoms
    1. Feelings of depression
    2. Poor appetite
    3. Weight loss
    4. Insomnia
    5. Guilt associated with deeds done or not done at time of death
    6. Thoughts of death related to being better off dead
    7. Preoccupation with worthlessness, marked psychomotor retardation or functional impairment is uncommon.
    8. Reaction to loss may not be immediate but is time-limited; rarely occurs after 2–3 months.
    9. Duration of ''normal'' bereavement varies among different cultural groups.

Suicide

- Definition: A self-directed act to end one's life associated with:
    1. Major Depression
    2. Bipolar Disorder
    3. Schizophrenia (command hallucinations)
    4. Alcohol and Drug Use or Withdrawal
    5. Impulse Control Disorders
- Involves:
    a. Behavior Changes
    b. Anxiety
    c. Insomnia
    d. Anorexia
    e. Expression of anger, helplessness, or hopelessness
    f. Giving away personal possessions, closing bank accounts
    g. Sudden calmness or improvement in a depressed client
    h. Questions about guns, poisons or other lethal instruments

i. Social withdrawal/isolation (physical or social)

j. Stress (i.e. loss of health, significant other, job)

k. Feelings of worthlessness (i.e. everyone would be better off without me)

- See Table 2

Table 2

Risk Factors Related to Suicide

- History of Suicidal Ideation and/or Attempts
- Hopelessness
- Physical Illness
- Family History of Substance Abuse
- Family History of Depression or Suicide
- Caucasian Race
- Male Gender
- Advanced Age
- Depression
- Living Alone/Isolation
- Presence of Psychotic Symptoms
- Lethality of Suicide Plan

Etiology of Mood Disorders

- Genetic/Biologic Theories

1. Neurotransmitter Hypothesis

a. Imbalances in nerve cells whose neurotransmitters are biogenic amines (e.g.) serotonin (5 HT), norepinephrine (NE) and other related modulating neurohormones, acetylcholine and gamma acetyl buteric acid (GABA); the feedback between messenger hormones and target organs suggest many types of defective neuro-endocrine secretion.

b. Overactivity of the limbic hypothalamic-pituitary-adrenal axis (LHPA) leading to hypercortisolism

2. Circadian Rhythm Hypothesis

a. A disturbance in regulation of biological rhythms that synchronize body functions is congruent with rhythmical cyclical nature of mood disorders.

b. Depressed persons may be in a chronic state of sleep satiety (arousal) leading to REM sleep abnormalities. Acetylcholine may be involved in shortened REM latency in depression (phase advance of circadian rhythms) leading to advances in cortisol secretion (which normally surges in early morning to prepare for wakefulness).

c. Depressed persons may dispense earlier with central nervous system (CNS) programs that promote vegetative functions or overcome the restraints of arousal systems sooner than non-depressed persons.

d. The phase delay hypothesis posits that for individuals with seasonal affective disorder (SAD) circadian rhythms occur at a later time relative to sleep onset and temperature, and predicts an antidepressant response to morning photo-therapy. This shifts the onset of melatonin production and secretion to an earlier time in the evening, which results in a correction of the disrupted relationship between sleep, temperature and circadian rhythms.

e. Bipolar patients in the manic phase may have phase shifting, loss of patterning, and disorders of amplitude.

3. Kindling and Behavioral Sensitization Hypothesis

a. Kindling refers to electrical stimulation (shock) leading to nerve depolarization and seizure activity, which can later occur spontaneously when animals are placed in the environment in which original electrical stimulation occurred; animals also exhibit dysphoria.

b. Stress, like shock, is hypothesized to lower the threshold for stimulant induced sensitization, especially inescapable stress, resulting in behavioral and neurochemical abnormalities associated with depression.

c. Bipolar patients in the manic phase may have repeated daily subthreshold electrical stimulation producing seizure-like activity. Features of this seizure are irritability, rapid mood swings, and epileptic auras.

4. Genetic Hypothesis

a. Data consistently demonstrate higher rates of depression among lst degree relatives of people with unipolar depression and bipolar disorder and among monozygotic versus dizygotic twins.

b. Prevalence
   (1) Unipolar
      (a) General population—7%
      (b) First-degree relatives—18%
   (2) Bipolar
      (a) General population—1–2%
      (b) First-degree relatives—8%
   (3) Any major affective disorder
      (a) General population—8–9%
      (b) First-degree relatives—24%

c. No genetic factor consistently identified

- Psychoanalytic Theory
  1. Object Loss Hypothesis—infants experiencing loss of the maternal love object in infancy experience separation anxiety and grief related to loss of the primary love object; early loss is thought to predispose the adult to respond dysfunctionally to losses that occur later in life, becoming depressed significantly more often than those not experiencing such early losses.
  2. Aggression-Turned-Inward Hypothesis—depression is proposed to be a turning inward of the aggressive instinct that is not directed at the appropriate object, with accompanying feelings of guilt.
     a. This process is initiated by loss of an object toward whom a person feels love and hate (ambivalence).
     b. The person is unable to express the angry feelings because they are thought to be irrational or inappropriate and are unacceptable to the superego.
     c. The person may develop a pattern of containing angry/aggressive feelings and directing them inward against the self leading to self-hatred.
     d. Suicide viewed as a strike against the hated and loved object as well as the self; manic episode viewed as a defense against depression

- Cognitive Theory
  1. Depression is a cognitive problem originating from disturbed thinking in which the depression-prone person explains an adverse event as a personal shortcoming.
  2. Developmental experiences sensitize certain people and make them vulnerable to depression. The constellation of negative thoughts that characterize depression remains dormant until a person becomes depressed. When depression occurs after a life stressor, the dormant cognitive set appears; negative cognitive processes replace objective thinking.
  3. Cognitive Elements of Depression
     a. Cognitive triad—the person's negative view of self, the world and the future, which is a distortion of reality
     b. Silent assumptions—irrational beliefs or rules that significantly affect the depressed person's cognitive, affective, and behavior patterns
     c. Logical errors—faulty information processing and errors in thinking that maintain the person's belief in the validity of his/her negative concept despite contradictory evidence
- Hopelessness Theory of Depression (Learned Helplessness)
  1. Based on attribution theory—a chain of perceived negative life events are hypothesized to be the "occasion setter" for people to become hopeless and depressed.
  2. Depression consists of four classes of deficits: motivational, cognitive, self-esteem, and affective.
  3. Three types of influences determine whether a person will become hopeless, and, in turn depressed, when negative life events are experienced.
     a. When highly desired outcomes are believed improbable or when highly aversive outcomes are perceived probable, and the person anticipates that no response in his or her repertoire will positively affect the outcome (helplessness), depression occurs.
     b. When negative life events are attributed to stable versus unstable and global versus specific causes, and are viewed as important, helplessness, low self-esteem and depression ensue.

c. Inferred negative consequences are most likely to lead to depression. The consequence is viewed as important, not remediable, likely to change, and affecting many areas of life. When inferred characteristics about the self (self-worth, abilities, desirability, etc.) are negative and will interfere with attainment of important outcomes, hopelessness and depression may ensue.

- Family Theory

1. Developmental experiences within the family system (abuse, conflict, divorce, death) can be antecedents of depression.

   a. Nodal events (significant exits and entries of people, places, objects, activities, and roles in a family system), especially those perceived as undesirable, can precipitate depression, especially when an event generates stress or anxiety not openly dealt with in the family system.

   b. Multiple nodal events occurring within a brief period may escalate the likelihood of stress (cluster stress) and depression.

   c. Anniversary reactions (affective responses around anniversary of nodal event), which reactivate feelings associated with original nodal event, can take form of depression, suicidal thoughts, gestures attempts, and other stress-related symptoms.

2. Family precursors of mood disorders include early developmental family experiences related to strong nurturing in early childhood followed by cutting off of nurturing supplies in early childhood, coupled with unrealistic expectations, unquestioning acceptance of parental values, and frustrated efforts to obtain family approval and love. Underlying resentment toward parents may erupt briefly, followed by quiet and fear of rejection. Manic episode masks guilt, loss, and rejection. Depressive episode represents internalization of disappointment, loss, and perceived failure.

Nursing Diagnoses (See Table 3)

Table 3

Comparison of DSMIII-R Criteria and Nursing Diagnosis Related to Mood Disorders

DSMIII-R Criteria	Nursing Diagnoses
Depression	
1. Psychomotor retardation or agitation	Mobility, alteration in
2. Loss of interest in usual pleasures	Coping, ineffective individual/impaired social interaction

Table 3 - Continued

DSMIII-R Criteria	Nursing Diagnoses
3. Decreased ability to concentrate	Thought processes, alteration in
4. Feelings of worthlessness, guilt	Self-concept, disturbance in
5. Insomnia or hypersomnia	Sleep pattern disturbance
6. Fatigue or loss of energy	Fatigue/self-care deficit
7. Recurrent thoughts of death or suicide	Potential for self-harm Dysfunctional grieving
8. Appetite disturbance	Nutrition, alteration in less than body requirements more than body requirements
9. Depressed mood with psychotic features (hallucinations, delusions)	Alteration in perception or cognition
Mania	
1. A distinct period of abnormally elevated, expansive, or irritable mood	Emotional lability
2. Grandiosity	Self-concept, disturbance in
3. Hyperverbal, pressured speech	Communication, impaired verbal
4. Distractibility	Thought process, alteration in
5. Poor Judgement	Sensory perceptual alteration; potential for self-harm
6. Decreased need for sleep	Sleep pattern disturbance
7. Racing thoughts, flight of ideas	Thought processes, alteration in
8. Increased activity	Impaired social interaction/self-care deficit
9. Excessive involvement in pleasurable activities	Altered impulse control/manipulation
10. Mania with psychotic features (delusions, hallucinations)	Alteration in perception/cognition

Nursing Interventions

- Pharmacological Interventions
    1. Objectives
        a. Symptom reduction (initial objective)
        b. Improved function
        c. Recurrence prevention
    2. Role of the nurse
        a. Collection of pretreatment assessment data
        b. Coordination of treatment modalities
        c. Client education
            (1) Provide information about medication and its side effects (See Tables 4, 5, 6 and 7)
            (2) Clarify misinformation
            (3) Explore perceptions and feelings about medication

(4) Medication management strategies

d. Monitoring drug effects/minimize side effects

e. Prescribing and/or administering medications

3. Antidepressant drugs

a. First-line treatment modality for depressive disorder when:

(1) Depression is moderate to severe

(2) Presence of psychotic, melancholic, or atypical (overeating, hypersomnia, weight gain) symptom features

(3) Client requests medication

(4) Medication and psychotherapy are planned treatment strategy

(5) Psychotherapy not available

(6) Prior positive response to medication

(7) Maintenance/treatment is planned

b. Mode of action

(1) Exact mechanism of action unknown

(2) Equilibrate effects of biogenic amines through various mechanisms

(a) Blocks uptake of neurotransmitters (norepinephrine, serotonin) at presynaptic neuron

(b) Inhibits metabolism of neurotransmitters (norepinephrine, serotonin)

(c) Regulates the locus ceruleus, the part of the brain where most norepinephrine is made

(3) Pharmacology outlined in Table 4

(4) MAOIs—inhibit the action of monoamine oxidase, an enzyme that metabolizes neurohormones responsible for stimulating physical and mental activity (serotonin, norepinephrine, and epinephrine). Usually used when client is unresponsive to non-MAOI anti-depressants.

Table 4

Pharmacology of Antidepressant Medications

Drug	*Therapeutic Dosage Range* (mg/day)	*Increase in Neuro-transmitter Function* 5–HT	NE	*Sedative Effect*	*Therapeutic Blood Levels* ng/ML	*Elimination Halflife (h)*
Tricyclics						
Amitriptyline (Elavil, Endep)	75–300	3	2	4	150–250	10–46
Clomiprimine (Anafranil)	75–300	3	1	2	100–250	17–28
Desipramine (Norpramin, Pertoframe)	75–300	0	4	1	125–300	12–76
Doxepin (Sinequan, Adapin)	75–300	2	2	4	150–250	8–36
Imipramine (Tofranil, Janimine)	75–300	2	3	3	150–250	4–34
Nortriptyline (Aventyl, Pamelor)	40–200	2	3	2	50–150	13–88
Protriptyline (Vivactil)	20–60	2	4	1	70–250	54–124
Trimipramine (Surmontil)	75–300	2	3	4	150–250	7–30
Heterocyclics						
Amoxapine (Ascendin)	100–600	1	4	3	200–600	8
Bupropion (Wellbutrin)	225–450	1	1	1	25–100	10–14
Maprotiline (Ludiomil)	100–225	0	4	3	200–600	27–58
Trazodone (Desyrel)	150–600	4	0	4	800–1600	4–9
Selective Serotonin Reuptake Inhibitors (SSRIs)						
Fluoxetine (Prozac)	10–40	3	1	1	200–700	24–96
Paroxetine (Paxil)	20–50	3	1	2	100–400	24
Sertraline (Zoloft)	50–200	3	1	2	20–500	24
MAOIs						
Isocarboxazid (Marplan)	Recently withdrawn from market					
Phenelzine (Nardil)	45–90	u	u	3	u	
Tranylcypromine (Pamate)	10–60	u	u	2	u	

High = 4 5HT = Serotonin
Moderate = 3 NE = Norepinephrine
Low = 2
Slight = 1
None = 0
Potency Unknown = u

c. Administration

(1) Oral route

(2) Begin with low dosage administered at bed time to minimize side effects (e.g., 25 to 50 mg/day of desipramine).

(3) Increase dosage in increments over 1 to 3 weeks (except fluoxetine).

(4) Fluoxetine and protriptyline administered in morning, others at night

(5) Note time lag in onset of therapeutic effect, 7–28 days.

(6) Monitor blood levels and side effects weekly/biweekly and adjust dosage after 3 days.

(7) Evaluate side effects weekly/biweekly.

(8) Assess outcomes at 6 weeks and 12 weeks.

(9) Continue medication for 4–9 months.

(10) Continuation of medication may be indicated if depression is recurring.

d. Side/adverse/toxic effects of non-MAOIs

(1) Incidence of side/adverse effects most common at beginning of treatment subside over time and/or clients adapt to many side effects over time (See Table 5) and/or develop tolerance

Table 5

Adverse/Side Effects of Antidepressants and Nursing Interventions

Side Effect	*Nursing Intervention*
Neurological	
Sedation, psychomotor slowing, difficulty concentrating and planning	Inform the client, especially if he operates machinery or must perform mental tasks; tolerance can develop and thus side effects do decrease or dose can be lowered
Muscle weakness, fatigue, nervousness, headaches, vertigo neuropathies, tremors, ataxia, paresthesias, twitching	Not common; tolerance can develop and thus side effects do decrease or dose can be lowered
Lowered seizure threshold	Start drugs at lower dose and increase more gradually with seizure disorder clients
Extrapyramidal side effects (EPS): acute dystonic reactions, akathisia, Parkinson's syndrome, tardive dyskinesia	Rare, since they do not block dopamine; amoxapine, the exception, can cause all the common EPS reactions, possibly tardive dyskinesia with long-term use
Psychiatric symptoms: increased anxiety, depression, insomnia, nightmares, psychotic reactions, or confusional states with delusions, hallucinations, and disorientation; mania	Uncommon, may have to discontinue drug; mania may be precipitated if client has prior history of mania in self or family (avoid tricyclics if possible in patients predisposed to mania)
Gastrointestinal	
Heartburn, nausea, vomiting	Take with meals; switch medication if discomfort becomes severe or vomiting occurs
Decrease in intestinal motility, paralytic ileus	Monitor elimination patterns
Dry mouth	Increase fluids
Hematological	
Leukopenia and thrombocytopenia	Monitor; rarely clinically significant

Table 5 - Continued

Side Effect	*Nursing Intervention*
Agranulocytosis: Allergic response of sudden onset; appears 40 to 70 days after initiation of drug (low WBC, normal RBC, infection of the pharynx, fatigue, malaise)	Very rare; discontinue drug and place patient in reverse isolation immediately; never administer drug again; try antidepressant with a different chemical structure and follow client closely
Cardiovascular	
Postural hypotension: light-headedness or dizziness on rising due to decrease in blood pressure on rising	Occurs frequently; take vital signs sitting and then standing ½ hour after dose; rise slowly, dangle feet, tolerance can develop in first few weeks; not dose related, can continue to raise dose
Tachycardia: rapid heart beat	
EKG changes	Occurs frequently; tolerance usually develops; can increase symptoms of angina in clients with coronary artery disease; very frightening to panic disorder clients; worsening of intraventricular conduction problems; take a careful cardiac history and do a pretreatment EKG, especially with clients over 40 years of age
Sudden death	Rare; clients at risk for cardiac heart block; over 50 years of age, family history of heart disease, preexisting cardiac disease or recent myocardial infarction, or bundle-branch block
Opthalmological	
Blurred vision caused by ciliary muscle relaxation	Tolerance can develop over the first few weeks of treatment; distant vision is usually intact; do not use with clients with narrow-angle glaucoma
Hepatic	
Liver toxicity within first 8 weeks of treatment: abdominal pain, anorexia, fever, mild transient jaundice, abnormal liver function tests	Rare hypersensitivity response; discontinue drug; switch to another type of antidepressant
Endocrine	
Amenorrhea, galactorrhea	Due to increased prolactin caused by amoxapine; rare with other tricyclics
Menstrual irregularities	Rare and reversible; decrease dose; change to a different tricyclic
Cutaneous	
Maculopapular rashes, petechiae, photosensitivity	Rare; can give an antihistamine; anti-depressant
Genitourinary	
Increased or decreased sexual desire, delayed ejaculation	Decrease dose, change to a less anticholinergic drug; take daily dose after sexual intercourse, not immediately before, for delayed ejaculation
Urinary retention	Lower dose, change to a less anticholinergic drug, try bethanechol; rare: acute renal failure following an atonic bladder

Table 5 - Continued

Side Effect	*Nursing Intervention*
Miscellaneous Tinnitus, weight loss, increased appetite and weight gain, psychomotor stimulation, parotid swellling, alopecia, allergic response: edema, generalized on face, tongue, and orbits	Very rare; weight control; decrease dose; may have to discontinue drug and try an antidepressant that is structurally different
Pathological sweating	Occurs in 25% of patients; head, neck, and upper extremities; episodic, or occurs only at night
Withdrawal syndrome Mild withdrawal after sudden discontinuation: malaise, muscle aches, coryzia, chills, nausea, dizziness, anxiety	Taper client off drug gradually (one to several weeks)
Intoxication syndromes Poisoning: usually seen in overdose CNS depression and/or cardiotoxicity: hallucinations delirium, agitation, sensitivity to sounds, dilated pupils, hypothermia, hyperpyrexia, seizures, coma, arrhythmias, respiratory arrest	Treat aggressively; recovery can be slow; induce emesis, gastric lavage, cardiac monitoring, respiratory support, blood chemistry, arterial blood gases, monitor tricyclic plasma levels, carefully administer physostigmine, valium, mannitol, lidocaine, and other symptomatic treatments
Anticholinergic syndromes Confusion, delirium, disorientation, agitation, hallucinations, anxiety, motor restlessness, seizures, delusions, constipation, urinary retention, decreased sweating, increased pupillary size, dry mouth, increased temperature, motor incoordination, flushing, tachycardia	Usually occurs with high doses of psychoactive drugs with anticholinergic effects; physostigmine, cardiac monitoring, respiratory support; in sensitive or aged clients, may occur at normal, therapeutic levels

(2) Toxic effects same as side effects but intensified

(a) Anticholinergic, CNS stimulation followed by CNS depression

(b) Cardiac irregularities (except fluoxetine and fluroxamine); extends duration of QRS complex ≤ 0.125)

e. Side/Adverse Effects of MAOIs

(1) Most common effects are: constipation, anorexia, nausea, vomiting, dry mouth, urinary retention, skin rash, transient impotence, drowsiness, headache, dizziness, orthostatic hypotension

(2) Occasional stimulant effect (insomnia, restlessness, anxiety)

(3) Hypomania in patients with bipolar disorders (35%)

(4) Parasthesias (tingling at periphery, electric-shock-like sensations)

(5) Hypertensive crisis (See Tables 6 & 7)

4. Mood Stabilizers

a. Lithium

(1) First-line treatment modality for bipolar disorders

(a) In manic and depressive episodes

(b) As prophylaxis against further episodes

(c) In other disorders with an affective component

- Recurrent unipolar depression
- Schizo affective disorder
- Catatonia
- Alcoholism

(d) In non-affective disorders

- Aggressive conduct disorder
- Eating disorders
- Borderline personality disorder

(2) Mode of Action

(a) Exact mode of action not fully understood

(b) Corrects anion exchange abnormality

(c) Alters sodium transport in nerves and muscle cells

(d) Normalizes synaptic transmission of norepinephrine, serotonin, and dopamine

(e) Increases reuptake and metabolism of norepinephrine

(f) Changes receptor sensitivity for serotonin

(3) Administration

(a) 10–14 days before complete effect is observed

(b) Acute mania often initially treated with neuroleptics to manage psychotic symptoms and/or behavioral excitement until lithium is effective.

Table 6

Signs and Symptoms of Hypertensive Crisis and Nursing Interventions

Signs and Symptoms	*Nursing Intervention*
Warning Signs	
Increased blood pressure	Hold next MAOI dose
Palpitations	Do not lie client in supine or prone position (elevated BP in head)
Frequent Headaches	
Symptoms of Hypertensive Crisis	
Sudden elevation of blood pressure	Monitor vital signs
Explosive headache (occiptal radiating frontally)	Chlorpromazine 100 mg IM (blocks Norepinephrine, repeat if necessary)
Palpitations; chest pain	
Sweating	Phentolamine slowly administered in 5 mg IV doses (binds with norepinephrine receptor sites, blocking norepinephrine)
Fever	
Nausea; vomiting	
Dilated pupils	Manage fever with external cooling techniques
Photophobia	Assess intake of tyramine containing foods
Neck stiffness	
Nosebleed	
Intracranial bleeding	

Table 7

Dietary Restrictions for Patients Taking MAOIs

Food and Beverages to Avoid	*Safe Food, Beverages and Medication*
Cheese, especially aged or matured (Cheddar, Mozzarella, Parmesan, Gruyre, Stilton, Brie, Swiss, blue, Camembert)	Cottage Cheese
	Farmer's Cheese
Fermented or aged protein (salami, mortadella, sausage, bologna, pepperoni)	Cheese Whiz
	Ricotta
Pickled or smoked fish	Havarti
Beer, red wine, Sherry, Cognac, liqueurs	Boursin
Yeast or protein extracts (Marmite, Oxo, Bovril)	Fresh fruits
Broad bean pods	Bread products raised with yeast (bread)
Beef or chicken liver	
Yogurt	
Sauerkraut	
Over ripe fruit	
Foods and Beverages to be Consumed in Moderation	
Chocolate	
Sour cream	
Avocado	
Clear spirits and white wine	
Soy sauce	
Caffeine drinks	
Medications to Avoid	*Safe Medications*
Cold Medications	Aspirin, Tylenol
Nasal and sinus decongestants	Pure steroid asthma inhalants
Allergy and hay fever remedies	Codeine
Narcotics, especially meperidine	Plain Robitusin or Terpin-hydrate with codeine
Inhalants for asthma	All laxatives
Local anesthetics with epinephrine	All antibiotics
Weight reducing pills	Antihistamines

(c) Dose guided by plasma level; increase slowly to minimize side effects until symptoms are reduced, side effects are too great as upper limit of therapeutic blood level is reached.

(d) Acute treatment: 900–2400 mg daily (.08–1.2 mEq/L) (300 mg tid)

(e) Maintenance: 400–1200 mg daily (0.6–1.0 mEq/L) (tid, bid, or bid if sustained release form is used)

(f) Blood levels drawn

- 7 days after tx begins (12 hours after last dose)
- 2× weekly × 2 weeks
- 1× weekly × 2 weeks
- q 3 months × 6 months
- q 6 months thereafter

(g) Therapeutic Range 0.6–1.4 mEq/L for adults; 0.6–0.8 mEq/L in geriatric clients or those with medical illness

(4) Side/adverse/toxic effects of Lithium

(a) Incidence of side effects most common at beginning of treatment disappear after a few weeks (See Table 8)

(b) Symptoms coincide with peaks of lithium concentration due to rapid absorption of lithium ion

(c) Lithium toxicity—usually dose related (see table 9)

b. Anticonvulsants

(1) Second-line treatment modality for mood stabilization bipolar disorder

(a) Prevention of recurrence

(b) Lithium is contraindicated or ineffective

(c) For rapid cyclers (> 4 episodes/year)

Table 8

Lithium Side Effects and Nursing Interventions

Side Effect Symptom	*Nursing Intervention*
Polyuria, with possible progression to diabetes insipidus. Urine output is large in volume and so dilute that it may be colorless.	Reassure client that increased urination is common and benign.
Client may complain of urinating so frequently that it interferes with activities of daily living, including sleep.	Urine volume may diminish if the physician reduces the lithium dose or changes to a slow release form or a single daily dosage. When severe, the physician usually orders 24-hour urine volume. If volume is greater than 3 L, a further renal workup is usually requested. When severe, polyuria is often treated by the physician with a thiazide or potassium-sparing diuretic (taking care to reduce the lithium dose). Lithium is contra-indicated for clients with renal dysfunction.
Increased thirst	Recommend that clients quench their thirst and maintain a fairly stable intake of liquids from day to day. The best thirst quencher is water or a low-calorie beverage that will not cause weight gain when taken in large amounts. Gum or hard candies may help moisten the mouth.
Tremor: A fine tremor that worsens with intentional movements. It can make writing, drinking hot beverages, and many other motor tasks difficult.	Reassure that this is benign and may be temporary. In some clients it is persistent. The physician may order a reduction in dose, more frequent doses, or a change to a slow-release form. When the tremor is severe or incapacitating, the physician may treat it with a beta blocker, usually propranolol (Inderal). Recommend that the client reduce or eliminate caffeine-containing beverages.
Nausea, abdominal discomfort, diarrhea, or soft stools	Reassure that this is benign and usually temporary. Recommend that the client take lithium with meals, a glass of milk, or a snack. If symptom persists, the physician may change to another lithium preparation.
Muscle weakness or fatigue	Reassure that this is benign and usually temporary. Since this is not a very common side effect of lithium, ascertain whether it is being caused by another medication being taken by the client. Encourage the client to remain active and get regular physical exercise. If symptom persists, the physician may reduce the dose, order more frequent divided doses, change to slow-release, or reduce the dose and more gradually increase to the present dose level.
Edema of the feet or other body parts	Reassure that this is benign and may be temporary. A moderate salt restriction may reduce the edema. If moderate salt restriction is undertaken, the serum lithium level usually rises somewhat. It then becomes necessary to monitor for signs of toxicity and keep the physician informed in case it becomes necessary to reduce the lithium dose.
Hypothyroidism (5%)	Explain that this is reversible and treatable. The physician usually orders thyroid hormone replacement, such as levothyroxine (Synthroid) or desiccated thyroid.

Table 8 - Continued

Side Effect Symptom	*Nursing Intervention*
Weight gain (60%)	Explain that this is fairly common and benign. Moderate calorie restriction and increased exercise usually help. Advise against fluid restriction or sodium restriction unless undertaken with knowledge of the physician and nurse, since either intervention can cause the serum lithium level to rise.
Hair thinning or loss	Explain that this may be temporary. Since hair loss can be a symptom of hypothyroidism, inform the physician so that thyroid functioning can be checked. If hair does not return, lithium is usually stopped so that hair can regrow. During periods of hair loss, encourage the client to consider wearing a wig.
Benign, reversible granulocytosis	Explain that this is benign. This side effect is the basis for its use as a treatment in some granulocytopenic conditions.
Decreased Libido	Suggest timing sexual activity to not coincide with peak action time of medication. Explore strategies for continuing relationship intimacy.

Table 9

Lithium Toxicity and Related Treatment

Mild
- At lithium levels of 1.5–2 mEq/L; occasionally occurs at normal levels
- Develops gradually over several days
- Symptoms: ataxia, coarse tremor, confusion, diarrhea, drowsiness, fasciculation, slurred speech

- Treatment: Hold all lithium doses
  Obtain lithium blood level
  Check vital signs
  Patient education

Moderate to Severe
- At lithium levels > 2 mEq/L
- Gradual or sudden onset
- Symptoms: muscle tremor, hyperreflexia, pulse irregularities, hyper or hypotension, EKG changes, visual or tactile hallucinations, oliguria or anuria, seizures, coma, death

- Treatment: Rapid assessment of clinical signs and symptoms of lithium toxicity
  Hold all lithium doses
  Monitor vital signs and LOC
  Protect airway and provide standby oxygen
  Obtain lithium level stat; BUN, creatnine, urinalysis; CBC; monitor electrolytes EKG; monitor cardiac states
  Limit lithium absorption; provide an emetic; N–G suctioning may be appropriate
  Vigorously hydrate 5 to 6 L/day IV; indwelling catheter; monitor intake and output; ROM; deep breathing
  Maintain bed rest

(2) Mode of Action
   (a) Structurally related to tricyclic antidepressants
   (b) Anticonvulsant activity mediated through a "peripheral" type benzodiazepine receptor
   (c) Effective in inhibiting seizures kindled from repeated stimulation of limbic structures
   (d) GABA antagonist activity

(3) Administration
   (a) Fourteen days before peak effect
   (b) Dose guided by plasma levels (See Table 10)
   (c) Complete laboratory tests prior to beginning therapy
      - CBC
      - Liver function tests
      - Serum electrolytes
      - EKG
   (d) Blood tests q 2 weeks × 3 months; q 3 months thereafter to monitor hematopoetic suppression and hyponatremia

(4) Reinforce teaching after each treatment.

- Electroconvulsive Therapy
  1. Mode of action
     a. Largely unknown
     b. Therapeutic effect may be due to seizure activity in brain producing changes in post-synaptic response to neurotransmitters similar to antidepressants.
  2. Indications
     a. Emergency therapy for suicidal or hyperactive clients who are in physical danger
     b. Clients unresponsive to or cannot tolerate medications

Table 10

Anticonvulsant Used in Treatment of Bipolar Disorder

Drug	*Dose*	*Effects Side/Adverse/Toxic*
Carbamezapine (Tegretol)	Begin at 200 mg/day in divided doses and increase progressively by 100 mg 2×/wk to as much as 1600 mg/day until attaining serum levels of 6–12 mg/l. First serum level drawn > 5 days after starting therapy Usual dose 300–1200 mg daily (less in Orientals and elderly) Slow-release tablets available; may decrease side effects due to peak levels of drug	skin rash sore throat mucosal ulceration low-grade fever drowsiness vertigo ataxia diplopia blurred vision nausea vomiting hepatotoxicity benign ↓ in WBC agranulocytosis
Valproate/Valproic Acid (Depakene, Depakote)	Begin at 500–1000 mg/day untile serum level of 50–125 μg/ml is achieved Response occurs in 1=2 weeks	anorexia nausea vomiting diarrhea tremor sedation ataxia increased appetite pancreatitis
Clonazepam (Klonapin)	4–24 mg/day	ataxia drowsiness cognitive impairment increased salivation behavioral dyscontrol (disinhibition) blurred vision paradoxical agitation

c. During time lag between initiation of pharmacotherapy and establishment of therapeutic medication level

3. Treatment
   a. 6–12 treatments on alternate days
   b. Atropine sulfate administered for vagolytic effect 30 minutes prior to treatment
   c. Short-acting barbiturate (Brevital Sodium) administered IV to induce anesthesia

d. Succinyl choline (Anectine) administered IV as muscle relaxant after anesthetic

e. 100% O_2 administered 1–2 min. to prepare for apneic period from muscle relaxant and convulsion

f. Client positioned in supine position; mouth gag inserted; jaw supported; suctioning, prn

g. Electrodes applied unilaterally (less amnesia) at non-dominant side temple or bilaterally (more amnesia) at temples

h. Fingers and toes observed for twitching

i. O_2 administered by bag breathing when twitching stops until spontaneous respiration resumes.

j. Patent airway maintained; client positioned on side

k. Vital signs monitored until stable

l. Patient begins to respond in 10–15 minutes.

4. Side Effects

   a. Anoxia during seizure

   b. Memory loss—temporary

   c. Cardiac arrhythmias

   d. Mortality 1:10,000 patients

5. Nursing intervention

   a. Complete physical assessment including EKG, EEG, X-rays of spine and chest

   b. Provide opportunity to express feelings about ECT.

   c. Assess client's response.

   d. Client education

      (1) Assess patient and family anxiety level and ability to understand.

      (2) Individualize amount of information shared (i.e., treatment, post ECT confusion, memory loss, etc.).

      (3) Provide time to discuss concerns and answer questions.

(4) Instruct accompanying adult in dealing with post ECT effects.

(a) Orienting to time, place, and person

(b) Headache

(c) Nausea

e. Treatment responsibilities

(1) Check emergency equipment.

(2) Maintain NPO status.

(3) Remove harmful objects (dentures, jewelry, etc.).

(4) Monitor vital signs.

(5) Position on side until reactive.

(6) Maintain airway.

(7) Assist to ambulate.

(8) Orient to environment.

(9) Offer antiemetic or analgesea as needed.

f. Ethical considerations

(1) Provide patient/family education.

(2) Obtain informed consent.

(3) Act as patient/family advocate.

- Monitoring Physical Needs

1. Alteration in nutrition

a. Record intake and output.

b. Weigh clients daily.

c. Monitor electrolytes.

d. Assist clients in identifying food preferences.

e. Offer small, frequent high calorie meals and fluids.

f. Provide nutritional meals that can be ''eaten on the run'' by manic clients.

g. Assist as needed with feeding.

   h. Promote weight management strategies for clients who overeat.

2. Alteration in Sleep Patterns
   a. Discourage daytime sleeping.
   b. Administer antidepressants hs (except Prozac, which may increase insomnia).
   c. Teach bedtime relaxation techniques.
      (1) Relaxation exercises
      (2) Hot baths
      (3) Back rub
      (4) Soft music
   d. Provide rest periods for manic clients.
   e. Decrease environmental stimuli.
   f. Limit intake of caffeinated drinks.
   g. Administer sedatives hs prn.
3. Alteration in elimination
   a. Monitor intake and output.
   b. Promote fluid intake.
   c. Promote high fiber diet.
   d. Promote exercise.
   e. Administer laxatives prn.
   f. Catheterize prn.
4. Alterations in Hygiene
   a. Matter-of-factly assist with bathing, dressing, grooming as needed.
   b. Promote independence in activities of daily living (ADLs).
   c. Set limits on neglect of self-care.
   d. Positively reinforce self-care behaviors.

- Psychotherapeutic Interventions
  1. Intervening in Uncomplicated Grief Reaction
     a. Objective to assist individuals experiencing loss resolve grieving and prevent dysfunctional coping
     b. Self-awareness necessary to understand own feelings and responses to loss
     c. Communicate open and directly but respect need for denial
     d. Assess prior losses and coping patterns to determine:
        (1) Stresses previously experienced
        (2) Coping style/resources
        (3) Support systems
        (4) Nature of current relationship
        (5) Persons at high risk for dysfunctional coping behaviors
     e. Provide anticipatory guidance prior to loss
        (1) Discuss impending loss.
        (2) Review and analyze significance of past losses and responses in relation to impending loss.
        (3) Teach about mourning process.
        (4) Assist family in formulation of coping strategies.
     f. Support patient and family.
        (1) Consider cultural, religious and social customs of mourning.
        (2) Provide private place for expression of feelings.
        (3) Do not leave alone until a support system is available.
     g. Assist in grief work.
        (1) Help patient experience and express feelings of loss.
        (2) Normalize intensity of feelings.
        (3) Non-judgmentally accept hostility, anger, guilt, ambivalence, crying, testing and withdrawal

(4) Respond empathetically yet communicate hope for future

(5) Initially, assist in immediate decision-making if necessary

(6) Initially, support defenses such as denial, dependence, reaction formation, over-identification, etc.

(7) Encourage exploration and analysis of dysfunctional coping patterns.

(8) Support and reinforce development of functional coping patterns, gradual release of attachment bonds, and eventual investment in new relationships and interests.

(9) Promote social network support.

(a) Family

(b) Friends

(c) Clergy

(d) Community agency

(e) Self-help groups

2. Cognitive interventions

a. Objectives

(1) Increase client's sense of control over his/her goals/behavior.

(2) Increase self-esteem.

(3) Assist client in modifying negative expectations.

b. Assist in exploring feelings to elicit patient's view of problem(s).

c. Assist client in identifying negative thoughts.

d. Accept client perceptions, not conclusions.

e. Teach thought interruption or substitution.

f. Encourage client to increase realistic thinking by appraising personal assets, strengths, accomplishments, and opportunities.

g. Encourage formulation of realistic versus unrealistic goals.

3. Behavioral interventions
   a. Objectives
      (1) Activating clients in a realistic goal-directed way
      (2) Develop alternative problem-solving and coping strategies.
      (3) Increase self-esteem.
      (4) Instill hope.
      (5) Increase client responsibility for change.
      (6) Gradual redirection of self-preoccupation to interests in outside world
   b. Assess client strengths and weaknesses and personal and environmental factors that maintain depression.
   c. Work with client to develop a structured daily program of activities which
      (1) Considers probability of succeeding
      (2) Considers attention span, distractibility and motivation
      (3) Contains realistic goals and expectations
      (4) Provides opportunities for performance-based positive reinforcement
   d. Involve clients in:
      (1) Assertiveness training
      (2) Role playing
      (3) Social skills training
      (4) Stress management
         (a) Relaxation exercises
         (b) Meditation
         (c) Physical fitness/exercise
   e. Increase client's present versus past or future orientation.
4. Interpersonal interventions
   a. Objectives

(1) Increase appropriate expression of thoughts and feelings.

(2) Increase self-esteem.

(3) Increase social interaction.

b. Facilitate expression of feelings.

(1) Acknowledge client pain and despair.

(2) Reinforce that depression is self-limiting.

(3) Convey hope for future.

(4) Do not give false reassurance.

(5) Engage in active listening.

(6) Demonstrate acceptance of thoughts and feelings.

(7) Facilitate expression of positive and negative thoughts and feelings.

(8) Assist client in identifying strategies for expressing and coping with negative feelings (anger, guilt, aggressiveness, etc.).

(9) Provide objective feedback and positive reinforcement.

c. Increasing Self-Esteem

(1) Schedule regular sessions with client.

(2) Accept negativism without judgement.

(3) Minimize time focused on real or perceived failures.

(4) Focus on identifying strengths and accomplishments.

(5) Collaborate with client in identifying factors maintaining low self-esteem.

(a) Interpersonal deficits

(b) Role transitions

(c) Role disputes

(d) Marital conflict

(e) Grief

(6) Collaborate with client in areas to change.

(7) Collaborate on goals and problem-solving strategies.

(8) Involve in activities that produce immediate success.

(9) Provide realistic positive feedback.

(10) See Cognitive and Behavioral Interventions.

- Family Interventions
  1. Objectives
     a. Family participation in discharge planning
     b. Increased functional family interaction patterns
     c. Increase family effectiveness in coping with grief, loss, stress.
  2. Assess family functioning.
  3. Family education including:
     a. Client's diagnosis and treatment plan, including medications
     b. Relapse signs and symptoms and what to do should they reappear
     c. Community resources (medical, social, vocational, support groups)
     d. Positive support and knowledge to anticipate and avoid problems
     e. Resocialization issues
  4. Explore dysfunctional family interaction patterns that maintain depressive or manic symptoms.
     a. Dependency/codependency
     b. Dysfunctional communication patterns
     c. Unrealistic expectations
     d. Reinforcement of secondary gains of depressive or manic behavior
     e. Dysfunctional role patterns/strain
     f. Stress and grief coping patterns
     g. Sources of conflict
        (1) Demandingness
        (2) Manipulation

(3) Testing

(4) Impulsivity

(5) Underfunctioning/overfunctioning

5. Refer to or conduct family therapy sessions.
6. Family intervention when suicide is attempted or completed
   a. Explore family response to stress.
   b. Explore family relationships re: isolation, scapegoating, estrangement.
   c. Explore family communication patterns.
   d. Promote grief rituals and customs.
   e. Facilitate open expression of feelings (guilt, anger, sadness, helplessness, etc.).
   f. Refer to or conduct family therapy. Refer to support groups.

- Group Interventions
  1. Objectives
     a. Increase self-esteem through identification with group.
     b. Increase awareness of personal strengths.
     c. Increase social support.
     d. Increase shared humanness.
     e. Modify dysfunctional communication and interaction patterns.
     f. Learn functional ways to cope with stress.
     g. Decrease social withdrawal.
  2. Gradually involve clients in:
     a. Psychotherapy groups
     b. Assertiveness training groups
     c. Social skills training groups
     d. Occupational therapy
     e. Art therapy
     f. Activity groups

3. Group interventions
    a. Devise a structured plan of therapeutic activities that considers client's level of depression or mania.
    b. Encourage attendance at group sessions and activities.
    c. Accept non-verbal participation.
    d. Set limits on disruptive behavior.
    e. Positively reinforce appropriate participation.
    f. Encourage sharing of common feelings, thoughts, behaviors, life experiences among clients.
    g. Promote problem-solving within group.
    h. Promote modification of dysfunctional expectations of self and others.
    i. Teach stress management strategies.
    j. Instruct and model social skills.
    k. Use role playing and rehearsal of social interactions.
    l. Encourage initiation of socialization in an expanded social environment.

- Milieu Interventions
    1. Objectives
        a. Maintain client safety.
        b. Decrease manipulation.
        c. Increase self-responsibility.
    2. Interventions to maintain client safety
        a. Complete assessment of suicidal risk.
        b. Determine level of precautions.
            (1) Level of observation
            (2) Removal of dangerous objects
            (3) Limits in freedom and activity
        c. Initiate no harm contract with client.

d. Establish rapport and communicate expectations related to safety issues.

e. Use seclusion and restraints as last resort to maintain safety.

3. Interventions to decrease manipulation

a. Develop coordinated limit setting plan that presents a united front.

b. Set consistent, realistic limits and consequences.

c. Set expectations for personal responsibility.

(1) Obeying rules

(2) Cleaning room

(3) Dressing modestly, etc.

d. Give positive feedback for appropriate behavior.

e. Avoid defensive personal responses.

f. Explore purpose and meaning of behavior with client.

g. Engage client in learning how to make decisions and accept responsibility.

4. Structuring the environment

a. Establish a structured daily program of activities.

b. Monitor environmental stimuli.

c. Involve client in unit activities appropriate to level of functioning.

d. Provide appropriate positive reinforcement.

e. Avoid reinforcing negative or inappropriate behavior.

f. Set agreed upon limits on manipulative, demanding and testing behaviors.

g. Engage client in developing functional coping strategies.

(1) Stress management

(a) Exercise

(b) Relaxation response

(c) Meditation

(d) Nutritional diet

(e) Adequate sleep

(f) Differentiating normal mood response and stress from illness symptoms

- Community Resources

1. Objectives

   a. Facilitate reintegration of client in community through coordination of services.

   b. Increase use of support systems.

   c. Expand social interactions.

   d. Maximum independent functioning.

2. Interventions

   a. Collaborate discharge planning to include:

      (1) Appropriate living arrangements

         (a) Family

         (b) Solo

         (c) Halfway house

         (d) Group home

      (2) Employment/vocational planning

      (3) Referral to psychoeducation programs

         (a) Vocational rehabilitation

         (b) Social skills training

         (c) Mental health education programs

      (4) Referral to day treatment programs

      (5) Referral to support/self help groups

         (a) National Alliance for the Mentally Ill (NAMI)

         (b) Manic-Depressive and Depressive Association

         (c) Recovery, Inc.

b. Professional involvement in advocacy groups, community and professional organizations, self-help groups, political coalitions lobbying for mental health resources and rights

Questions
Select the best answer

1. Susan Z, age 20, was at a bar in the town where she went to college. Always an outgoing, life-of-the-party type, Susan became loud and abusive to people at the bar, jumped on the bar and began doing a strip dance, singing loudly, knocking over everything in sight. The police were called and at the station house, Susan loudly rambled on about how all the women in her family were life-of-the-party types. The community mental health nurse interviewing Susan understands that:

   a. Bipolar disorder does not have a higher rate in families with relatives who have the disorder.
   b. Bipolar disorder does have a higher rate in families with relatives who have the disorder.
   c. Bipolar disorder is inherited.
   d. Bipolar disorder is not recurring.

2. People at highest risk for suicide are:

   a. Married, white males below age 60
   b. Single, white males above age 60
   c. Black males
   d. Males below age 24 and above age 50

3. What percentage of the annual suicides are associated with depression?

   a. 20%
   b. 30%
   c. 50%
   d. 80%

4. Mr. B. has experienced depressed mood and difficulty sleeping over the past six weeks. He reports having no appetite and has lost 15 pounds during this time. Mr. B. describes a loss of interest in most of the activities he used to find pleasurable and a diminished ability to concentrate. Although this is the first time he has felt this way, Mr. B. states that he frequently thinks about taking his life. The Clinical Nurse Specialist would probably give him which of the following diagnoses?

   a. Bipolar disorder, depressed
   b. Major depression, recurrent
   c. Major depression

d. Seasonal affective disorder

5. Mrs. C., age 42, is brought to the hospital by her husband who reports that she has been neglecting her housework and family responsibilities and eating very little. She has not left the house in the past two months and has lost 30 pounds. Mrs. C's history reveals that her 7-month-old daughter recently died of Sudden Infant Death Syndrome (SIDS). She is admitted to the psychiatric unit with a diagnosis of:

   a. Major depression
   b. Bereavement, uncomplicated
   c. Melancholia
   d. Bereavement, complicated

6. In addition to assessment for specific signs and symptoms of major depressive disorder, it is essential for the Clinical Nurse Specialist to assess the patient's ____________ in order to make an accurate differential diagnosis.

   a. prior episodes of unipolar depression or bipolar disorder
   b. risk for suicide
   c. concurrent substance abuse
   d. non-psychiatric physical health problems

7. A priority feature of the assessment process with the depressed patient is:

   a. Assessment of family history
   b. Assessment of suicide risk
   c. Assessment of concurrent substance abuse
   d. Assessment of stressful life events

8. When assessing the depressed patient, a frequently used patient self report questionnaire is:

   a. The Beck Depression Inventory
   b. Hamilton Rating Scale for Depression
   c. Schedule for Affective Disorders and Schizophrenia
   d. Minnesota Multiphasic Personality Inventory

9. An experimental laboratory test to assess levels of norepinephrine in depressed patients prior to initiating pharmacotherapy is:

   a. CBC test
   b. Urinary MHPG test
   c. TRH stimulation test

d. Dexamethasone suppression test

10. Which laboratory test is proposed to differentiate unipolar depression from bipolar disorder?

    a. Urinary MHPG test
    b. Dexamethasone suppression test
    c. TRH and CRH stimulation test
    d. SMAC test

11. At an appointment with the Clinical Nurse Specialist in private practice, Edward K. reports that for the past 3 or 4 years he becomes depressed in October after golf season is finished, begins to feel better in April, and feels totally normal and happy again by May. He says to the nurse, ''Maybe I need other meaningful things in my life.'' The CNS would probably give him which of the following diagnoses?

    a. Major depression, recurrent
    b. Major depression
    c. Uncomplicated bereavement
    d. Seasonal Affective Disorder

12. Marcia S., age 53, describes herself as being depressed for as long as she can remember. She describes it as ''living under a gray cloud.'' Three weeks ago, Marcia describes waking up feeling like the gray cloud turned black. She feels sad, hopeless, worthless, guilty about something she cannot identify, and pessimistic about things getting better for her. The nurse would probably give her which of the following diagnoses?

    a. Dysthymia
    b. Double depression
    c. Depression, recurrent type
    d. Depression, melancholic type

13. Karen K. called the office of the Clinical Specialist in private practice saying she had to have an appointment now or she was going to fall apart. During the assessment interview, Karen described herself as becoming increasingly depressed following the birth of her first child nine months ago in April. At first she felt blue, then increasingly despondent, sleeping a lot, hardly able to get out of a chair, crying all the time. She is now fearful that she might hurt the baby if she doesn't get some help. The CNS would probably give her which diagnosis?

a. Major depression
b. Major depression, melancholic type
c. Major depression, psychotic type
d. Major depression, postpartum type

14. Carl W., 60 years old, has been hospitalized on a medical unit for various aches and pains he has been experiencing for several weeks. He feels depressed, tense and unable to sleep at night. In talking to the nurse, he reveals that his wife died 8 months ago and he has not adjusted to the loss. To maximize the opportunity to determine the extent of Mr. W's bereavement versus depression, the nurse should:

    a. Ask the internist for a psychiatric consultation for Mr. W. as soon as possible
    b. Continue the discussion about his wife's death
    c. Explore his ambivalence toward his wife
    d. Inform the head nurse about Mr. W's feelings

15. D, age 33, is brought to the local hospital by her husband who tells the nurse that she has been involved in a whirl wind of activity that began several months ago when she quit her job to write the "Great American Novel." At the same time, she began painting her house. When he tried to get her to slow down, her activity just increased, taking little time to sleep or eat, and began spending huge amounts of money. Her husband brought her to the hospital following a call from the bank informing him that she had just tried to cash a check for $500,000. On admission, D. is agitated, speaking loudly and challenging the nurse.
    The nurse would probably give D. which of the following diagnoses?

    a. Bipolar Disorder: Depressed Phase
    b. Bipolar Disorder: Manic Phase
    c. Bipolar Disorder: Hypomanic Phase
    d. Bipolar Disorder: Recurrent Type

16. Two days ago, G. arrived on the psychiatric unit in a manic episode, exhibiting extreme excitement, disorientation, incoherent speech, agitation, frantic, aimless physical activity, and grandiose delusions. Which assessment finding is most characteristic of this stage of mania?

    a. Expansive mood
    b. Depressed mood
    c. Hypersomnia
    d. Low self-esteem

17. Jason King, age 55, is admitted to the psychiatric unit of the general hospital. His wife states that he has gradually become withdrawn over the last month, refusing to bathe or change clothes, eating little, failing to go to work and sleeping only 3 to 4 hours per night. This evening Mrs. King heard a shot from the basement and found Mr. King bleeding from a superficial chest wound.
To assess Mr. King's current potential for suicide, the nurse should:

    a. Ask Mr. King why he feels like killing himself
    b. Observe Mr. King for scars on his wrists or other signs of previous attempts
    c. Ask Mrs. King about any previous suicide attempts or threats by Mr. King.
    d. Determine if there is a family history of suicide

18. To further assess Mr. King's suicide potential, the CNS should be particularly alert to his expression of:

    a. Frustration and impatience
    b. Anger and resentment
    c. Anxiety and loneliness
    d. Helplessness and hopelessness

19. The neurotransmitter hypothesis proposes that depression occurs as a result of:

    a. Depletion of dopamine at the post-synaptic receptor site
    b. Depletion of norepinephrine at the post-synaptic receptor site
    c. Disturbance in regulation of biological rhythms
    d. Shift in melatonin production and secretion

20. The kindling hypothesis proposes that in bipolar disorder, manic phase, patients have daily subthreshold electrical stimulation producing seizure like activity including all of the following, except:

    a. Tonic movements
    b. Auras
    c. Irritability
    d. Rapid mood swing

21. The circadian rhythm hypothesis proposes that people with unipolar depression may:

    a. Be in a chronic state of sleep satiety
    b. Have chronic hypo arousal
    c. Have REM phase delay

d. Be in an acute state of hypersomnia

22. The circadian rhythm hypothesis proposes that people with unipolar depression may:

    a. Be in a chronic state of somnolence
    b. Have a disturbance in regulation of biological rhythms
    c. Have circadian rhythms that occur at a time late for sleep onset
    d. Be in a chronic state of under arousal

23. Based on an understanding of the psychoanalytic theory of depression, the nurse can best help a patient develop more healthy coping mechanisms by:

    a. Promoting interpersonal relationships with peers
    b. Allowing her to assume responsibility for her decisions
    c. Promoting the external expression of anger
    d. Setting realistic limits on her maladaptive behavior

24. When assessing a depressed person's premorbid personality characteristics, the nurse would expect that he/she demonstrated:

    a. Vulnerability to loss
    b. Overmeticulousness
    c. Stubbornness
    d. Vulnerability to anger

25. Blanche, 26 years old, is admitted to the psychiatric unit with a diagnosis of bipolar disorder, manic episode. She is brought in by her husband, who states that she was fine until 3 days before admission. At that time she decided to plan a huge high school reunion and began calling all her classmates. Her speech became louder, more rapid, and insulting when the idea was not greeted with enthusiasm. Yesterday she went on a shopping spree and charged clothing worth $7000. This morning she went into her husband's office and began reorganizing his files. She became quite agitated, and her husband brought her to the emergency room.
    In assessing Blanche, the nurse is aware that the manic episode is in reality an:

    a. Attempt to block unconscious feelings of depression
    b. Incorrect interpretation of environmental stimuli
    c. Exaggerated response to an elating situation
    d. Uncontrolled acting out of uncensored id drives

26. Laurie M., age 32, is married and is a very successful attorney. She and her

husband have a Victorian house they have restored. They ski, play tennis and have an active social life. Yet Laurie reports feeling depressed all the time. She perceives her self as ''never measuring up.'' Despite having friends, she thinks they are only nice to her because they like her husband. She never enjoys the sports she does, because she never performs as well as she thinks she should. According to cognitive theory, Laurie's symptoms are most likely related to:

a. Logical errors
b. Negative feedback
c. Developmental trauma
d. Distorted self-concept

27. Laurie's cognitive, affective, and behavior patterns are maintained by irrational beliefs and rules called:

a. Logical errors
b. Silent assumptions
c. Cognitive distortions
d. Developmental trauma

28. Ted H., age 26, dropped out of college once, failed out twice, and currently works nights as a janitor in a factory. Both Ted and his family regard him as the family disappointment. Ted calls the mental health clinic because he feels depressed and very worried that he is going to lose his job. He states that his company is laying people off, and despite good evaluations, he knows that he will, as usual, be one of the unlucky who get fired.
According to the Hopelessness Theory of Depression, the Clinical Nurse Specialist understands that Ted's symptoms are most likely to occur when negative life events are perceived to be:

a. Stable, global, important
b. Unstable, global, important
c. Stable, specific, important
d. Unstable, global, important

29. Ted's ability to affect the outcome of potentially negative life events, like losing his job, is perceived by him to be:

a. Nonexistent
b. Low
c. Moderate
d. High

30. Fran S., age 57, is brought to the hospital Emergency Department by her daughter. She sits crying in a chair saying, ''how much can a person take? I cannot take anymore.'' Her daughter reports that Mrs. S's husband was killed in a car accident 3 years ago and her 80-year-old mother was diagnosed with Alzheimers last year. Six months ago, her son revealed that he is homosexual and last week told the family that he has been HIV positive for 3 years and was just diagnosed as having Kaposi's sarcoma. Since that time, Fran has been mute other than when she is crying and muttering. She refuses to eat, bathe, or change her clothes. She has not slept more than 3 hours a night and says she just wants to crawl under a cover and not come out.
The Clinical Nurse Specialist understands that Fran's depression may be precipitated by:
    a. Cluster stress events
    b. Anniversary reaction
    c. Stress reaction
    d. Lack of social support

31. If Fran S. began to feel depressed around the time of year when her husband was killed, this would be called a(n):
    a. Nodal event
    b. Stress reaction
    c. Anniversary reaction
    d. Life cycle stressor

32. Bipolar patients frequently report family relationship patterns that consist of:
    a. Open communication patterns
    b. Realistic expectations
    c. Closed communication patterns
    d. Unrealistic expectations

33. When a manic patient exhibits extreme excitement, disorientation, frantic, aimless physical activity and grandiose delusions, which nursing diagnostic category would hold the highest priority?
    a. Ineffective individual coping
    b. Hopelessness
    c. Potential for self-harm
    d. Personal identity disturbance

34. Carl W., age 70, is hospitalized for depression. His wife died one year ago. He

has felt sad and tense ever since. He has lost 40 pounds this year, has difficulty getting up in the morning, has missed numerous days of work and says to the nurse, ''What's the use of talking? I'd rather be dead. I can't go on without my wife.''

The Clinical Nurse Specialist makes the nursing diagnosis of dysfunctional grieving associated with the loss of his wife. She makes this nursing diagnosis because of Mr. W's:

a. Prolonged period of grief and mourning after his wife's death
b. Difficulty expressing his loss
c. Inability to talk about his loss
d. Inability to sleep and symptoms of depression

35. The initial objective of pharmacological intervention in unipolar depression or bipolar disorder:

a. Symptom reduction
b. Improved function
c. Recurrence prevention
d. All of the above

36. The role of the nurse in pharmacological interventions that facilitates post discharge compliance with the medication regimen is:

a. Collection of assessment data
b. Coordination of treatment modalities
c. Monitoring of side effects
d. Patient education

37. M., a depressed patient, is started on imipramine (Tofanil) 75 mg orally at bedtime. The nurse should tell the patient that:

a. The medication may be habit forming, so it will be discontinued as soon as she feels better.
b. The medication has no serious side effects.
c. She should avoid eating such foods as aged cheese, yoghurt and red wine while taking the medication.
d. The medication may initially cause some tiredness, which should become less bothersome over time.

38. M., a depressed patient, will be started on a tricyclic antidepressant. The Clinical Nurse Specialist understands that this type of medication:

a. Decreases reuptake of neurotransmitters

b. Increases reuptake of neurotransmitters
c. Increases metabolism of neurotransmitters
d. Regulates the frontal cortex where norepinephrine is made.

39. D., a severely depressed patient, has not responded to tricyclic antidepressants. Prior to beginning ECT, a decision is made to initiate a trial of another antidepressant. The drug family of choice would be:

a. Heterocyclics
b. Monoamine oxidase inhibitors (MAOIs)
c. Selective Serotonin Reuptake Inhibitors (SSRIs)
d. Lithium

40. The physician orders tranylcypromine sulfate (Parnate) for D. The nurse would be aware that D. understood the teaching about the drug when the patient states, "While taking the medicine, I should avoid eating":

a. Fish
b. Red meat
c. Citrus fruit
d. Processed cheese

41. The nurse should teach a depressed patient on MAOIs that failure to adhere to dietary restrictions can result in:

a. Hyperglycemic episodes
b. Bradycardia
c. Hypertensive crisis
d. Snycope

42. A Clinical Nurse Specialist orders lithium carbonate 300 mg four times a day and chlorpromazine 100 mg four times a day for a manic patient who has just been admitted to the inpatient psychiatric unit exhibiting extreme excitement, disorientation, frantic, aimless activity, and grandiose delusions. Which statement best explains the reason for ordering chlorpromazine?

a. A lower dose of lithium can be given.
b. Chlorpromazine helps control the manic symptoms until the lithium takes effect.
c. Joint administration makes both drugs more effective.
d. Joint administration decreases the risk of lithium toxicity.

43. The physician plans to order lithium carbonate for a manic patient. Before beginning the lithium treatment regimen, the nurse performs a physical assessment. She is aware that lithium is contraindicated when a patient exhibits dysfunction of the:

    a. Renal system
    b. Reproductive system
    c. Endocrine system
    d. Respiratory system

44. Early signs of lithium toxicity include:

    a. Coarse tremors, ataxia, drowsiness, diarrhea
    b. Ataxia, confusion, and seizures
    c. Elevated white blood cell count and orthostatic hypotension
    d. Restlessness, shuffling gait, and involuntary muscle movements

45. One week after a manic patient begins taking lithium, this nurse notes that his serum lithium level is 1 mEq/liter. How should the nurse respond?

    a. Call the physician immediately to report the laboratory results.
    b. Observe the patient closely for signs of lithium toxicity.
    c. Withhold the next dose and repeat the blood work.
    d. Continue administering the medication as ordered.

46. A second-line pharmacologic treatment modality for mood stabilization of bipolar disorder is:

    a. Benzodiazapines
    b. Neuroleptics
    c. Anti-Convulsants
    d. Hypnotics

47. Two weeks after a manic patient begins taking carbamezapine (Tegretol), the nurse notes that her serum Tegretol level is 14 mg/l. How should the Clinical Nurse Specialist respond?

    a. Call the physician immediately to report the laboratory results.
    b. Observe the patient closely for signs of toxicity.
    c. Withhold the next dose and notify the physician.
    d. Continue administering the medication as ordered.

48. M., a patient with severe depression, does not respond to several trials of antidepressant medications. At a team conference, a decision is made to initiate a

series of electro convulsive therapy (ECT) treatments. When should nursing intervention begin?

a. As soon as the patient and family are presented with this treatment alternative
b. The night before ECT is scheduled
c. Immediately after ECT is administered
d. When the patient returns to the unit after ECT therapy

49. The interdisciplinary team is considering electro convulsive therapy (ECT) treatments for M., a patient with severe depression. The Clinical Nurse Specialist knows that which of the following are appropriate indications for ECT as a treatment approach:

a. Emergency therapy for suicidal patients.
b. Patients who are unresponsive to antidepressants.
c. Use during time lag between initiation of pharmacotherapy and onset of effectiveness.
d. All of the above.

50. The most distressing side effect of ECT is:

a. Memory loss
b. Ataxia
c. Hypotension
d. Hyponatremia

51. The most serious side effect of ECT is:

a. Memory loss
b. Cardiac arrhythmias
c. Hypotension
d. Agitation

52. The most effective approach to meeting a manic patient's hydration and nutrition needs would be to:

a. Leave finger foods and liquids in her room and let her eat and drink as she moves about.
b. Bring her to the dining room and encourage her to sit and eat with calm, quiet companions.
c. Explain mealtime routines and allow her to make her own decisions about eating.
d. Provide essential nutrition through high-calorie tube feedings.

53. A depressed patient has difficulty sleeping at night. She reports feeling fatigued and unrefreshed. The nurse should NOT encourage the patient to:

   a. Limit intake of caffeinated drinks
   b. Take sedatives hs
   c. Take daytime naps
   d. Receive back rubs

54. The nursing staff request a consultation with the Clinical Nurse Specialist about a manic patient who demonstrates resistive behavior in relation to hygiene activities. He refuses to bathe, brush his teeth, or change his clothes. The CNS suggests which of the following interventions?

   a. Matter of factly assist with hygiene activities
   b. Ignore the behavior
   c. Confront the patient about his behavior
   d. Suggest that his medication be augmented with a neuroleptic

55. Andrew M., age 42, is brought to the psychiatric unit by his parents and a sister who states, ''He's just not himself since his wife died two years ago. He has no interests and doesn't care for himself any more, just sitting alone when he's not working. The nurse discusses the plan of care with Andrew. The nurse recognizes that it would be most helpful to:

   a. Involve him in outdoor group games each day.
   b. Encourage him to do relaxation exercises.
   c. Encourage him to talk about and plan for the future.
   d. Talk with him about his wife and the details of her death.

56. Andrew attends group therapy in which the Clinical Nurse Specialist is the leader. During one session, another client talks about his wife leaving and his feeling of abandonment. When the members are leaving the session, the CNS notices that tears are running down Andrew's face.
Considering his problems, the CNS should:

   a. Ask the group members to return and discuss Andrew's feelings.
   b. Observe Andrew's behavior carefully over the next few hours.
   c. Go to Andrew's room and ask him to discuss his thoughts and feelings.
   d. Ask another patient to stay and spend time talking with Andrew.

57. In planning activities for Mr. R., a depressed patient, the nurse finds him very resistive and complaining about his inadequacies and worthlessness. The best approach by the nurse would be to:

a. Involve Mr. R. in activities in which he will be assured of success.
b. Listen to Mr. R. and delay the planned activity for another time.
c. Schedule activities that Mr. R. can complete independently.
d. Encourage Mr. R. to select an activity in which he has some interest.

58. Which of the following responses reflects a cognitive approach to dealing with low self-esteem?

    a. For each negative trait you list about yourself, I will ask you to give me a positive trait.
    b. Can you recall six positive things about yourself?
    c. What do you think interferes with your ability to view yourself in a positive manner?
    d. What do you think would enable you to see yourself in a positive way?

59. D., age 33, was brought to the hospital by her husband following a call from the bank informing him that she had just tried to cash a check for $500,000 in an account that had a $5 balance. D.'s husband states that she has hardly slept or eaten in the past two weeks. On admission, D. is agitated, speaking loudly and challenging the nurse. Which approach would be most therapeutic in working with D.?

    a. Teaching the patient about banking procedures.
    b. Confronting the patient about her unappropriate behavior.
    c. Kindly but firmly guiding the patient into such activities as bathing and eating.
    d. Showing the patient that she is in a controlled environment.

60. When consulting with the nursing staff about the development of a standardized care plan for manic clients that reflect behavioral interventions, the CNS suggests that the following are important to consider when designing interventions EXCEPT:

    a. Attention span
    b. Distractability
    c. Unit resources
    d. Medication supply

61. Ms. W. is admitted to the psychiatric unit with a diagnosis of severe depression. One morning, Ms. W. said to the nurse, "God is punishing me for my past sins." The nurse's best response is:

    a. "God is punishing you for your sins, Ms. W.?"

b. ‘‘Why do you think that, Ms. W.?’’
c. ‘‘You really seem upset about this’’
d. ‘‘What sins would he be punishing you for?’’

62. Ms. W. tells the nurse that she has an unhappy marriage and has had several affairs. Although she feels that her husband ignores her, she blames herself for having had these affairs. The most appropriate response to assist Ms. W. in exploring her thoughts and feelings is:

a. ‘‘Help me to understand how these affairs are all your fault?’’
b. ‘‘Tell me why the affairs are your fault.’’
c. ‘‘It sounds like your husband ignores you. Who could blame you for having an affair?’’
d. ‘‘Tell me about your husband.’’

63. James R., a manic patient, is approaching discharge. He is to be discharged on lithium carbonate. In the family teaching plan for discharge, the nurse should stress the importance of:

a. Watching his diet to avoid aged cheese, yogurt, and caffeinated beverages.
b. Taking the pills with milk
c. Having a CBC done once a month
d. Having his blood levels checked as ordered.

64. The Clinical Nurse Specialist is meeting with a group of recurrent bipolar patients and their families. A key preventive intervention designed to maintain family function is:

a. Recognition of relapse signs and symptoms
b. Referral for family therapy
c. Referral to NAMI
d. Recognition of early signs of lithium toxicity

65. Mrs. K. is admitted to the psychiatric unit following a suicide attempt. Mrs. K. does not answer any of the nurses’ questions. To assess Mrs. K’s current potential for suicide, the nurse should:

a. Ask Mrs. K. why she feels like killing herself.
b. Observe Mrs. K. for scars on her wrists or other signs of previous attempts.
c. Ask Mr. K. about any previous suicide attempts or threats by Mrs. K.
d. Determine if there is a family history of suicide.

66. In teaching an orientation group about nursing care of the suicidal patient, the Clinical Nurse Specialist teaches that the suicidal risk for a depressed patient is often greatest:

    a. When the depression is most severe.
    b. Before any kind of somatic treatment is started.
    c. When the patient begins to express anger.
    d. When the patient makes a sudden and dramatic improvement.

67. A manic patient is assigned to a private room that is somewhat removed from the nurse's station. The primary reason for this room assignment is:

    a. Decreased environmental stimuli
    b. Prevent the patient's excessive activity from disturbing others
    c. Deter the patient from disturbing the nurses
    d. Provide the patient with a quiet environment for thinking about his problems

68. On the unit, a manic patient is elated and sarcastic. She is constantly cursing and using foul language. She has the other clients on the units terrified. The Clinical Nurse Specialist, who has been asked to consult in the management of this patient, advises the staff to:

    a. Demand that she stop what she is doing.
    b. Firmly tell her that her behavior is unacceptable.
    c. Ask her what is bothering her.
    d. Increase her medication or have additional medication ordered.

Answers

1. b
2. b
3. c
4. c
5. a
6. b
7. b
8. a
9. b
10. c
11. d
12. a
13. d
14. b
15. b
16. a
17. c
18. d
19. b
20. a
21. a
22. b
23. c
24. a
25. a
26. a
27. b
28. a
29. a
30. a
31. c
32. d
33. c
34. d
35. d
36. d
37. d
38. a
39. b
40. d
41. c
42. b
43. a
44. a
45. d
46. c
47. c
48. a
49. d
50. a
51. b
52. a
53. c
54. a
55. d
56. c
57. a
58. a
59. c
60. d
61. c
62. a
63. d
64. a
65. c
66. d
67. a
68. b

Bibliography

Agency for Healthcare Policy and Research (1993). *Depression in primary care,* vol. 1. Detection and diagnosis and vol. 2. *Treatment of major depression.* Rockville, MD: U.S. Department of Health and Human Services. AHCPR Publication No. 93-0551.

American Psychiatric Association (1993). *DSM-IV draft criteria.* Washington, DC: American Psychiatric Association.

Arana, G. W., & Hyman, S. E. (1991). *Handbook of psychiatric drug therapy* (2nd ed.). Toronto, Canada: Little, Brown and Company.

Bertrus, P. A., & Elmore, S. K. (1991). Seasonal affective disorder, part I: A review of the neural mechanisms for psychosocial nurses. *Archives of Psychiatric Nursing.* 5(6), 357–364.

Bezchlibnyk-Butler, K. Z., & Jeffries, J. J. (1991). *Clinical handbook of psychotropic drugs* (3rd ed.). Lewiston, NY: Hogrefe & Huber Publishers.

Gold, P. W., Goodwin, F. K., & Chrousos, G. P. (1988). Clinical and biochemical manifestations of depression—part one. *New England Journal of Medicine.* 319, 348–353.

Goodwin, F. K., & Jamison, K. R. (1990). *Manic-depressive illness.* New York: Oxford University Press.

Haber, J., Leach-McMahon, A., Price-Hoskins, P., & Sideleau, B. F. (1992). *Comprehensive psychiatric nursing* (4th ed.). St. Louis: C. V. Mosby Co.

Simmons-Ailing, S. (1987). New approaches to managing affective disorders. *Archives of Psychiatric Nursing.* 1(4), 219–224.

Stuart, G. W., & Sundeen, S.J. (1991). *Principles and practice of psychiatric nursing* (4th ed.). St. Louis: C. V. Mosby Co.

Ugarriza, D.N. (1992). Postpartum affective disorders. *Journal of Psychosocial Nursing.* 30(5), 29–31.

Behavioral Syndromes and Disorders of Adult Personality

Richardean Benjamin-Coleman

Eating Disorders

Fear of obesity and the pursuit of thinness represent the driving force in both Anorexia and Bulimia Nervosa, two of the most common eating disorders (Abraham & Llewellyn-Jones, 1992; Meades, 1993).

Anorexia Nervosa

- Definition/Symptoms
    1. Refusal to eat
    2. Intense fear of gaining weight or becoming fat
    3. Weight less than 85% of expected weight
    4. Distorted body image
    5. At least 3 consecutive missed menstrual periods
    6. Excessive exercising
    7. Preoccupation with food
    8. Bodily changes
        a. Emaciated appearance
        b. Lanugo growth on face, extremities and trunk
        c. Bradycardia, hypotension, arrhythmias
        d. Delayed gastric motility
        e. Dry skin, dry and falling hair
    9. Laboratory changes
        a. Leukopenia
        b. Mild anemia
        c. Low serum potassium
        d. Elevated blood urea nitrogen
        e. High serum calcium levels that may indicate that osteoporosis is occurring, and renal calculi may result
- Mental status variations
    1. Mood and affect
        a. Dysphoric mood with crying spells

   b. Emotionally labile
2. Sleep disturbance (insomnia or hypersomnia)
3. Thought processes
   a. Distorted body image
   b. Delusional thinking about body size
   c. Concrete thinking
   d. Overpowering fear of losing control
   e. Hypochondriasis
   f. Obsession with food and cooking
   g. Compulsive
4. Appearance—emaciated
5. Defense mechanisms
   a. Repression
   b. Regression
   c. Denial
   d. Manipulation—untruthful about food intake and methods of losing weight
6. Impaired judgment related to food
7. Impaired insight
   a. Intellectualization
   b. Perfectionistic

- Psychotherapeutic interventions
  1. Individual psychotherapy
     a. Establish realistic thinking process.
     b. Increase self-esteem.
     c. Establish a healthy sense of control and autonomy.
     d. Deal with underlying psychologic conflicts.
  2. Cognitive/behavior therapy
     a. Establish contract.

   b. Describe expected behaviors.
   c. Eliminate power struggle.
   d. Need consistency from staff to coordinate treatment.
   e. Confront if client caught cheating.
3. Teach relaxation.

- Family dynamics/family therapy
  1. Family systems dysfunction
     a. Rigidity
     b. Enmeshment
     c. Overprotectiveness
     d. Psychosomatic symptoms maintained to avoid conflict
  2. Power and control issues
  3. High value placed on perfectionism
  4. Parental criticism promotes perfectionistic and obsessive behavior in child
  5. Feelings of helplessness and ambivalence
  6. Perceived loss of control in life
  7. Family unable to resolve problems which arise with the family
  8. Need "sick" member to enable the other family members to communicate with each other

- Milieu approaches
  1. Provide for safety and physical needs.
  2. Sit with and observe during and 60 minutes after meals.
  3. Counteract effects of starvation by promoting weight gain and restoring normal nutritional balance.
  4. Include dietitian in treatment plan.
  5. Encourage client to share feelings with staff.
  6. Maintain consistency among staff members.
  7. Document intake and output.

8. Avoid discussing food or eating with client once protocol established.
9. Use behavioral reinforcement.
10. Provide group interaction with peers.
11. Adolescent development issues

- Treatment objectives

1. Increase weight to normal range.
2. Help client re-establish normal eating behavior, avoid excessive exercise, self-induced vomiting or laxative abuse.
3. Explain physical symptoms in a way which is understood by the client.
4. In hospital, give client opportunity to be responsible for own weight gain and reward for conforming to treatment regimen.

Bulimia Nervosa

- Symptoms

1. Recurrent episodes of binge eating
2. Self-induced vomiting or abuses laxatives/diuretics
3. Dieting/fasting or excessive exercise to control weight
4. Weight usually within normal range
5. Dehydration, electrolyte imbalance
6. Gastric acid in vomitus contributes to erosion of tooth enamel
7. Psychoactive substance abuse/dependence
8. Perceived inability to control binging
9. Average of at least 2 binges a week for at least 3 months
10. Depressed mood and self-deprecatory thoughts following binges
11. Exaggerated concern about body shape and weight
12. Enlargement of face and cheeks due to swelling of salivary glands
13. Changes in EKG—cardiac arrhythmias leading to renal problems

- Mental status variations

1. Judgment and insight
    a. Recognizes eating behavior is abnormal
    b. Problems with impulse control (stealing, drug and/or alcohol abuse, self-mutilation, suicide attempt)
    c. Manipulative and untruthful
    d. Difficulty identifying and dealing with emotions
2. Thought processes
    a. Overly concerned with body shape and weight
    b. Obsessional ideas
3. Mood—depressed (feels sad and lonely, empty and isolated with self-criticism and guilt feelings)
4. Orientation—lethargy and confusion due to extreme dehydration caused by self-induced vomiting and excessive use of laxatives

- Psychotherapeutic interventions
    1. Cognitive therapy
    2. Family therapy
    3. Relaxation
    4. Supportive psychotherapy
    5. Behavior therapy
        a. Positive reinforcement
        b. Informational feedback
        c. Progressive desensitization focusing on feelings prior to an episode of binge eating
- Family dynamics—family environment chaotic, conflictual with marital discord and hostility
- Milieu interventions
    1. Behavioral diaries
    2. Express feelings—gain insight into eating behavior.
    3. Reinforce healthy coping.
    4. Teach to recognize cues for hunger and satiation.

5. Limit exercising in treatment to decrease in-hospital stays and cost of treatment.
6. Avoid keeping food records, weighing frequently, constantly counting calories, cooking for others and reading recipes.

- Differential Diagnoses for Anorexia and Bulimia
    1. Depressive disorders
        a. Absence of distorted body image
        b. Absence of intense fear of obesity
        c. True loss of appetite
    2. Schizophrenic disorders
        a. Bizarre eating patterns present without eating disorder syndrome or concern with the caloric content of food
        b. Absence of hyperactivity seen in anorectic client
        c. True loss of appetite
    3. Medical illnesses
        a. Hyperthyroidism
        b. Neoplasms
        c. Anemia
        d. Diabetes mellitus
    4. Borderline personality disorder
- Nursing Diagnoses for Anorexia and Bulimia (Krupnick & Wade, 1993)
    1. Body image disturbance
    2. Fluid volume deficit—high risk
    3. Anxiety (moderate to severe)
    4. Altered nutrition—less than body requirements
        a. Nursing interventions
            (1) Implement behavioral modification protocol for gradual weight gain.
            (2) Supervise meals to ensure adequate intake of nutrients.

(3) In collaboration with dietitian, determine number of calories required to provide adequate nutrition and weight gain.

(4) Sit with client during mealtime for support and to observe amount ingested.

(5) Strictly document intake and output.

(6) Weigh client daily upon arising.

(7) Once nutritional status is stable explore with client feelings associated with fears.

(8) Observe weighing activity to assure that client is not secreting weights to falsify data.

b. Outcome criteria

(1) Client has achieved and maintained at least 85 percent of expected body weight.

(2) Vital signs, blood pressure, and laboratory serum studies are within normal limits.

(3) Client verbalizes importance of adequate nutrition.

- Genetic/Biological Theories for Anorexia and Bulimia
  1. Decreased hypothalamic norepinephrine activation
  2. Dysfunction of lateral hypothalamus
  3. Abnormal dexamethasone suppression test findings
  4. Bulimics may have a low serum serotonin level.
  5. Hereditary predisposition
  6. Excess endorphins shutting down the feeding system and inhibiting release initiating amenorrhea
  7. Chronic deficit of endorphins initiating feeding to stimulate this down regulated system
- Biochemical Approaches for Anorexia and Bulimia
  1. No specific medications for eating disorders
  2. Medications may be given for associated symptoms such as depression or anxiety
  3. Bulimia with Atypical Depression—Parnate 30 to 40mg/day

- Intrapersonal Theories for Anorexia and Bulimia
  1. Unresolved conflicts during childhood
  2. Inconsistent parental response to child's needs
  3. Disturbance of self-esteem
  4. Food serves as a means to express feelings.
  5. Anorexia—separation, individuation, and control issues
  6. Independence/dependence struggle between woman and parent(s)
  7. Avoidance of sexuality
- Group Approaches for Anorexia and Bulimia
  1. Types
     a. Supportive
     b. Self-help
     c. Small group therapy
     d. Support group for parents
  2. Group functions
     a. Foster self-esteem
     b. Gain insight
     c. Share concerns
     d. Provide constructive support from peers
- Family therapy for Anorexia and Bulimia
  1. Education of members about the disorder
  2. Support family as they deal with guilt and stigma of having member with disorder.
  3. Focus on fostering open, healthy interaction patterns.
- Community resources for Anorexia and Bulimia
  1. Eating disorder groups
  2. Family support groups
  3. Twelve-step programs

Sexual and Gender Identity Disorders

Paraphilias

Repetitive or preferred sexual fantasies or behaviors that involves giving or receiving pain, or activity with a nonconsenting partner, to experience full sexual arousal and satisfaction (Wilson & Kneisl, 1992)

- Definitions
  1. Fetishism—uses clothing as source of sexual arousal
  2. Exhibitionism—exposes genitals in public
  3. Frotteurism—body contact with strangers in public places
  4. Pedophilia—sexual contact with prepubescent child
  5. Sexual masochism—receives physical/mental pain from sexual partner
  6. Sexual sadism—inflicts physical/mental pain on sexual partner
  7. Transvestic fetishism—recurrent cross-dressing by heterosexual male
  8. Voyeurism—watching others undressing/engaged in sexual activity
- Differential diagnoses
  1. Nonpathogenic sexual experimentation
  2. Rule out public urination
  3. Rule out exposure as prelude to sexual activity with child
  4. Rule out poor judgment due to
     a. Mental retardation
     b. Organic personality syndrome
     c. Alcohol intoxication
     d. Schizophrenia
- Mental status variations
  1. Inadequate social skills
  2. Depressed mood and anxiety accompany the behaviors.
- Genetic/biological theories

1. Limbic system or temporal lobe abnormalities
2. Abnormal levels of androgens

- Biochemical approaches
  1. Antiandrogenics—Medroxyprogesterone—5mg to 10mg/day induces a reversible chemical castration
- Intrapersonal theories
  1. Unresolved Oedipal Complex leading to identification with opposite gender parent or object for libido cathexis
  2. Castration anxiety
- Psychotherapeutic interventions
  1. Psychodynamic psychotherapy
     a. Explore thoughts, feelings, and behavior that precede paraphiliac behavior in order to control occurrences
     b. Eliminate anxiety or depression that accompanies behavior
  2. Behavior therapy
     a. Systematic desensitization
     b. Aversive techniques
  3. Combination of psychodynamic and behavioral techniques
- Milieu approaches—nurse's role is primarily associated with prevention of problems, which focuses on the development of adaptive coping strategies to deal with stressful life events.

Gender Identity Disorder

- Definition: Persistent discomfort with one's assigned gender and a feeling that it is inappropriate or inaccurate (Blanchard & Steiner, 1990)
- SIgns and Symptoms—DSM-IV Criteria (APA, 1993)
  1. A strong and persistent cross-gender identification (not merely a desire for any perceived cultural advantages of being the other sex)
     a. In children, manifested by at least four of the following:
        (1) Repeatedly stated desire to be, or insistence that he or she is, the other sex

(2) In boys, preference for cross-dressing or simulating female attire; in girls, insistence on wearing only stereotypical masculine clothing

(3) Strong and persistent preferences for cross-sex roles in make-believe play or persistent fantasies of being the other sex

(4) Intense desire to participate in the stereotypical games and pastimes of the other sex

(5) Strong preference for playmates of the other sex

b. In adolescents and adults, manifested by symptoms such as

(1) Stated desire to be the other sex

(2) Frequent passing as the other sex

(3) Desire to live or be treated as the other sex

(4) The conviction that one has the typical feelings and reactions of the other sex

2. Persistent discomfort with one's sex or sense of inappropriateness in the gender role of that sex.

a. In children, manifested by any of the following:

(1) In boys, assertion that his penis or testes are disgusting or will disappear or assertion that it would be better not to have a penis

(2) Aversion toward rough-and-tumble play and rejection of male stereotypical toys, games, and activities

(3) In girls, rejection of urinating in a sitting position or assertion that she does not want to grow breasts or menstruate, or marked aversion toward normative feminine clothing.

(4) In adolescents and adults, manifested by symptoms such as preoccupation with getting rid of one's primary and secondary sex characteristics (e.g., request for hormones, surgery, or other procedures to alter physically sexual characteristics to simulate the other sex) or belief that one was born the wrong sex.

3. Not concurrent with a physical intersex condition

4. Clinically significant distress or impairment in social, occupational, or other important areas of functioning.

- Mental status variations
  1. Dysphoric mood
  2. Anxiety
- Genetic/biological theories
  1. Prenatal estrogen and androgen levels favor development of the disorder
  2. Chromosomal abnormalities
- Intrapersonal theories
  1. Physical or psychological loss of the mother that results in separation anxiety in the child
  2. Severe disruption or distortion in mother-son relationship that results in the mother's withdrawal which leads to separation anxiety and feminine behavior
  3. Feminine behavior and/or identification caused by excessive closeness to mother
- Psychotherapeutic interventions
  1. Psychotherapy
     a. Assist to individuate from mother.
     b. Aid in developing diverse perceptions of men and maleness.
     c. Work through loss of the attachment figure.
  2. Behavioral therapy
     a. Systematically arrange that rewards follow sex-appropriate behaviors.
     b. Target behaviors, such as selection of toys and dress-up play, exclusive affiliation with opposite sex, and mannerism.
     c. Enhance behavior deficiencies such as poor athletic ability.
     d. Focus on overt sex-type behaviors rather than gender identity or gender dysphoria.
     e. Provide social attention or social reinforcement

f. Encourage self-monitoring procedures.

- Family dynamics/family therapy
  1. Strong interest in opposite-gender role behavior and weak reinforcement of normative gender-role behavior by parents
  2. Extreme physical and psychological closeness with son by the mother
  3. Parental encouragement of cross-gender behavior—mothers of feminine boys themselves had gender identity conflicts as children which led them to devalue men and masculinity.
  4. Father is physically absent or psychologically peripheral—no counterforce to pathogenic mother-son relationship

Sexual Dysfunctions

- Definitions (APA, 1993)
  1. Male Erectile Disorder—persistent or recurrent inability to maintain an erection until completion of sexual activity
  2. Female Sexual Arousal Disorder—persistent or recurrent inability to attain or maintain an adequate lubrication-swelling response of sexual excitement until completion of the sexual activity
  3. Dyspareunia—pain before, during, and after sexual intercourse
  4. Vaginismus—recurrent or persistent involuntary spasm of the musculature of the outer third of the vagina that interferes with sexual intercourse
  5. Orgasmic Disorder—persistent or recurrent delay in, or absence of, orgasm following a normal sexual excitement phase
  6. Premature Ejaculation—persistent or recurrent ejaculation with minimal sexual stimulation before, upon, or shortly after penetration and before the person wishes it
  7. Hypoactive Sexual Desire Disorder—persistently or recurrently deficient (or absent) sexual fantasies and desire for sexual activity
  8. Sexual Aversion Disorder—persistent or recurrent extreme aversion to and avoidance of all (or almost all), genital sexual contact with a sexual partner
- Differential diagnoses

1. Central nervous system tumors
2. Mood disorder
3. Rape trauma syndrome
4. Neuroendocrine disorders
5. Penile, prostate, or testicular cancer
6. End-stage renal disease

- Mental status variations—affect may be sad, depressed, or anxious
- Genetic/biological theories
  1. Decreased levels of serum testosterone
  2. Elevated levels of prolactin
  3. Physical changes due to
     a. Surgery, aging, or trauma
     b. Drug abuse or medication side effects
     c. Neurological disorders
     d. Infection and poor hygiene
- Intrapersonal theories
  1. Religious orthodoxy
  2. Gender identity or sexual preference
  3. Sexual phobias
  4. Depression
  5. Fear of becoming pregnant
  6. Traumatic sexual experiences in childhood
  7. Negative conditioning that sex is dirty
- Psychotherapeutic interventions
  1. Cognitive therapy—change maladaptive beliefs
  2. Psychodynamic therapy—resolve intrapsychic conflicts
  3. Behavioral therapy
     a. Systemic desensitization
     b. Sensate focus exercises

   c. Masturbatory training
   d. ''Squeeze'' technique for premature ejaculation
4. Marital/sex therapy to treat dysfunctions of sexual response cycle
5. Hypnotherapy

- Milieu approaches
  1. Use nondirective approach in completing assessment.
  2. Use language that is understandable to the client.
  3. Convey attitude of warmth, openness, honesty and objectivity.
  4. Remain nonjudgmental.
- Nursing Diagnoses for Sexual and Gender Identity Disorders (Wilson & Kneisl, 1992)
  1. Altered sexuality patterns
  2. Personal identity disturbance
  3. Sexual dysfunction
     a. Nursing interventions
        (1) Encourage partners to express feelings.
        (2) Help client and partner to learn means of clear and open communication (primary intervention).
        (3) Explore with couple information about sex positions or habits.
        (4) Assist to identify relationship problems.
        (5) Contract to work on problems.
        (6) Provide information about sexual techniques.
        (7) Refer for sex therapy with trained counselor.
     b. Outcome criteria
        (1) Client identifies conflicts that contribute to loss of sexual desire.
        (2) Client resumes sexual activity at level satisfactory to self and partner.

- Family Therapy—Couples/Marital Therapy for Sexual and Identity Disorders
    1. Homework assignments for exercises
    2. Observing and responding to homework
- Group Approaches for Sexual and Identity Disorders
    1. Discussion of problems and concerns
    2. Homework for individual and couple exploration
    3. Group support and reassurance
- Community Resources for Sexual and Identity Disorders
    1. Sex Addicts Anonymous
    2. American Association of Sex Educators, Counselors, and Therapists (AASECT)

Personality Disorders

An enduring pattern of perceiving, relating to, and thinking about the environment and oneself to the extent that it leads to inflexible and maladaptive and either significant functional impairment or subjective distress (APA, 1993)

Antisocial Personality Disorder

- Symptoms
    1. More common in men
    2. History of irresponsibility and impulsiveness
    3. Lacks remorse for actions
    4. Exploits and manipulates others
    5. Self-centered
    6. Anger that leads to hostile outbursts
- Differential diagnoses
    1. Conduct disorder—if person younger than 18 years with characteristic features present

2. Psychoactive substance abuse—episodic behavior associated with alcohol/drug intake
3. Mental retardation—may exhibit remorse due to actions or behavior
4. Schizophrenia—presence of prolonged psychotic episodes
5. Manic episode—mood changes
6. Cyclothymia disorder—alternating hypomanic periods with euthymic periods

- Mental status variations
  1. Absence of anxiety or depression
  2. Suicide threats and somatic preoccupation
  3. Absence of delusions or other signs of irrational thinking
  4. Highly manipulative and untrustworthy
  5. Lacks remorse
- Genetic/biological theories
  1. Hereditary predisposition
  2. Low cortical arousal and reduced level of inhibitory anxiety may play a role
  3. Biochemical approaches (Stein, 1992)
     a. Lithium carbonate—900mg to 1200mg/day
     b. Inderal—160mg to 240mg/day
     c. Side effects—medications are seldom prescribed outside a structured setting because of high risk of abuse by clients with antisocial personality disorder
- Intrapersonal theories—arrest in normal psychologic development with failure to integrate ambivalent feelings originally aroused against the primary caretaker
- Psychotherapeutic interventions
  1. Confrontation of inappropriate behavior
  2. Individual psychotherapy
  3. Structured living with supervision
  4. Outpatient supportive therapy

- Family dynamics/family therapy
    1. Chaotic home environment
    2. Parental deprivation during the first 5 years of life
    3. Presence of intermittent appearance of inconsistent, impulsive parents
    4. Traumatic abandonment experiences
    5. Physical and sexual abuse
- Group therapy
    1. Help client assume responsibility for behaviors.
    2. Confront inappropriate and manipulative behaviors.
    3. Allow client to receive parenting not previously received.
    4. Allow client to tolerate feelings of emptiness, depression, and anxiety.
    5. Develop socially appropriate behavioral responses.
- Community resources
    1. Alcoholics Anonymous
    2. Emotions Anonymous
    3. Narcotics Anonymous

Borderline Personality Disorder

- Symptoms
    1. Two-thirds of those diagnosed are female
    2. Self-mutilation, labile mood
    3. Impulsivity
    4. Outbursts of intense anger and rage
    5. Unstable relationships
    6. Identity confusion
    7. Frantic efforts to avoid real or imagined abandonment

- Differential diagnoses
    1. Cyclothymia—presence of hypomania
    2. Schizophrenia—presence of prolonged psychotic episodes, thought disorder or other signs
    3. Paranoid personalities—extreme suspiciousness
    4. Schizotypes—show marked peculiarities of thinking, strange ideation, and recurrent ideas of reference
- Mental status variations
    1. Affect—mood swings, anxious, depressed
    2. Thought processes
        a. Difficulty concentrating
        b. Suicidal gestures and attempts
    3. Insight lacking—poor judgment
    4. Defense mechanisms
        a. Manipulation
        b. Splitting
        c. Projection
        d. Denial
        e. Rationalization
        f. Idealization
        g. Devaluation
    5. Memory—recent memory disturbance
- Intrapersonal theories
    1. Inconsistent and unpredictable parenting
    2. Unmet need for love
    3. Separation/individuation phase not accomplished
- Psychotherapeutic interventions
    1. Reality oriented therapy favored over in-depth unconscious interpretations

2. Long-term psychotherapy with supportive modifications to develop trust
3. Behavioral therapy—structured living under supervision

- Biochemical approaches
  1. Anticonvulsants—Carbamazepine—200mg bid with food
  2. Antidepressants—Parnate—10-20mg/day maintenance dose
  3. Anti-anxiety—Prozac—20mg/day not to exceed 80mg/day
  4. Antipsychotic
     a. Chlorpromazine 150-500mg/day
     b. Haloperidol 7-12mg/day
- Family dynamics/family therapy
  1. Parent may be critical and rejecting, or
  2. Parent may be suffocating and smothering and interferes with optimal progression of attachment-separation sequences
- Community resources
  1. Day hospital programs
  2. Halfway houses
- Milieu Approaches for Borderline and Antisocial Personality Disorders
  1. Staff develops self-awareness to avoid negative counter-transference.
  2. Establish trusting relationship with client.
  3. Institute safety precautions.
  4. Provide structured supportive and consistent environment.
  5. Apply behavioral limits judiciously.
  6. Assist patient in taking responsibility for consequences of actions.
  7. Assist the client in identifying feelings and in learning how to express them in a socially acceptable manner.
  8. Enhance the client's self-esteem and sense of self-worth.
- Nursing Diagnoses for Borderline and Antisocial Personality Disorders (Haber, McMahon, Price-Hoskins & Sideleau, 1992)

1. Impaired social interaction
2. High risk for violence—directed at others
3. High risk for self-directed violence
    a. Nursing interventions
        (1) Observe client for unsafe behavior.
        (2) Determine suicidal potential.
        (3) Obtain contract not to harm self or others.
        (4) Assist client to recognize and accept consequence of own behavior.
        (5) Act as role model for appropriate expression of feelings.
        (6) Remove all dangerous objects from client's environment.
        (7) Provide physical outlets to redirect anger.
        (8) Provide restrictive measures (e.g., medication, restraints to ensure client safety).
    b. Outcome criteria
        (1) Anxiety level maintained to avoid aggressive acts
        (2) Client recognizes, verbalizes and accepts consequences of own behavior.

- Definitions only will be provided for the following less frequently treated personality disorders (Kaplan, 1988):
    1. Paranoid Personality Disorder—characterized by long-standing suspiciousness and mistrust of people in general
    2. Schizoid Personality Disorder—diagnosed in patients who display a lifelong pattern of social withdrawal—often described as eccentric
    3. Schizotypal Personality Disorder—individuals are strikingly odd or strange, even to laypersons. Magical thinking, peculiar ideas, ideas of reference, illusions, and derealization are part of their everyday world.
    4. Histrionic Personality Disorder—characterized by colorful, dramatic, extroverted behavior in excitable, emotional persons—accompanying their flamboyant presentation, however, is often an inability to maintain deep, long-lasting attachments.

5. Narcissistic Personality Disorder—characterized by a heightened sense of self-importance and grandiose feelings that they are unique in some way
6. Avoidant Personality Disorder—persons show extreme sensitivity to rejection, which may lead to a socially withdrawn life. Behavior is due to shyness rather than desire to be asocial.
7. Dependent Personality Disorder—persons with the disorder subordinate their own needs to those of others, get others to assume responsibility for major areas in their lives, lack confidence, and may experience intense discomfort when alone for more than a brief period of time.
8. Obsessive-Compulsive Personality Disorder—characterized by emotional constriction, orderliness, perseverance, stubbornness, and indecisiveness

Sleep Disorders

Primary Insomnia

- Definition: The inability to obtain adequate sleep not due to any other cause (e.g., psychiatric illness, medical illness, or drug use)
- Differential diagnoses
  1. Physical conditions
  2. Medication—withdrawal from CNS stimulants
  3. Dysthymia—mood disturbance
  4. Cyclothymia—insomnia due to hypomania
  5. Normal aging—changes in sleep pattern
  6. Psychiatric disorder
- Mental status variations
  1. Anxiety
  2. Depression
  3. Appears tired (e.g., tired, sleepy, dark circles under eyes)
- Nursing diagnoses
  1. Ineffective individual coping

2. Sleep pattern disturbance
    a. Nursing Interventions
        (1) Discuss reasons for disturbance.
        (2) Provide a comfortable safe environment.
        (3) Encourage expression of emotions that may affect sleep.
        (4) Provide a variety of stimuli during waking hours.
        (5) Promote self-management of sleep by planning with client sleep-inducing activities.
    b. Outcome criteria
        (1) Express anxieties, worries, and stress.
        (2) Accept that minor interruptions to sleep may exist and not dwell on them.
        (3) Learn techniques to reduce tension.

- Genetic/biological theories
    1. Increased autonomic activity
    2. Increased physiologic activation as evidenced by increased heart rate, core body temperature, skin conductance
    3. Increased levels of stress
    4. Other psychopathology
        a. Mood disorders
        b. Psychoactive substance abuse disorder
    5. Physical disorders that cause pain/discomfort such as arthritis
    6. Hormonal disturbances—angina
    7. Lifestyle that includes frequent changes or irregular sleep-wake patterns
    8. Febrile illness in childhood associated with sleep terror disorder and sleep walking disorder
- Biochemical approaches
    1. Benzodiazepines
        a. Triazolam—.125mg to 0.5mg at hs

   b. Temazepam—15mg to 30mg at hs
2. Barbiturates—Secobarbital 100 to 200mg at hs
3. Nonbenzodiazepine—Meprobamate 800mg at hs
4. Nonbarbiturates—Buspirone 15 to 25mg at hs
5. Chloral derivatives—Chloral hydrate 500 to 2000mg at hs
6. Side effects
   a. Daytime sedation and drowsiness
   b. Decrease in mental and physical responsiveness and efficiency
   c. Dizziness
   d. Fatigue
   e. Light-headedness
   f. Incoordination
   g. Impaired motor performance, judgment and attention
   h. Paradoxical excitement
   i. Antegrade amnesia
   j. Headache, blurred vision, nausea and vomiting, epigastric distress and diarrhea, or weight gain

- Intrapersonal theories
  1. Higher levels of depressed mood and anxiety than normal individuals
  3. Increased cognitive activity for clients without medical or psychiatric disorder other than anxiety caused by stress
- Psychotherapeutic interventions (Bootzin & Perlis, 1992)
  1. Sleep hygiene training
  2. Stimulus control instructions
  3. Sleep restriction
  4. Chronotherapy
  5. Bright light therapy
  6. Relaxation, meditation, biofeedback

7. Cognitive therapy
    a. Alter view of sleep problem
    b. Paradoxical intention with thought stopping and identification of irrational beliefs about sleep

- Family dynamics/family therapy—none described
- Group approaches
    1. Self-hypnosis
    2. Autogenic training
    3. Share concerns.
    4. Gain insight.
- Milieu approaches
    1. Decrease caffeine and alcohol intake during afternoon and evening.
    2. Increase exercise during morning and afternoon.
    3. Encourage use of relaxation techniques.
    4. Discourage daytime naps.
    5. Encourage expression of emotion that might affect sleep.
    6. Eliminate or diminish environmental factors that may disturb sleep.
    7. Encourage patient to get out of bed for alternative activities when unable to fall asleep.
- Community resources
    1. Stress management training
    2. Biofeedback training
    3. Yoga classes
- Definitions only will be provided for the following sleep disorders (APA, 1993):
    1. Narcolepsy—excessive daytime sleepiness and abnormal manifestations of REM sleep
    2. Breathing-related Sleep Disorder—sleep disturbance due to sleep-related breathing difficulties (e.g., sleep apnea or central alveolar hypoventilation syndrome)

3. Circadian Rhythm Sleep Disorder (Sleep-Wake schedule Disorder)—sleep disruption due to mismatch between the sleep-wake schedule required by a person's environment and his/her circadian sleep-wake pattern
4. Sleep Terror Disorder—recurrent episodes of abrupt awakening from sleep without dream recall
5. Sleepwalking Disorder—repeated episodes of arising from bed during sleep and walking about
6. Primary Hypersomnia—excessive sleepiness that resulted in impairment in social, occupational, or other important areas of functioning

Impulse Control Disorders

Characterized by a need or desire that must be satisfied immediately regardless of the consequences (Kaplan & Sadock, 1988)

Intermittent Explosive Disorder

- Definition: Those individuals who have discrete episodes of losing control of aggressive impulses resulting in serious assault or the destruction of property
- Differential diagnoses
  1. Psychotic disorders—violent behavior may result in response to delusions and hallucinations, and there is gross impairment of reality testing.
  2. Organic mental disorder—violent behavior results from confusion.
  3. Antisocial or borderline personality disorder—aggressiveness and impulsivity are part of the client's character and are present between outbursts.
  4. Conduct disorder—presents with a repetitive and resistant pattern of behavior as opposed to an episodic pattern
  5. Intoxication with a psychoactive substance
- Mental status variation
  1. Uncontrolled anger
  2. Impulsivity
  3. Poor judgment

- Genetic/biological theories
  1. Prenatal trauma, infantile seizures, head trauma, encephalitis, and hyperactivity
  2. Disordered brain physiology in the limbic system
  3. Hereditary predisposition
- Biochemical approaches
  1. Lithium—300mg tid—qid
  2. Carbamazepine—200mg bid with food
  3. Oxazepam—10 to 30mg tid or qid
  4. Propranolol—60 to 640mg/day
- Nursing diagnoses for impulse control disorders
  1. Ineffective individual coping
  2. High risk for violence directed toward others
     a. Nursing interventions
        (1) Convey an accepting attitude toward the client.
        (2) Maintain low level of stimuli in client's environment (low lighting, few people, simple decor, low noise level).
        (3) Help client recognize the signs that tension is increasing and ways in which violence can be averted.
        (4) Explain to client that should explosive behavior occur, staff will intervene in whatever way is required (e.g., tranquilizing medication, restraints, isolation) to protect the client and others.
        (5) Help client identify the true object of his/her hostility.
     b. Outcome criteria
        (1) Client will not cause harm to self or others.
        (2) Able to verbalize the symptoms of increasing tension.
        (3) Able to verbalize strategies to avoid becoming violent.
- Intrapersonal theories—early frustration, oppression and hostility as predisposing factors

- Psychotherapeutic interventions—individual psychotherapies have met with little success.
- Family dynamics/family therapy
    1. Early chaotic and violent family environment with heavy drinking, by one or both parents
    2. Parental brutality, child abuse, and emotional and physical unavailability of a father figure
    3. Family therapy helpful when client is adolescent or young adult
- Group approaches/group therapy
    1. Foster group loyalty.
    2. Peer pressure to reinforce expectations and provide confrontation
- Milieu approaches
    1. Provide structured outlets for the energy of anger.
    2. Encourage physical activity that allow large muscle involvement.
        a. Punching bag
        b. Jogging, swimming, weight lifting
    3. External controls
        a. Physical restraints
            (1) Monitor frequently.
            (2) Remove dangerous articles.
            (3) Provide fluids and food.
        b. Indications for use
            (1) Physical assault—self, others, and environment
            (2) Physical and verbal threats
    4. Teach appropriate expression of anger.
    5. Reduce sources of undue anxiety or high levels of anxiety to prevent angry outbursts.
- Community resources—mental health centers

Pathological Gambling

- Definition: Chronic and progressive failure to resist impulses to gamble and gambling behavior that compromises, disrupts, or damages personal, family or vocational pursuits (Kaplan & Sadock, 1988).
- Differential diagnoses
    1. Social gambling—associated with gambling with friends, on special occasions, and with predetermined acceptable and tolerable losses
    2. Manic episode—history of marked mood change and loss of judgment preceding the gambling
    3. Antisocial personality disorder—marked mood changes and loss of judgment preceding the gambling
- Mental status variations
    1. Anxious
    2. Impulsive
    3. Lacks insight
- Genetic/biological theories—fathers of men and mothers of women more likely to have the disorder than the general population
- Biochemical approaches—none recommended
- Intrapersonal theories—inappropriate parental discipline (absence, inconsistency, or harshness)
- Psychotherapeutic interventions
    1. Psychodynamic psychotherapy
    2. Behavior therapy
- Family dynamics—absent, inconsistent, or harsh discipline
- Group approaches
    1. Gamblers Anonymous (GA)
        a. Inspirational group therapy
        b. Public confession
        c. Peer pressure
        d. Reformed gamblers as sponsors to help individuals resist the impulse of gambling

- Milieu approaches—remove client from the environment in order to assist them to gain insight into the problem
- Community resources—Gamblers Anonymous
- Definitions only will be provided for the following impulse control disorders:
  1. Kleptomania—recurrent inability to resist the impulse to steal objects not needed for personal use or their monetary value
  2. Pyromania—the deliberate and purposeful fire setting on more than one occasion; tension or an affective arousal before setting the fires; and intense pleasure, gratification, or relief when setting the fires or seeing the fires burn
  3. Trichotillomania—recurrent failure to resist impulses to pull out one's own hair

Questions

1. The characteristics most typical of bulimia are
    a. Unsuccessful efforts to control weight normally
    b. Persistent overconcern with body shape and weight combined with periods of strict dieting
    c. Self-induced vomiting alternating with periods of normal eating
    d. Episodes of binge eating and self-induced vomiting or other severe weight control methods

2. The clinical nurse specialist is giving an inservice on Bulimia Nervosa. Which of the following would be valid information to present? Families with a member with Bulimia Nervosa are:
    a. Rigid and inflexible
    b. Chaotic
    c. Overprotective
    d. Abusive

3. To assess Constance's eating patterns, what strategy might the nurse use? Ask
    a. "Do you often feel fat?"
    b. "Who plans the family meals?"
    c. "What do you eat in a typical day?"
    d. "What do you think about your present weight?"

4. Based on what is known about Constance, what nursing diagnosis can be established? Alteration in nutrition: less than body requirement related to
    a. Abuse of laxative as evidenced by electrolyte imbalances.
    b. Physical exertion in excess of energy produced through caloric intake as evidenced by weight loss.
    c. Self-induced vomiting as evidenced by swollen glands.
    d. Refusal to eat as evidenced by loss of 15% of body weight.

5. When the clinical nurse specialist engages the family of a client with a diagnosis of Anorexia Nervosa in family therapy, what type of family dynamics might she/he expect to see:
    a. Enmeshment, rigidity, conflict avoidance
    b. Overprotective, abusive, rigid
    c. Impulsive, rigid, perfectionistic
    d. Controlling, impulsive, abusive

6. All of the following would be areas for milieu management of Bulimia Nervosa *except:*
   a. Maintain behavioral diary
   b. Promote exercise
   c. Promote expression of feelings
   d. Develop adaptive coping

7. While conducting an initial assessment the nurse gathered the following sex history; pain before, during and after sexual intercourse. Which of the following nursing diagnoses would be most appropriate for the data described?
   a. Transvestic fetishism
   b. Sexual Arousal Disorder
   c. Sexual Dysfunction
   d. Altered Sexuality Patterns

8. According to the premise of cognitive therapy, which of the following would represent an example of cognitive restructuring in the treatment of the client with a Sexual Dysfunction?
   a. Maintain a diary of all stressful events
   b. Asks someone else to validate negative thoughts
   c. Identify irrational thoughts and counter thoughts with rational explanations
   d. Practice affirmations

9. In psychosocial development models, the term ''gender identity'' refers to the:
   a. Personal perception of being male or female
   b. Outward expression of socially accepted masculine or feminine traits
   c. Sexual classification assigned at birth
   d. Congruence of hormone levels and sexual behavior

10. Which of the following is true about a person with Paraphilia?
    a. Paraphilia is a sexual dysfunction.
    b. Persons with Paraphilia do not have normal sexual habits.
    c. Erotic pleasure is received from the activity.
    d. The Paraphilia tends to be obsessional in nature.

11. The initial intervention in assessment at the initiation of sex therapy is:
    a. Clarification of each member's perceptions of the other

b. Exploration of each member's beliefs about sexuality
c. Separate assessments to enhance free expression
d. Assessment of the couple's communication patterns

12. The nurse is assessing a client's sexual problem. In order to assess the client's feelings and attitudes about sex, the nurse might ask:

    a. The client's beliefs about alternative sexuality
    b. How the client's religion views sex
    c. For a description of the client's earliest sexual experiences
    d. Their perception of the client's parent's relationship

13. As the nurse plans treatment for a sexual problem, it is important to focus the interventions toward:

    a. The couple
    b. The identified client
    c. Each member individually
    d. The partner

14. The primary intervention by the nurse in sex therapy is:

    a. Activities for the couple
    b. Homework assignments
    c. Communication clarification
    d. Values clarification

15. Which of the following mental status variations would the nurse expect to see in a patient with a medical diagnosis of gender identity disorder:

    a. Dysphoric mood
    b. Poor insight
    c. Hallucinations
    d. Memory loss

16. Gender identity disorder can be manifested by:

    a. Fetishism
    b. Cross-dressing
    c. Sexual sadism
    d. All of the above

17. Mr. Cartwright tells the nurse that his sexual functioning is normal when his wife wears gold pumps. He states, "Without the gold pumps. I'm not interested in sex." The clinical nurse specialist assess this as:

    a. Pedophilia
    b. Exhibitionism
    c. Voyeurism
    d. Fetishism

18. Which of the following question would be best to use when the nurse wished to assess a client's sexual functioning?

    a. "Have you recently experienced a change in your self-esteem."
    b. Has anything such as illness, pregnancy, or a health problem interfered with your role as a wife/husband."
    c. "Has anything such as a heart attack or surgery changed the way you feel about yourself as a man/woman?"
    d. "Has anything such as surgery or disease changed your body's ability to function sexually?"

19. A new nurse tells the clinical nurse specialist "I'm unsure about my role when clients bring up sexual problems." The clinical nurse specialist should give clarification by saying.

    a. "All nurses qualify as sexual counselors because of their knowledge about biopsychosocial aspects of sexuality throughout the life cycle."
    b. "All nurses should be able to screen for sexual dysfunction and give limited information about sexual feelings, behaviors, and myths."
    c. "All nurses should defer questions about sex to other health care professionals because of their limited knowledge."
    d. "All nurses who are interested in sexual dysfunction can provide sex therapy for individuals and couples."

20. The nurse is caring for a client who presents with a medical diagnosis of Antisocial Personality Disorder. Which of the following nursing diagnoses would be most appropriate?

    a. Ineffective family coping
    b. Impaired social interaction
    c. Anxiety
    d. Altered sensory perception

21. Joan, who has a history of conflictual relationships, expresses the desire for friends but acts in alienating ways with people who befriend her. Which of the following would be an important nursing intervention for Joan?

    a. Help her find friends who are patient and extra caring.
    b. Establish a therapeutic relationship in which role-modeling and role-playing may occur.
    c. Accept her as she is, because she can't change.
    d. Point out her difficulties in relationships and suggested areas for improvement.

22. Mr. Grady constantly bends rules to meet his needs and then gets angry when other patients and staff confront him on his behavior. He threatens patients and manipulates staff to get what he wants. Which is the best nursing approach to use with Mr. Grady?

    a. Administer p.r.n. medication every time Mr. Bradley does not follow the rules.
    b. Ignore his behavior and privately tell the other patients to let Mr. Grady switch the television channels as much as he wants.
    c. Encourage the other staff to take turns watching Mr. Grady.
    d. Set firm limits for Mr. Grady and be consistent in confronting behaviors and enforcing unit rules.

23. The affect most commonly found in the client with Borderline Personality Disorder is one of:

    a. Happiness and elation
    b. Apathy and flatness
    c. Sadness and depression
    d. Anger and hostility

24. The action by the nurse that would be most appropriate when Mr. Smith states, *''I'm no good, I'm better off dead.'' would be:*

    a. Stating, ''I will stay with you until you are less depressed.''
    b. Stating, ''I think you are a good person, who should think about living.''
    c. Alerting all staff to provide 24-hour observation of the client
    d. Removing all articles that may be potentially dangerous

25. Limit setting is an intervention strategy to be utilized with which of the following behaviors?

    a. Manipulation

b. Repression
c. Reaction formation
d. Projection

26. Conrad, 29 years old, is admitted for psychiatric observation after being arrested for breaking windows in the home of his former girlfriend, who refuses to see him. His history reveals abuse as a child by a punitive step-father, torturing family pets, and one arrest for disorderly conduct. Which nursing diagnosis should be considered?

a. Impaired social interaction
b. Altered thought processes
c. High risk for trauma
d. High risk for violence directed at others

27. Under which of the following circumstances is restraint appropriate?

a. To encourage adherence to unit rules.
b. To control difficult interpersonal situations.
c. To establish the consequence of behaviors.
d. To prevent harm to self and others.

28. Which of the following mental status variations would the nurse expect to see in a client with a diagnosis of Borderline Personality Disorder:

a. Euphoria
b. Good insight and judgment
c. Mood lability
d. Hallucinations

29. While you are caring for Jennifer she tells you that she's afraid her husband will leave her because she has no interest in sex anymore. Jennifer asks the nurse if anything can be done about her lack of interest in sex. The most appropriate referral by the nurse for this client is:

a. Marriage counselor
b. Psychiatrist
c. Psychoanalyst
d. Sex therapist

30. The psychiatric nurse clinical specialist is asked to assess a 24-year-old female who reports that she is unable to have intercourse because of involuntary contractions of her vagina. The term is described as:

a. Arousal disorder
b. Dyspareunia
c. Orgasmic dysfunction
d. Vaginismus

31. The nurse is evaluating the outcome of measures to promote sleep. Which of the following would indicate that these measures have been successful?

    a. Client able to sleep at least 4 hours each night
    b. Client states he felt rested the next day
    c. Client accepts minor interruptions to sleep as normal
    d. Client able to verbalize anxieties

32. The sleeping disorder that can be described as excessive daytime sleepiness is which of the following disorders

    a. Sleep Terror Disorder
    b. Primary Hypersomnia
    c. Circadian rhythm sleep disorder
    d. Narcolepsy

33. The nurse is admitting a client with a diagnosis of Primary Insomnia. Which of the following assessment findings would be essential to confirm the diagnosis?

    a. Inability to obtain sleep not due to any other cause
    b. Inability to obtain sleep due to a medical disorder
    c. Disturbance of sleep-wake cycle
    d. Excessive daytime sleepiness

34. You are the psychiatric clinical specialist on a sleep disorder unit. Which of the following is the key aspect of a psychotherapeutic intervention program:

    a. Verbalize feelings
    b. Gain insight
    c. Thought stopping
    d. Sleep hygiene training

35. Which of the following nursing diagnosis is most appropriate for a client with a sleep disorder?

    a. Perceptual disturbances
    b. Impaired thought processes
    c. Sleep pattern disturbance
    d. Ineffective family coping

36. All of the following would be examples of milieu approaches for Primary Insomnia except:

    a. Decrease alcohol and caffeine intake during afternoon and evening.
    b. Thought stopping
    c. Discourage daytime naps.
    d. Increase exercise during morning and afternoon.

37. Before making a diagnosis of Primary Insomnia, the clinical specialist would need to consider all of the following phenomena *except:*

    a. Medication withdrawal
    b. Situational/Environmental changes
    c. Normal aging
    d. Mood disorders

38. The clinical specialist is implementing a behavior modification plan with a client with a diagnosis of pathological gambling. Which of the following family dynamics might he/she expect to observe?

    a. Absent, inconsistent or harsh discipline
    b. Chaotic and violent environment
    c. Rigid and overprotective parents
    d. Heavy drinking

39. Ferman, a 15 year-old female has complained of an intense impulse to pull his hair out, followed by a sense of relief on having carried out the act. Which of the following medical diagnoses would be most appropriate for the clinical nurse specialist to make?

    a. Obsessive-Compulsive Personality Disorder
    b. Tinea capitis
    c. Trichotillomania
    d. Autism

40. All of the following mental status variations are associated with pathological gambling except?

    a. Anxiety
    b. Impulsivity
    c. Sadness
    d. Poor insight

41. Johnson C. Smith is diagnosed with Pyromania. Which of the following behaviors would the nurse expect to observe in Mr. Smith?
    a. Aggressiveness
    b. Sadness
    c. Obsessive-compulsiveness
    d. Intense pleasure when watching fires

42. John is pacing the hall near the nurses station swearing loudly. An appropriate initial intervention for the nurse would be to say
    a. "John, please quiet down."
    b. "Hey, John, what's up?"
    c. "John, you seem pretty upset. Tell me about it."
    d. "John, you need to go to your room to get control of yourself."

43. Each of the following interventions is appropriate for the nurse in the above situation except:
    a. Telling the client that violence is not acceptable
    b. Speaking in a loud, urgent tone of voice
    c. Standing with arms relaxed at sides
    d. Listening attentively to the client

44. It becomes necessary to give an intramuscular injection of psychotropic medication to a client who is becoming increasingly more aggressive. The client is in the television room. The nurse should
    a. Enter the room; say, "Would you like to come to your room and take some medication your doctor has ordered for you?"
    b. Take three staff members with you to the room as a show of solidarity; say, "Mr. Summer, please come to your room so I can give you some medication that will help you feel more comfortable."
    c. Take a male staff member to the television room; tell Mr. Summer, "Mr. Summer, you can come to your room willingly to take your shot or Mr. Crinshaw and I will take you there."
    d. Enter the television room; place Mr. Summer in a basket hold; say, "I'm going to take you to your room to give you an injection of medication to calm you."

45. Following an incident in which staff intervention was required to control a client's aggressive behavior, staff should evaluate all of the following *except:*

a. The client's behavior preceding and during the incident
b. Intervention techniques used
c. The environment
d. The staff's views about theories of the etiology of aggression

46. Based on the client's potential for violence toward others and inability to cope with anger, which short-term goal would be most appropriate? The client will

a. Acknowledge his angry feelings.
b. Describe situations that provoke angry feelings.
c. List how he's handled his anger in the past.
d. Practice expressing anger

47. The impulse control disorder that is characterized as the deliberate and purposeful setting of fires is which of the following

a. Pyromania
b. Kleptomania
c. Trichotillomania
d. Intermittent explosive disorder

48. The impulse control disorder that is characterized as the inability to resist the impulse to steal objects is which one of the following

a. Pyromania
b. Kleptomania
c. Trichotillomania
d. Intermittent explosive disorder

Answers

1.d	17. d	33. a
2. b	18. d	34. d
3. c	19. b	35. c
4. d	20. b	36. b
5. a	21. b	37. b
6. b	22. d	38. a
7. c	23. c	39. c
8. c	24. c	40. c
9. a	25. a	41. d
10. c	26. d	42. c
11. d	27. d	43. b
12. b	28. c	44. b
13. a	29. d	45. d
14. c	30. d	46. b
15. a	31. c	47. a
16. b	32. d	48. b

Bibliography

Abraham, S., & Llewellyn-Jones, D. (1992). *Eating disorders: The facts.* NY: Oxford University Press.

American Psychiatric Association (1994). *Diagnostic and statistical manual of mental disorders.* (4th ed.). Washington, DC: American Psychiatric Association.

Blanchard R., & Steiner, B. W. (Eds.) (1990). *Clinical management of gender identity disorders in children and adults.* Washington, DC: American Psychiatric Press, Inc.

Bootzin, R. R., & Perlis, M. L. (1992). Nonpharmacologic treatments of insomnia. *Journal of Clinical Psychiatry, 53*(6), 37–41.

Haber, J., McMahon, A. L., Price-Hoskins, P., & Sideleau, B. F., (1992). *Comprehensive psychiatric nursing.* Baltimore: Mosby Year Book.

Kaplan, H. J., & Sadock, B. J.,(1988). *Synopsis of psychiatry.* Baltimore: Williams & Wilkins.

Krupnick, S., & Wade, A. (1993). *Psychiatric care planning.* Springhouse, PA: Springhouse Corp.

Meades, S. (1993). Suggested community psychiatric nursing interventions with clients suffering from anorexia nervosa and bulimia nervosa. *Journal of Advanced Nursing, 18,* 364–370.

Stein, G. (1992). Drug treatment of the personality disorder. *British Journal of Psychiatry, 161,* 167–184.

Wilson, H. S., & Kneisl, C. R. (1992). *Psychiatric nursing.* NY: Addison-Wesley Nursing.

Organic Mental Disorders

Anita Thompson-Heisterman
Jane Bryant Neese
Ivo L. Abraham

Organic Mental Disorders are associated with or caused by disturbance in the physiological functioning of brain tissue—structural, hormonal, biochemical, electrical, etc.—which causes cognitive deficits; ranges along continuum from acute (delirium) to chronic (primary degenerative dementia of the Alzheimers type).

Delirium

- Definition: A transient, reversible, confusional state resulting from a gross disruption in brain physiology and developing from a wide variety of factors (Inaba-Roland & Maricle, 1992); can progress to permanent dementia if identifying causes are not diagnosed and treated.
- Signs and Symptoms
  1. Disturbance of consciousness
  2. Change in cognition (memory deficit)
  3. Disturbance in sleep-wake cycle and level of psychomotor activity
  4. Disorientation to time, place, or persons
  5. Reduced ability to focus, shift, or maintain attention
  6. Disorganization of thinking (may manifest as irrelevant, rambling, or incoherent speech)
  7. Perceptual disturbances resulting in illusions and hallucinations;
  8. Emotional disturbances constituting lability of affect
  9. Transient, occurs abruptly, and fluctuates throughout the day (APA, 1993; Francis, 1992; Lipowski, 1989)
- Differential Diagnosis
  1. Schizophrenia—due to perceptual, affective, and behavioral similarities
  2. Schizophreniform Disorder and other psychotic disorders
  3. Dementia—onset of delirium is abrupt and duration is shorter than dementia with symptoms lasting a day to no longer than one month (Francis, 1992; Lipowski, 1989). Refer to Table 1 for differentation of symptoms.

Table 1
Differentiation of Symptoms

Factors	*Delirium*	*Dementia*
Level of consciousness	Fluctuates throughout the day	Alert; clear sensorium
Mood/affect	Irritable; fluctuates; can be volatile or depressed	Depends on situation
EEG	Diffusely abnormal, slowing	Focal points lower range of normal
Onset	Rapid; abrupt	Insidious; slow
24 Hour Course	Fluctuates	Stable
Duration	Short—from less than a week to no more than a month	long term; years
Behavior	Agitated; lethargic; fluctuating	"sundowning"; more confused at night
Thought processes	Thoughts may be slow or accelerated; somewhat dreamlike; presence of hallucinations (illusions); sometimes delusions, but they are poorly organized	Slow thought processes; impoverished; Delusions may be present but often absent
Orientation	Usually impaired, especially to time and place, but not usually to person	May be impaired or intact; may tend to confabulate
Memory	Recent and remote impaired; common knowledge intact	Recent memory impaired; remote memory may be intact; loss of common knowledge
Perceptions	Misperceptions often, especially visual	Misperceptions are absent
Speech	Slow or rapid, often incoherent	Normal
Involuntary movements	Asterixis or course tremor often present	Absent
Physical illness or drug toxicity	One or both are present	Often absent

Note. From "Depression in the General Hospital" by J. B. Neese, 1991, *Nursing Clinics of North America, 26*(3), p. 615. Copyright 1991 by W. B. Saunders. Adapted from "Transient cognitive disorders (delirium, acute confusion states) in the elderly" by Z. J. L. Lipowski, 1983. *American Journal of Psychiatry, 140*, p. 432. Copyright 1991 by W. B. Saunders. Adapted by permission.

4. Depression—sluggishness and depressed affect when delirious, similar to major depressive episode or an adjustment disorder with depressed mood, however, depression is not the underlying pathology
5. Anxiety Disorder—due to affective and behavioral similarities
6. Definitive diagnosis based on constellation of findings, rapidity of onset, and associated medical and environmental risk factors (Inaba-Roland & Maricle, 1992)

- Mental Status
  1. Fluctuating cognitive impairment with lucid intervals

2. Inability to maintain attention or engage in goal-directed behavior; difficulty following questions upon examination and may perseverate in response to earlier questions
3. Disorganization of thought—difficulty maintaining coherent stream of thought, easily distracted; speech rambling, inconsequential, or illogical; faulty reasoning and lack of goal-directed behavior
4. Perceptual disturbances—illusions, hallucinations, delusions may be present, but they generally are poorly organized; can suffer acute paranoid delusions accompanied by fear, anxiety, attempts to escape or destructive rage episodes
5. Impairment in the level of consciousness—the client falls asleep during the interview
6. Disturbed sleep-wake cycle—hypervigilant during the night and sleeps during the day
7. Abnormally increased or decreased psychomotor activity; may pick at the bed linen or be sluggish, resembling catatonia-like movements; three clinical patterns (Lipowski,1990; Inaba-Roland & Maricle, 1992)
   a. Hypoalert-hypoactive client who is lethargic and drowsy
   b. Hyperalert-hyperactive client who is restless and agitated
   c. Mixed variant who shifts between lethargy and agitation
8. Disorientation in all spheres (place, time and/or person); disorientation to place and time is very common; however, disorientation to person is rare.
9. Memory impairment—usually short-term memory is impaired and both anterograde (memory for events just prior to onset of delirium) and retrograde (memory for events just after the episode) amnesia are present.
10. Emotional lability ranging from depressive to rage affects

- Nursing Diagnoses
  1. Alteration in thought processes is the major NANDA-approved nursing diagnosis for delirium (Rawlins, Williams and Beck, 1993).

2. Others include communication, impaired verbal; sensory/perceptual alterations (specify which one is disturbed); fatigue; high risk for injury; altered nutrition; altered role performance; self-care deficit; and sleep pattern disturbance.

3. Anxiety—acute anxiety, fear, and hypervigilant behavior may accompany delusions as a result of the delirium.

- Biological Theories: Usually delirium can be attributed to a wide range of organic disorders ranging from metabolic disturbances to withdrawal from substances such as alcohol or sedative-hypnotic agents (APA, 1987; Francis, 1992; Lipowski, 1989). Medication intoxication is the most common cause in the elderly.

  1. Risk factors associated with delirium:

     a. Severity of illness—the more severe the illness, the more likely delirium will occur.

     b. Age—the older the patient, the more likely delirium will occur (Francis, 1992); persons over age 80 most vulnerable.

     c. Impairment in cognition (Schor, Levoff, Lipsitz, Reily, Cleary, Rowe, & Evans 1992) or physical functioning, such as confinement in a restricted space or bed (Francis, 1992)

     d. Presence of dementia—approximately 25% to 50% of patients diagnosed with dementia have been found to have delirium superimposed upon the dementia (Francis, 1992).

     e. Chronic lesions on neuroimaging studies (Francis, 1992)

     f. Chronic brain diseases such as Parkinsonism (Francis,1992) or metastases to the brain

     g. Systemic infection (Schor et al., 1992)

     h. Narcotic use (Schor et al., 1992)

     i. Disruption of the sleep cycle

     j. Relocation—especially if rapid, sudden and unplanned

     k. Pain

     l. Hearing or visual impairment

     m. Amnesia as a result of drugs, surgery, or trauma

   n. Environment—sensory overload or deprivation such as critical care unit (Inaba-Roland & Maricle, 1992)

2. The following disorders have been credited with causing delirium:
   a. Primary intracranial diseases (Lipowski, 1989)
   b. Systemic infections or diseases that secondarily affect the brain—in the elderly, most often the causes of delirium are related to other illnesses such as cancer, congestive heart failure, myocardial infarction, uremia, diabetes, hypoglycemia, malnutrition, dehydration, sodium depletion, hypokalemia, stroke, and epilepsy (Lipowski, 1989).
   c. Metabolic disorders (hypoxia, hypercarbia, hypoglycemia, electrolyte imbalance, hepatic or renal disease, or thiamine deficiency (Inaba-Roland & Maricle, 1992)
   d. Post-operative states (Francis, 1992)
   e. Cerebrovascular events—thrombotic, embolitic, hemorrhagic (Inaba-Roland & Maricle, 1992)
   f. Postictal activity (Inaba-Roland & Maricle, 1992)
   g. Post head trauma (Inaba-Roland & Maricle, 1992)
   h. Substance intoxication and withdrawal (Francis, 1992; Lipowski, 1989) (Refer to Table 2 for drugs causing delirium.)

- Biochemical Interventions
  1. Dependent on determination of identifying causes which entails:
     a. Complete physical examination
     b. Complete neurological examination
     c. Complete battery of laboratory tests including but not limited to: SMA12, complete blood count, complete urine drug screen, electroencephalogram (EEG), B12 levels, thyroid profile, CT scan and MRI (Francis, 1992; Lipowski, 1989)
  2. Treatment of the underlying cause(s)
     a. Restore adequate fluid and electrolyte balance, nutrition, and vitamin supply (Lipowski, 1989).
     b. Eliminate medication(s) suspected to affect mental status. (Table 2 lists medications associated with causing delirium.)

Table 2

Drugs Associated with Delirium

Classification of Drugs	*Types*
Narcotics	Morphine, Meperidine, Oxycodone
General Anesthetic	Ketamine
Sedatives and Hypnotics	Alcohol, Phenobarbital, Dalmane
Antihistamines and 2 Receptor Blockers	Cimetidine, Ranitidine, Famotidine, Nizatidine, Clonidine
Drugs for the treatment of Parkinsonism	Amantadine, Levodopa/carbidopa, Dopamine agonists (pergolide, bromocriptine), Anticholinergics (benztropine)
Steroids	Prednisone
Antidepressants (especially in seriously medically ill patients)	Trazadone, Tricyclics
Anthelmintic	Quinacrine
Anticonvulsants	Dilantin, Zarontin, Mysoline
Alcohol deterrent	Disulfiram
Antihypertensive	Clonidine
Antibiotics	Amphotericin B, Tobramycin
Hemostatic	Aminocaproic acid
Anticholinergic drugs	Amitriptyline, Diphenhydramine, Thioridazine, Atropine, Scopolamine, Quinidine
Benzodiazepines	Diazepam, Alprazolam, Triazolam
Digatalis	Digoxin
Diuretics	Furosemide

(1) If toxicity from cimetidine or ranitidine is suspected, the use of physostigmine reverses the delirium for ''15 to 60 minutes following a 1 to 2 mg intravenous dose'' (Francis, 1992, p. 836).

(2) Caution, however, should be taken when administering physostigmine for antidepressant overdoses due to the potentiation action of physostigmine with antidepressants.

c. Treat withdrawal from substances

(1) Alcohol withdrawal delirium develops after recent cessation or reduction of alcohol consumption. Marked autonomic activity occurs,usually within one week. The condition is also called ''delirium tremens.''

(2) Management of acute withdrawal with benzodiazepines is indicated. Chlordiazepoxide (Librium) 25 mgm prn for withdrawal symptoms is often chosen. It is important to monitor the withdrawal carefully, checking vital signs and mental status.

(3) Need to replace thiamine and other vitamins to prevent permanent organic disorder due to deficiency.

d. If client becomes agitated and restless, pharmacologic restraint may be necessary.

(1) Haloperidol—most commonly used sedative because of low anticholinergic side effects, quick sedation, and low incidence of orthostatic hypotension (Francis, 1992; Lipowski, 1989); potential for extrapyramidal symptoms such as "cog-wheel" rigidity in joints (can be seen in flexing and extending the elbow) and excessive salivation, and dystonic reactions such as torticollis (extreme turning of head to one side with the inability to correct posture). A low dose of 0.25 to 0.5 mg TID prn given by mouth in liquid suspension or intramuscularly usually diminishes agitation (Butler, Lewis & Sunderland, 1991).

(2) Droperidol—has a more rapid onset of sedation and can be given in the same dosages as haloperidol. Hypotension is side effect (Francis, 1992).

- Psychosocial Approaches

1. Be attentive to the client's concerns and fears, which may be expressed in the hallucinations and/or delusions (Lipowski, 1989).
2. Reorient the client to reality, especially when illusions are present.
3. Reduce fear and anxiety by providing a calm reassuring manner, assuring the client that you will be sure he is safe.
4. Explain all procedures to allay anxiety.
5. If client is extremely agitated, the use of physical restraints is not recommended as they may increase fear and agitation along with increasing the risk of problems associated with immobility. The use of "sitters" or enlisting the family's help is more efficacious.

- Family Dynamics/Family Therapy
    1. Involve the family in assessment, planning, intervention, and evaluation of the nursing care plan.
    2. Family can provide useful information as to the clients premorbid cognitive status, the possible causative factor of the delirium, history of the client and other critical data.
    3. Family can assist in planning psychosocial interventions which are likely to be most successful.
    4. Family can assist in interventions by helping to orient and reassure the client.
    5. Family needs to be provided with information and reassurance along with referral information for use post delirium.
- Group Approaches: For delirious clients, group intervention, of any kind, is contraindicated.
- Milieu Approaches
    1. Aimed at providing safety, support, and structure
    2. Environmental interventions help reestablish orientation by placing clock, calendar, and familiar belongings in the client's room.
    3. Encourage family visits to assist patient with orientation (Francis, 1992).
    4. Correct any sensory deficit that the patient may have by having eyeglasses or hearing aid made available and within close reach.
    5. Place the client in a room with windows to help orient to day and night.
    6. Keep outside, distracting noises to a minimum and keep a low light on at night.
    7. Reduce, but don't eliminate stimulation, as sensory deprivation also contributes to delirium.
- Community Resources: Not indicated during the acute episode but may be chosen as a referral for aftercare based on:
    1. Etiology of the delirium (i.e., Alcoholics Anonymous; Narcotics Anonymous; social support such as senior center, case management or home health services)

2. Need for the client and/or family to resolve the emotional trauma associated with the acute episode of delirium through participation in individual, group, or family counseling/therapy.

Dementia (Reversible and Irreversible)

- Definition
  1. Development of multiple cognitive deficits which cause significant impairment in social or occupational functioning, represent a significant decline from a previous level of functioning, do not occur during the course of a delirium, and are judged to be related to a causative factor (APA, 1993).
  2. Etiology
     a. Hereditary factors
     b. Cerebrovascular disease—in particular, stroke and cerebral blood flow problems
     c. Cerebral oxygenation problems
     d. Infectious diseases of, or affecting, the central nervous system
     e. Brain trauma
     f. Toxins
     g. Metabolic disturbances
     h. Hypoglycemia
     i. Normal pressure hydrocephalus
     j. Degenerative neurologic diseases
     k. Medications
  3. Criteria for severity of Dementia
     a. Mild—although work or social activities are significantly impaired, the capacity for independent living remains, with adequate personal hygiene and relatively intact judgment.
     b. Moderate—independent living is hazardous, and some degree of supervision is necessary.
     c. Severe—activities of daily living are so impaired that continual supervision is required, (e.g., unable to maintain minimal personal hygiene; largely incoherent or mute.)

4. Although dementia syndromes are commonly thought of as irreversible and progressively deteriorating, some syndromes may be reversible, non-progressive, or both.

Dementia (Reversible)

- Definition: A category of illnesses with (most notably, cognitive impairment) that can be resolved by addressing the underlying cause.
- Signs and Symptoms: May be alternating periods of lucidity, followed by episodes of global cognitive impairment with memory deficits.
- Diagnostic Criteria for Reversible
  1. Evidence of impairment in:
     a. Short-term memory (inability to learn new information) may be indicated by inability to remember three objects after five minutes.
     b. Long-term memory impairment (inability to remember information that was known in the past) may be indicated by inability to remember past personal information (what happened yesterday, birthplace, occupation) or facts of common knowledge (past presidents, well-known dates)''
  2. At least one of the following:
     a. Impairment in abstract thinking—indicated by inability to find similarities and differences between related works, difficulty in defining words and concepts, and other similar tasks
     b. Impaired judgment—indicated by inability to make reasonable plans to deal with interpersonal, family, and job-related problems and issues
     c. Other disturbances of higher cortical action, such as aphasia (disorder of language), apraxia (inability to carry out motor activities despite intact comprehension and motor function), agnosia (failure to recognize or identify objects despite intact senory function), and ''constructional difficulty'' (inability to copy figures)
- Differential Diagnosis: As summarized by APA (1987), Neese (1991), and Lipowski (1989), various types of dementia may show symptomatologic similarities with:
  1. Delirium (Refer to Table 1.)

2. Chronic schizophrenia
3. Acute psychotic episode
4. Major depressive episode
5. Factitious disorder with psychological symptoms

- Mental Status
  1. Impairment in short- and long-term memory
  2. Impairment in abstract thinking and judgment
  3. Other disturbances of higher cortical functioning including agnosia, apraxia, and constructional difficulty
  4. May be affective instability
  5. May be perceptual disturbances such as hallucinations and illusions
- Genetic/Biological Theories: Conditions that may cause reversible dementias include:
  1. Depression (''pseudo dementia'')—although depression superimposed upon dementia is more common than ''pseudodementia.''
  2. Endocrine-metabolic disorders (hypo or hyperglycemia, hypercalcemia, hyperthyroidism, Cushings, renal failure, liver failure)
  3. Brain disorders (tumor, normal pressure hydrocephalus, subdural hematoma, encephalitis)
  4. Infections
  5. Cardiopulmonary disorders (congestive heart failure, arrhythmias, hypoxemia)
  6. Nutritional deficiency (vitamin B_{12}, folate, thiamine, niacin, pernicious anemia)
  7. Medications are often the cause of reversible dementias (see Table 3); due to changes in pharmacodynamics and pharmacokinetics in later life, careful consideration and individualization in drug therapy is essential in caring for the elderly. Drug reactions occur two to three times more often in the elderly than in young adults (Montamat, Cusack, & Vestal, 1989).

Table 3

Drugs Causing Psychiatric Symptoms

Drug Classification	*Generic Drug Name*	*Reactions Similar in Symptomatology to Various Organic Mental Disorders*
Antiviral agents	Acyclovir, Amantadine	Visual hallucinations, depersonalization, confusion, insomnia
B-2 Antagonist	Albuterol	Hallucinations
Antianxiety	Alprazolam, Diazepam	Manic symptoms, insomnia, anxiety, paranoia, hallucinations, depression, suicidal thoughts
Antibiotics	Amoxicillin, Chloramphenicol, Cephalosporins, Dapsone, Erythromycin, Gentamicin, Penicillin G procaine	Confusion, auditory hallucinations, hyperactivity, disorientation, paranoia, insomnia
Stimulants	Amphetamines, caffeine, cocaine, Methylphenidate, and similar anoretic agents	Hallucinations, paranoia, anxiety, restlessness, confusion, paranoid delusions
Antineoplastics	Asparaginase, Cisplatin, Chorambucil, Vincristine, Vinblastine	Confusion, depression, paranoia, disorientation, hallucinations
Antihypertensives	Atenolol, Captopril, Methyldopa, Prazosin, Propranolol, Timolol	Confusion, disorientation, hallucinations, insomnia, severe depression, paranoia, hyperactivity
Relaxants	Baclofen, Cyclobenzeprine	Hallucinations, paranoia, depression, anxiety, confusion, manic psychosis, delusions, hyperactivity
Sedative/Hypnotics	Barbiturates, Triazolam, Ethchlorvynol	Excitement, hyperactivity, visual hallucinations, depression, paranoia, anterograde amnesia, anxiety
Dopamine agonist	Bromocriptine	Delusions, visual or auditory hallucinations, paranoia, depression, anxiety
Antimalarial	Chloroquine, Hydroxychloroquine	Confusion, delusions, hallucinations, difficulty concentrating
Anticonvulsant	Clonazepam	Hallucinations, paranoia
Narcotics	Codeine, Methadone, Morphine, Pentazocine, Propoxyphene	Psychosis, disorientation, dysphoria, agitation, euphoria, nightmares, paranoia, depression, auditory hallucinations, confusion
Steroids	Corticosteroids, Oxymetazoline	Depression, confusion, paranoia, hallucinations, anxiety
Antituberculars	Cycloserine, Ethionamide, isoniazid	Anxiety, depression, confusion, disorientation, hallucinations, paranoia
Immunosuppressant	Cyclosporine	Hallucinations, depression
Antidysrhythmics	Digitalis glycosides, Disopyramide, Quinidine, Lidocaine, Tocainide	Confusion, delusions, amnesia, visual or auditory hallucinations, paranoia, depression, disorientation
Adrenergics	Ephedrine, Pseudoephedrine	Hallucinations, paranoia

Table 3 — Continued

Drug Classification	*Generic Drug Name*	*Reactions Similar in Symptomatology to Various Organic Mental Disorders*
Nonsteroidals	Ibuprofen, Indomethacin, Naproxen, Sulindac	Paranoia, depression, inability to concentrate, confusion, hallucinations, disorientation, personality change
Antidepressants	Isocarboxazid, Phenelzine	Insomnia, anxiety, paranoid delusions, hyperactivity
Serotonin antagonist	Methysergide	Depersonalization, hallucinations
Cholinergic	Metoclopramide	Severe depression
Amebicides	Metronidazole, Pargyline	Depression, disorientation, manic psychosis, hallucinations
Urinary tract anti-infectives	Nalidixic acid, Trimethoprim sulfamethoxazole	Confusion, depression, hallucinations, psychosis
Calcium channel blocker	Nifedipine	Hyperexcitability, depression
Nasal decongestant	Phenylephrine	Depression, hallucinations, paranoia
Keratolytic	Podophyllin	Delirium, paranoia
Diuretics	Polythiazide, Trichlormethiazide	Depression, suicidal ideation
Local anesthetic	Procainamide	Paranoia, hallucinations
Nonnarcotic analgesic	Salicylates	Hallucinations, paranoia
Spasmolytic	Theophylline	Hyperactivity
Antihelmintic	Thiabendazole	Hallucinations
Hormone	Thyroid hormones	Depression, hallucinations, paranoia

Note. From "Some Drugs that Cause Psychiatric Symptoms" by M. Abramowiez, 1988, *The Medical Letter, 28*(721), pp. 81–86. Copyright 1986 by The Medical Letter Inc. Adapted by permission.

8. The following are physiological changes in old age that affect the absorption and elimination of medications:
   a. Multiple chronic diseases that are associated with reduced serum albumin levels (Montamat et al., 1989).
   b. Hepatic functioning that decreases with normal aging; drugs have been shown to have a longer half-life and decrease plasma clearance (Montamat et al., 1989). Drugs that require a high rate of hepatic extraction should be used judiciously (i.e., major tranquilizers, tricyclic antidepressants, and antiarrhythmic agents) (Montamat et al., 1989).
   c. Decline in renal functioning due to the decline in glomerular filtration and tubular secretion rates; "Creatinine clearance is a

useful guide to the rate of renal drug elimination in the elderly)'' (Montamat et al., 1989, p. 305). Lithium, digoxin, procainamide, chlorpropamide, cimetidine, and amantadine are drugs that are primarily eliminated by the kidneys.

d. Nutritional status in the elderly, a general decline in nutritional status that includes protein and vitamin intake is common.

e. Cigarette smoking affects hepatic functioning.

f. The central nervous system is more sensitive in the elderly; therefore, smaller doses of benzodiazepines are indicated to produce similar amount of sedation as in younger adults (Montamat et al., 1989).

g. The elderly are prone to postural hypotension, urinary retention, sedation, and falls associated with psychoactive medications (Montamat et al., 1989); therefore, beginning dosages should be lower than in young adults and close observation is indicated to protect the safety of this population.

Primary Degenerative Dementia of the Alzheimer Type (Irreversible)

- Definition
  1. This type of irreversible dementia is characterized by a gradual and insidious onset and a generally progressive deteriorating course for which all other specific causes have been excluded by the history, physical examination, and laboratory tests (APA, 1993). It is the most prevalent of the dementias.
  2. This disease can occur with the following variations:
     a. Senile or presenile onset, depending on whether after or before age 65
     b. Within senile and presenile variants, disease can be with delirium, with delusions, with depression or uncomplicated.
- Signs and Symptoms
  1. Characterized by multifaceted loss of intellectual abilities, such as memory, judgment, abstract thought, and other higher cortical functions, changes in personality and behavior, and significant decline and impairment in social and occupational functioning (APA, 1993)

2. The clinical aspects of Alzheimer's disease are summarized in Table 4.

Table 4

Clinical Aspects of Alzheimer's Disease

Symptom Category	*Signs and Symptoms*
Memory	Recent memory deficits Remote memory deficits Disorientation Forgetfulness Confusion Dementia
Concentration	Short attention span Inability to acquire new information
Language and Speech	Word finding deficits Agnosia Anomia Paraphrasia Aphasia Echolalia Paralalia Logoclia Mutism
Praxis	Inability to conceptualize Difficulty with complex tasks Inability to write
Thought Content	Simple delusions Persecutory delusions Suicidal ideation
Lability	Fear and fearfulness Anxiety Anger Irritability Crying spells Catastrophic reactions
Depressed Mood	Sadness Hopelessness Helplessness Feelings of worthlessness Guilt Depression Suicidality
Mania	Busy behaviors Meddlesome Interference in affairs of others Destructive behavior Violence

Table 4 — Continued

Symptom Category	*Signs and Symptoms*
Related to Personality Change	Stubbornness Angry outburst Verbal abuse Restlessness Combativeness Agitation Resistance to care Assaultive and violent behaviors Wandering Roaming through rooms Regressive behaviors Hiding and hoarding things
Related to Vegetative Disorders	Sleep disturbance Urinary incontinence Dietary changes: (binge eating, pica) Sexual disinhibition
Related to Neuromotor Dysfunction	Gait disorder Tremors Seizures Flexional contracture Primitive reflexes
Sensory Distortion	Misidentification of people Misidentification of places Confusion of people and places Inability to recognize mirror image Treating TV events/people as real illusions
Sensory Deception	Visual hallucinations Auditory hallucinations Olfactory hallucinations
Social Withdrawal	Withdrawal from family Withdrawal from close social groups Withdrawal from complex groups
Personal	Increased self-preoccupation Personal isolation
Activities of Daily Living	Instrumental ADLs Physical ADLs
Self-Care	Nutrition Sleep/Rest Medication behavior

Note. From "Alzheimer's Disease and Nursing: New Scientific and Clinical Insights" by E. S. Yi, I. L. Abraham amd S. Holroyd, 1994, *Nursing Clinics of North America, 29*(1), pp. 88–89. Copyright by W. B. Saunders. Adapted by permission.

- Differential Diagnosis

  Exclusion of all alternative specific causes of dementia by complete history, physical examination, and laboratory tests

1. Benign forgetfulness, common phenomenon among older adults
2. Subdural hematoma
3. Normal pressure hydrocephalus
4. Brain tumors
5. Parkinson's disease
6. Vitamin B_{12} deficiency
7. Hypothyroidism
8. Delirium
9. Acute psychotic episode
10. Major depressive episode
11. Multi-infarct dementia (see below)
12. Reversible dementias
13. Medication interactions
14. AIDS dementia complex (ADC)

- Mental Status: Manifestations include:
  1. Recent and remote memory deficits
  2. Short attention span and inability to concentrate
  3. Impairment in abstract thinking and judgment
  4. Other disturbances of higher cortical functioning, such as agnosia, apraxia, aphasia, and constructional difficulty
  5. Affective lability
  6. Perceptual disturbances such as hallucination
  7. Depressed mood
- Genetic/Biological Theories: According to APA (1987) and Yi, Abraham & Holroyd (1994):
  1. Cause(s) of disease still unknown
  2. Hereditary factors
     a. Familial patterns exist
     b. Genetic markers on chromosomes 14 and 21

c. Alzheimer's type lesions occur around age 40 in most if not all people with Down's Syndrome

3. Most recent evidence points to protein process involving beta-amyloid.

Vascular or Multi-Infarct Dementia

- Definition: Direct consequence of cerebrovascular disease, characterized by the often abrupt onset of a stepwise deterioration in intellectual functioning that, early in the course, leaves some intellectual functions relatively intact (patchy deterioration) (APA, 1993)
- Signs and Symptoms
    1. Multiple cognitive deficits manifested by memory impairment and disturbance in executive functioning (i.e., planning, organizing, sequencing, abstracting), aphasia, apraxia, and/or agnosia (APA, 1993)
    2. A stepwise deteriorating course with ''patchy'' distribution of deficits (affecting some functions, but not others) early in the course (APA, 1993)
    3. Since the cause is cerebrovascular disease, focal neurologic signs and symptoms (e.g., exaggeration of deep tendon reflexes are an important diagnostic determinant)
        a. (e.g., ''weaknesses in the limbs, reflex asymmetries, extensor plantar responses, dysarthria, and small-stepped gait'' (APA, 1993).
        b. Can present with delirium, delusions, or depression pseudobulbar palsy, gait abnormalities, weakness of an extremity
    4. Evidence of significant cerebrovascular disease that is judged to be etiologically related to the disturbance
- Differential Diagnosis (APA, 1993; and Abraham et al., 1994):
    1. General differential diagnosis of Dementia and Primary Degenerative Dementia of the Alzheimer Type (see above)
    2. Impairment due to single stroke
- Mental Status: Is differentiated from other primary dementias only by the fact that the cognitive manifestations may wax and wan, showing patchy or stepwise deterioration

- Genetic/Biological Theories: Cerebrovascular diseases, commonly referred to as "mini-strokes"

  The following information is relevant for reversible and irreversible dementias except where noted.

- Nursing Diagnoses

  1. Alteration in thought processes—a state in which an individual experiences a disruption in cognitive operations and activities is the most common nursing diagnosis approved by NANDA that applies to dementia (Rawlins et al., 1993, pp. 659–660)
     a. Defining characteristics include physical, emotional, and intellectual.
     b. Physical dimensions include altered sleep pattern and hyperactivity.
     c. Emotional dimensions include inappropriate or labile affect and anxiety.
     d. Intellectual dimensions include altered states of consciousness (disorientation to time, place, person), impaired memory, confabulation, distractibility, disturbed thought flow, disturbed thought content, impaired problem solving, impaired judgment, inability to follow conversation, alteration in perception, cognitive disturbance, suicidal/homicidal ideation, attention deficit, egocentricity, inappropriate/non-reality based thinking (Rawlins et al., 1993).
  2. Numerous other nursing diagnoses can also apply to clients with dementia due to the complexity of the illness and the level of care required.
     a. Self-care deficit—feeding, bathing, toileting
     b. Impaired verbal communication; Sensory/perceptual alterations; anxiety; fear.
     c. High risk for fluid volume deficit; high risk for injury; altered nutrition
     d. Sleep pattern disturbance; fatigue
     e. Personal identity disturbance; altered role performance; Social interaction—impaired; social isolation

f. Ineffective coping—individual and family; Caregiver role strain.

- Biochemical Interventions

1. Initially these depend on the etiologic factor causing the dementia as the need is to treat the underlying cause of the disturbance (e.g., treat diabetes with insulin, hypothyroidism with thyroid replacement, thiamine deficiency with replacement, and iatrogenic disorders by eliminating the causative drug).
2. If biochemical intervention is indicated for control of agitation or hallucination associated with dementia, drug treatment should be used cautiously, beginning with the lowest possible dose and tapering upward as needed. Haloperidol is the drug of choice for controlling agitation in dementias due to lower anticholinergic effects. Low dosage of O.25 mgm should be initiated. Side effects include dystonias (rigidity in joints & torticollis) and excessive salivation. Orthostatic blood pressures should be monitored and the client and his caregiver(s) should be taught the side effects.
3. Short-acting benzodiazepines such as oxazepam (Serax) or Lorazepam (Ativan) have been shown to be useful in treating behavioral agitation but are not as useful as low dose neuroleptics (Coccaro, Kramer, Zemishlany, Thorne, Rice, Giodani, Duvvi, Patel, Torres, Nora, Neufeld, Mohs & Davis, 1990). Must be used with extreme caution as side effects can increase confusion in elderly organically impaired clients while controlling agitation and irritability. May cause dizziness and drowsiness. Need to check orthostatic blood pressure (sitting and standing) and monitor mental status. Need to monitor withdrawal symptoms and assess for suicide if depressed.
4. No treatment available to stop or reverse the progression of Alzheimer's disease. Several drugs are used for management of symptoms of the disorder. Depression is often a feature of primary degenerative dementia, although it may be difficult to detect. It has multiple adverse effects on the demented patient, including aggravation of behavioral symptoms. The following medications can be used to treat depression occurring with dementia.

   a. Tricyclic antidepressants. All cause orthostatic hypotension, sedation, and anticholinergic effects. Nortriptyline (Aventyl) 25-150 mgm per day or Desipramine (Norpramine) 25 mgm per day as an initial dose are the tricyclics of choice in elderly patients since they have fewer side effects (Yi, Abraham & Holroyd, 1994). Serum levels of tricyclic antidepressants should be closely monitored. All antidepressants should be given at the lowest possible effective dose in the elderly or those with compromised medical conditions.

b. Selective serotonin re-uptake inhibitors (SSRIs). A new class of antidepressants including fluoxetine (Prozac) and sertraline (Zoloft). The most common side effects in the elderly are nausea, weight loss, nervousness, and agitation (Yi, et al, 1994). Usual fluoxetine dose is 20 mgm daily, although it can be given every other day in the elderly. Sertraline dose is generally 50 mgm per day.

c. Trazadone—a serotonin uptake blocker well tolerated in the elderly due to low anticholinergic effects. It can be very sedating, which may be a desired outcome if sleep disturbance exists. Use trazadone with extreme caution because of high orthostatic hypotensive side effects. Need to monitor orthostatic blood pressure. Other side effects include dry mouth, insomnia, headache, tremor, nausea, and rash (Yi et al., 1994). Trazadone (Desyrel) is usually given at 150 mgm per day in divided doses.

5. In vascular dementia biochemical approaches are directed at treating the cardiovascular factor causing the dementia and managing behavioral symptoms as with other forms of dementia. As Curl (1992) states, multi-infarct dementia is managed like thrombotic stroke or transient ischemic attacks with ASA 650 mgm twice a day.

6. Anticonvulsants such as carbamazepine (Tegretol) or phenytoin (Dilantin) may be used to control seizures. Phenobarbital may be avoided due to potential for abuse by alcoholic. Phenytoin is given in three divided doses of 100 mgm each for seizure prophylaxis. Side effects include agranulocytosis, leukopenia, aplastic anemia, drowsiness, dizziness, nausea, and vomiting. Need to assess blood levels, assess mental status, teach client not to d/c the drug abruptly, since seizures may occur and to use good oral hygiene to prevent gingival hyperplasia.

- Psychosocial Approaches

1. Based on careful nursing assessment of the patient.
2. Adaptations to interviewing techniques needed with cognitively impaired clients include; need to allow more time, speak slowly and clearly, and provide an environment free of distractions (Thompson-Heisterman, Smullen & Abraham, 1992).
3. Goal of nursing care regardless of the setting is to help the client maintain the highest level of independence possible through "enhancing his abilities and compensating for deficits" (Curl, 1992).
4. Use warm, caring, respectful approach.
5. Use clear, simple and direct communication.
6. Keep tasks within the client's abilities, using sequencing and cuing (i.e., laying out the client's clothing in the order in which he/she needs to put it on.)
7. Avoid over- or under-stimulation.
8. Provide adequate rest and nutrition.
9. If the dementia is vascular, provide information to the client regarding managing risk factors associated with cardiovascular disease (diet, exercise, decrease stress, medication, signs of impending stroke, etc.).

- Family Dynamics/Family Therapy
  1. Family needs to be included in the assessment as well as the intervention phase of treatment with cognitively impaired clients as they can provide much useful information regarding how to best care for their loved one.
  2. Family members are often the hidden victims of the illness, especially when the dementia is chronic rather than reversible.
  3. Family interventions always include providing support and education, and in some cases, such as when the dementia is due to substance abuse, counseling or therapy may be indicated.
- Group Approaches: In selecting elder group participants, as with young adults, extreme paranoia and severe cognitive impairment is usually contraindicated for effective group work. Therefore, elders who are experiencing the latter stages of Alzheimer's Disease or other dementias, will not benefit from most of the following groups while those with mild cognitive impairment can and do benefit from group therapy.

1. Reminiscence groups aim to increase self-esteem through positive affiliations and interactions with others (Neese & Abraham, 1991). These groups may be helpful for elders and individuals with mild cognitive disorders and depression.

2. Cognitive-behavioral groups assist clients in correcting negative thoughts and attitudes, as well as maladaptive ways in which clients process information (Neese & Abraham, 1991). This type of group can be helpful to elders who suffer from mild cognitive impairment with superimposed depression or who have one of the above disorders.

3. Educational groups seek to inform and emphasize learning and discussion instead of therapy (Neese & Abraham, 1992). For elders who have mild cognitive impairment and their families, educational groups addressing the various types of dementias are an excellent method to help alleviate the isolation that clients and families feel when faced with a chronic disorder.

4. Validation Groups have been found by Feil (1989) to benefit even severely impaired clients. The goals of validation are to stimulate communication in order to prevent withdrawal inward, to restore well-being, to facilitate the resolution of unresolved issues to prepare for death, and to reduce caregiver burnout by teaching empathy skills.

- Milieu Approaches

  1. Milieu interventions are a critical factor in the treatment of both acute and chronic dementias whether the client is at home or in an institution.
  2. Provide safety, structure, and support.
  3. Provide consistency of routine.
  4. Provide orientation and environmental cues.
  5. Explain procedures in clear, direct language to enhance understanding and allay anxiety.
  6. Provide for adequate rest, nutrition, and elimination.
  7. Ryden (1992) found that most aggression in demented clients occurs in response to an environmental trigger. Therefore, it is very important to assess and modify the environment. Aggression often

occurred as the client's responses to pain, need for control, need to feel safe, need for stimulation, and need to decrease stress.

8. Whall and Booth (1992), and Ryden (1992) caution regarding the need to avoid chemical and physical restraints through modification of the environment. Federal mandates, specified in the Omnibus Budget Reconciliation Act (OBRA) passed by Congress in 1989, stipulate that if neuroleptic drugs are used in nursing homes, there must be a specific medical reason. They cannot be used solely for chemical restraint. Both types of restraints have many complications including increasing agitation and confusion.

- Community Resources

1. Potential resources for clients and caregivers are extensive depending on the etiology, duration, and level of cognitive and functional impairment associated with the dementia.

2. Organizations related to organic factors causing the disorder would include Alcoholics Anonymous, The American Cancer, Diabetes, Lung Association, and the Alzheimer's Disease and Related Disorders Foundation.

3. Harper (1992) lists a wide array of community services that may be needed to maintain the client and family, including home health agencies, social services, outreach programs, homebound meals, church support, day care, respite care, hospice, nursing homes, and others.

Questions
Select the best answer

1. Ms. S, age 50, has been hospitalized for cholecystectomy. Two days postoperatively she develops pneumonia. The nurse notes that Ms. S. does not know where she is and that she is picking at the bedclothes. What is the most likely diagnosis?
   a. Hemorrhage
   b. Sensory deprivation
   c. Delirium
   d. Urinary tract infection

2. Ms. S is likely to be oriented to which of the following:
   a. The time of day
   b. The day of the week
   c. Her daughter
   d. The name of her medication

3. Which of the following is the hallmark indication of delirium?
   a. Fluctuation of sensorium and limited attention span
   b. Global cognitive impairment
   c. Severe agitation
   d. Dysphoria

4. What level of consciousness is Ms. S. likely to exhibit during delirium?
   a. Alert and oriented
   b. Hyper-vigilant
   c. Fluctuating
   d. Comatose

5. Ms. S is likely to exhibit what type of perceptual disturbance?
   a. Poorly organized delusions
   b. Hallucinations
   c. Illusions
   d. All of the above

6. The onset of delirium is characterized by:
   a. Onset occurring over several days

b. Abrupt onset
c. Occurrence within two days of exposure to a causative factor
d. Fluctuating onset

7. Ms. S. has an EEG. The findings are likely to show which feature?

a. Diffusely abnormal slowing
b. Normal
c. Focal points
d. Lower range of normal

8. Ms. S's nurse needs to write a care plan. Which is the major nursing diagnosis she would use?

a. Self-care deficit
b. Alteration in thought processes
c. High risk for violence
d. Alteration in role performance

9. One of the ways in which delirium is differentiated from dementia is that delirium is:

a. Characterized by sundowning
b. A progressive deteriorating disease
c. Characterized by fluctuating level of consciousness
d. Chronic

10. All of the following are risk factors for delirium except:

a. Use of narcotics
b. Family dynamics
c. Systemic illness
d. Presence of dementia

11. Delirium is most common in which age group?

a. Age 10–20
b. Age 20–40
c. Age 40–60
d. Age 60–80

12. All of the following physical disorders can cause delirium except:

a. Hypertension

b. Substance abuse and withdrawal
c. Metabolic disorders
d. Systemic infections

13. Ms. S was determined to have delirium. What intervention is most critical?
    a. Symptom management
    b. Treating the underlying cause
    c. Administering medication
    d. Education of the patient

14. Which intervention would be the second most important?
    a. Symptom management
    b. Treating the underlying cause
    c. Administering medication
    d. Education of the patient

15. Which of the following drugs could further complicate Ms. S's delirium?
    a. Antibiotics
    b. Antihistamines
    c. Antihypertensives
    d. All of the above

16. Mr. D is a 65-year-old widowed white male. He is brought to the emergency room by his family because he has become agitated, disoriented, and has been hallucinating. Family reports that Mr. D takes ranitadine for ulcer disease. What is the most likely cause of his symptoms?
    a. His age
    b. His ulcer disease
    c. His medication
    d. An undetected organic factor

17. The most important initial nursing intervention for Mr. D is to:
    a. Interview Mr. D without his family present
    b. Use chemical restraints to protect Mr. D
    c. Provide the family with a list of support groups
    d. Institute measures to clear the medication from Mr. D's body

18. Which of the following medications could the nurse anticipate for Mr. D.?

a. Chlordiazepoxide 25 mgm po
b. Physostigmine 2mgm iv
c. Chlorpromazine 100 mgm iv
d. Diazepam 10 mgm iv

19. In administering physostigmine the nurse would be concerned about which of the following classes of medications potentiating the drug?

a. Antiemetics
b. Antianxiety
c. Antidepressants
d. Anticonvulsants

20. If Mr. D continues to be agitated, what other pharmacological agent is the physician likely to order?

a. Haloperidol
b. Chlorpromazine
c. Thioridazine
d. Lithium

21. The nurse could anticipate which side effects of haloperidol?

a. Cogwheel rigidity
b. Excessive salivation
c. Dystonia
d. All of the above

22. The nurse in caring for Mr. D would make all of the following individual interventions except:

a. Reorienting Mr. D to day, place, situation
b. Being attentive to Mr. D's fears
c. Telling Mr. D that he needs to eat to get better
d. Offering fluids every 2 hours

23. The nurse would make all of the following environmental interventions except:

a. Limiting family visits as these may be overstimulating
b. Providing orientation devices (clocks, calendars) in Mr. D's room
c. Keeping a low light on at night
d. Having Mr. D wear his glasses during the day

24. All of the following interventions are indicated for Mr. D at this time except:

a. Individual
b. Group
c. Family
d. Milieu

25. Organic mental disorders include all of the following except:

a. Affective disorders
b. Primary degenerative dementia
c. Vascular dementia
d. Psychoactive substance-induced delirium

26. Ms. T, who is 85, is unable to perform several of her ADLs due to her inability to conceptualize and complete tasks. Her level of dementia is:

a. Mild
b. Moderate
c. Severe
d. Fluctuating

27. Ms. T.'s nurse notes that she has short-term memory loss. An example would be:

a. Inability to remember what happened yesterday
b. Inability to remember current president
c. Inability to remember three objects after five minutes
d. Inability to remember an anniversary

28. A disorder of language is also noted. What would it be called?

a. Agnosia
b. Anhedonia
c. Apraxia
d. Aphasia

29. Ms. B., a 68-year-old African American, has a B/P of 220/110. She has had several episodes of dizziness and temporary loss of consciousness. Her family notes that she has had difficulty remembering in the past few months. The most likely diagnosis would be:

a. Primary degenerative dementia of Alzheimers type
b. Delirium
c. Vascular or Multi-infarct dementia
d. Organic mood disorder

30. Mr. A is an 82-year-old white married male. He has been diagnosed as having probable primary degenerative dementia. He has withdrawn from his activities at the senior center but continues to perform his ADLs. The level of severity of his dementia could be characterized as:

   a. Mild
   b. Moderate
   c. Severe
   d. None of the above apply

31. All of the following are needed to make a diagnosis of dementia except:

   a. Impairment in short-term memory
   b. Transient confusion
   c. Impairment in long-term memory
   d. Significant changes in social relationships

32. Which nursing diagnosis would be used for Mr. A's condition?

   a. Self-care deficit
   b. Social isolation
   c. Sensory/perceptual alterations
   d. Alteration in thought processes

33. Various types of dementias may have symptoms similar to all of the following except:

   a. Acute psychotic episode
   b. Delirium
   c. Major depressive episode
   d. Adjustment disorder

34. Etiologic factors for dementia include all except:

   a. Heredity and degenerative neurologic disease
   b. Cerebral vascular disease and normal pressure hydrocephalus
   c. Lack of education, social isolation
   d. Toxins and metabolic disturbances

35. Mr. W is a 68-year-old widowed white male with a history of alcohol abuse. On interview he is able to remember in detail an incident which occurred 20 years ago but cannot remember 3 objects after 5 minutes on the mental status

exam. He has no change in personality and his judgment is good. Mr. W's condition is probably caused by:

a. A deficiency of thiamine
b. Heredity
c. Situational stress
d. A tumor

36. Ms. C is a 70-year-old widowed female. Recently she has become very suspicious about her neighbor, whom she believes is an FBI agent. On a recent CT scan a right cerebral lesion was discovered. Her suspiciousness is most likely related to:

a. Her neighborhood
b. Her family relationships
c. Her cerebral tumor
d. A grief reaction

37. Ms. C is brought to the emergency room by the police after locking herself in her apartment and making threatening phone calls to her neighbor. The best nursing response to her is:

a. Tell her not to worry, her neighbor is not an FBI agent
b. Take measures to allay her anxiety and protect her from harm
c. Agree that the FBI does intrude into our lives
d. Conduct a complete nursing assessment including physical examination

38. Nursing diagnoses for Ms. C include all of the following except:

a. Altered thought processes
b. Fear related to persecutory delusions
c. High risk for violence
d. Knowledge deficit

39. Which is always associated with dementia?

a. Ataxic gait
b. Impaired memory and judgement
c. Delusions
d. Affective disturbances

40. Alzheimers disease is primarily characterized by:

a. Progressive memory decline

b. Emotional distress
c. Dysphoria
d. Hallucinations

41. Assessment of Alzheimers disease is best done by a:

a. Physician
b. Nurse
c. Multidisciplinary team
d. Psychologist

42. Senile onset refers to:

a. The development of the disease before age 65
b. The development of the disease after the person is determined to be senile.
c. The disease occurs after age 65
d. None of the above

43. Mr. Y, an 80-year-old married male, has been diagnosed with primary degenerative dementia and placed on Haldol 10 mgm at night which is his only medication. He has become more agitated in the past week. His agitation is probably due to:

a. His illness
b. A change in his environment
c. His medication
d. A urinary tract infection

44. Mr. Y's wife, to whom he has been married for 50 years, dies 2 years after he is first diagnosed with dementia. Several months later he experiences weight loss, crying spells, and sleep disturbance. The most likely diagnosis would be:

a. Primary degenerative dementia with delusions
b. Primary degenerative dementia with depression
c. Primary degenerative dementia with delirium
d. None of the above

45. Mr. Y's affect is likely to include all of the following except:

a. Sadness
b. Hopelessness
c. Euphoria
d. Helplessness

46. Mr. Y may have all of the following hallucinations except:
    a. Tactile
    b. Visual
    c. Auditory
    d. Olfactory

47. Mr. Y develops praxis. This refers to:
    a. Inability to conceptualize
    b. Difficulty with complex tasks
    c. Inability to write
    d. All of the above

48. Which of the following medications might be used to treat Mr. Y's depression?
    a. Prozac
    b. Zoloft
    c. Trazadone
    d. All of the above

49. Which of the following is classified as a selective serotonin re-uptake inhibitor (SSRI)?
    a. Trazadone
    b. Desipramine
    c. Fluoxetine
    d. Lithium

50. Alzheimers disease is considered to result from:
    a. Aluminum intoxication
    b. Alcohol abuse
    c. Tumors
    d. Causes are still unknown

51. Most recent evidence for the cause of Alzheimers disease involve which substance?
    a. Amino acids
    b. Carotene
    c. Beta-amyloid
    d. Serotonin

52. Multi-infarct dementia is characterized by which of the following:

    a. Stepwise and patchy deterioration in intellectual functioning
    b. Global cognitive impairments
    c. Retrograde amnesia
    d. Headaches and fainting spells

53. The causes of "reversible dementias" include all of the following except:

    a. Medications
    b. Metabolic and endocrine imbalances
    c. Sensory deprivation
    d. Infectious diseases

54. Which of the following is the most prevalent form of dementia?

    a. Reversible dementia
    b. Organic amnestic disorder
    c. Alzheimers disease
    d. Multi-infarct dementia

55. The second most prevalent dementia is

    a. Reversible dementia
    b. Organic amnestic disorder
    c. Alzheimers disease
    d. Multi-infarct dementia

56. Ms. T has dementia and resides in a nursing home. Which of the following individual interventions are indicated to enhance her care?

    a. Provide balance between stimulation and rest
    b. Provide structure and support
    c. Provide clear and direct communication
    d. All of the above

57. Which of the following should be avoided in providing care to Ms. T.:

    a. The use of chemical and physical restraints
    b. Having family members visit
    c. Reminiscence groups as they would be too stimulating
    d. Orientation measures

58. The nurse is considering starting a group for residents of Ms. T's nursing home with mild cognitive impairment. Which type of group would be indicated?

    a. Reminiscence
    b. Cognitive-behavioral
    c. Educational
    d. All of the above

59. The primary purpose of cognitive behavioral group interventions is to:

    a. Increase self-esteem through positive affiliations with others
    b. Correct negative thoughts and attitudes
    c. Provide information
    d. Explore unconscious motivations of behavior

60. Mr. B, two days post admission for esophageal varices, develops delirium tremens. This state is most associated with which of the following conditions?

    a. Cocaine withdrawal
    b. Parkinson's disease
    c. Alcohol withdrawal delirium
    d. Hypoxia

61. Which of the following community resources would be most helpful to Mr. B's family?

    a. Alanon
    b. Alzheimers Disease and Related Disorders Foundation
    c. American Heart Association
    d. All of the above

62. Validation is a method to:

    a. Stimulate communication
    b. Restore well-being
    c. Facilitate resolution of unresolved issues
    d. All of the above

Answers

1. c	22. c	43. c
2. c	23. a	44. b
3. a	24. b	45. c
4. c	25. a	46. a.
5. d	26. c	47. c
6. b	27. c	48. d
7. a	28. d	49. c
8. b	29. c	50. d
9. c	30. a	51. c
10. b	31. b	52. a
11. d	32. d	53. c
12. a	33. d	54. c
13. b	34. c	55. d
14. a	35. a	56. d
15. d	36. c	57. a
16. c	37. b	58. d
17. d	38. d	59. b
18. b	39. b	60. c
19. c	40. a	61. a
20. a	41. c	62. d
21. d	42. c	

Bibliography

Abraham, I. L., Holroyd, S., Snustad, D. G., Manning, C. A., Brashear, H. R., Diamond, P., & Thompson-Heisterman, A. A. (1994). Multidisciplinary assessment of Alzheimer's disease. *Nursing Clinics of North America,* 29(1), 113–128.

Abramowiez, M. (1986). Drugs that cause psychiatric symptoms. *The Medical Letter on Drugs and Therapeutics, 28*(721), 81–86.

American Psychiatric Association (1987). *Diagnostic and statistical manual of mental disorders* (3rd ed. rev.). Washington, DC: American Psychiatric Association.

American Psychiatric Association (1993). *Diagnostic and statistical manual of mental disorders,* DSM-IV Draft cirteria. Washington, DC: American Psychiatric Association.

Butler, R. N., Lewis, M., & Sunderland, T. (1991). *Aging and mental health,* (p. 149–183) (4th ed.). NY: Macmillan.

Coccaro, E. F., Kramer, E., Zemishlany, Z., Thorne, A. , Rice, C. M., Giordani, B., Duvvi, K., Bhupendra, M. P., Torres, J., Nora, R., Neufeld, R., Mohs, R. C., & Davis, K. L. (1990). Pharmacologic treatment of noncognitive behavioral disturbances in elderly demented patients. *American Journal of Psychiatry 147*(12), 1640–1645.

Curl, A. (1992). Nursing care of the dementia patient. In K. C. Buckwalter (Ed.), *Geriatric mental health nursing: Current and future challenges* (pp. 27–43). Thorofare, NJ: Slack.

Feil, N. (1989) Validation: An empathetic approach to the care of dementia. *Clinical Gerontologist,* 8, 89–94.

Francis, J. (1992). Delirium in older patients. *Journal of the American Geriatrics Society, 40,* 829–838.

Harper, M. (1992). Home and community based mental health services for the elderly. In K. C. Buckwalter (Ed.), *Geriatric mental health nursing: Current and Future Challenges* (pp. 122–129). Thorofare, NJ: Slack.

Inaba-Roland, K. E., & Maricle, R. A. (1992). Assessing delirium in the acute care setting. *Heart and Lung,* 21(1), 48–55.

Lipowski, Z. J. (1990). *Delirium: Acute confusional states.* New York: Oxford University Press.

Lipowski, Z. J. (1989). Delirium in the elderly patient. *The New England Journal of Medicine, 320*(9), 578–581.

Maletta, G. J. (1990). The concept of ''reversible dementia'': How nonreliable terminology may impair effective treatment. *Journal of the American Geriatrics Society, 38,* 136–140.

Montamat, S. C., Cusack, B. J., & Vestal, R. E. (1989). Management of drug therapy in the elderly. *The New England Journal of Medicine, 321*(5), 303–309.

Neese, J. B. (1991). Depression in the general hospital. *Nursing Clinics of North America, 26*(3), 613–622.

Neese, J. B., & Abraham, I. L. (1992). Group interventions with the elderly. In K. C. Buckwalter (Ed.), *Geriatric mental health nursing: Current and future challenges* (pp. 75–83). Thorofare, NJ: Slack.

Ramsay, R., Wright, P., Katz, A., Bielawska, C., & Katona, C. (1990). The detection of psychiatric morbidity and its effects on outcome in acute elderly medical admissions. *International Journal of Geriatric Psychiatry, 6,* 861–866.

Rawlins, R. P., Williams, S. R., & Beck, C. K. (1993). *Mental health-psychiatric nursing: A holistic life-cycle approach* (pp. 649–670) (3rd ed.). St. Louis: Mosby Year Book.

Ryden, M. B. (1992). Alternatives to restraints and psychotropics in the care of aggressive, cognitively impaired elderly persons. In K. C. Buckwalter (Ed.), *Geriatric mental health nursing: Current and future challenges* (pp. 84–93). Thorofare, NJ: Slack.

Schor, J. D., Levoff, S. E., Lipsitz, L. A., Reily, C. H., Cleary, P. D., Rowe, J. W., & Evans, D. A. (1992). Risk factors for delirium in hospitalized elderly. *JAMA, 267*(6), 827–831.

Thompson-Heisterman, A. A., Smullen, D. E., & Abraham, I. L. (1992). Psychogeriatric nursing assessment. In K. C. Buckwalter (Ed.), *Geriatric mental health nursing: Current and future challenges* (pp. 17–26). Thorofare, NJ: Slack.

Whall, A. L., & Booth, D. E. (1992). The use of neuroleptic drugs in nursing homes: Innovative strategies and implications for rehabilitation. In K. C. Buckwalter (Ed.), *Geriatric mental health nursing: Current and future challenges* (pp. 103–110). Thorofare, NJ: Slack.

Yi, E. S., Abraham, I. L., & Holroyd, S. (1994). Alzheimer's disease and nursing: New scientific and clinical insights. *Nursing Clinics of North America,* 29(1), 85–99.

Behavioral and Emotional Disorders of Childhood and Adolescence

Michelle L. Zimmerman

Child and Adolescent Psychiatric Mental Health Nursing

Issues

- 7.5 million children and adolescents suffer from some mental disorder in the U.S. (NIMH).
- Shortage of skilled child psychiatric nursing clinicians (Pothier, 1988)
- Child clinicians need to have excellent family assessment skills, physical assessment skills, and keen knowledge of normal growth and development.
- Child psychiatric mental health nursing requires gathering data from multiple informants and providing feedback to multiple agencies, such as schools and social service agencies.

Professional Standards

- Specialists in this area hold a master's or doctoral degree in child and adolescent psychiatric nursing and are certified as clinical specialists by the American Nurse's Credentialing Center in child and adolescent psychiatric nursing.
- Standards for the child and adolescent psychiatric mental health nurse are set forth in *Statement on Psychiatric-Mental Health Clinical Nursing Practice and Standards of Psychiatric Mental Health Nursing Practice* (1994).

Diagnoses

- Mental health nursing has changed significantly with the advancement of DSM IV (1993).
    1. Axis II no longer used for developmental disorders, such as Mental Retardation, Pervasive Developmental Disorders and specific Developmental Disorders.
    2. New categories and reorganization of Learning Disorders, Motor Skills Disorder, and Communication Disorders have occurred.
    3. Eating Disorders and Gender Identity Disorders (moved)
    4. Attention Deficit Hyperactivity Disorder has been significantly modified to reflect both inattention and impulsivity.

Mental Retardation

Mental retardation (MR) involves significantly subaverage general intellectual functioning, with a tested I.Q. of <70. There are significant deficits in areas of work, daily living, socializing and self-sufficiency, and the onset is prior to age 18.

There are four degrees of severity, reflecting the degree of intellectual impairment (APA, 1993).

Mild Mental Retardation (formerly referred to as "educable")

- Signs and Symptoms
  1. IQ 50-55 to approximately 70
  2. 85% of those with this disorder are in this category.
  3. Can develop social and communication skills
  4. Can acquire academic skills to sixth grade level
  5. Can acquire skills for minimum self-support
  6. Can live in the community
  7. May need guidance and support during stress

Moderate Mental Retardation (formerly referred to as "trainable")

- Signs and Symptoms
  1. IQ 35-40 to 50-55
  2. 10% of the population with MR
  3. Can talk and communicate
  4. Can profit from vocational training, but are unlikely to progress beyond second grade level
  5. May have difficulties with social conventions
  6. Can live in supervised group homes
  7. Need supervision and guidance under stress

Severe Mental Retardation

- Signs and Symptoms

1. IQ 20-25 to 35-40
2. 3%-4% of the people with MR
3. Little or no communicative speech during pre-school; may learn speech during school-age years
4. Can be taught limited hygiene skills
5. Can ''sight-read'' some survival words, such as ''EXIT,'' ''STOP,'' ''MEN,'' ''WOMEN''
6. May perform simple tasks under close supervision
7. May live in the community in group homes or with families in the absence of an associated handicap

Profound Mental Retardation

- Signs and Symptoms
    1. 1% -2% of people with MR
    2. These children have minimal capacity for sensorimotor functioning.
    3. Motor development, self care and communication skills may improve if appropriate training is provided.
    4. May live in the community, in group homes, in intermediate care facilities, or with families
    5. Need day programs or sheltered workshop

Mental Retardation Severity Unspecified

- Signs and Symptoms
    1. This category used when formal testing cannot be accomplished due to impairment or lack of cooperation
    2. The younger the age, the greater the difficulties in diagnosing mental retardation, except for those with profound impairment
    3. This category not used when the intellectual level is presumed to be above 70

The following is pertinent to Mild, Moderate, Severe, and Profound Mental Retardation

- Differential Diagnosis

1. Schizophrenia
2. Autism
3. Tic Disorder
4. Depression

- Associated Disorders
    1. Prevalence of mental disorders at least three or four times higher than in the general population
        a. Pervasive developmental disorders
        b. Attention Deficit Hyperactivity Disorder (ADHD)
        c. Stereotypy/Habit Disorder
- Mental Status (formal Mental Status not evaluated under age 10) needs to be adjusted to level of retardation
    1. Passivity
    2. Dependency
    3. Low self-esteem
    4. Low frustration tolerance
    5. Aggressiveness
    6. Poor impulse control
    7. Stereotyped self-stimulating and self-injurious behavior
    8. Poor social skills (exception is Down Syndrome where social skills much higher than expected for level of retardation)
- Nursing Diagnoses
    1. Impaired verbal communication
    2. Aggression
    3. Impaired social interaction
    4. Altered growth and development
    5. Self care deficit(s)
    6. Self concept disturbance
    7. Powerlessness

- Genetic/Biological Origins
    1. Hereditary factors (5% of cases)
        a. Inborn metabolism errors (Tay-Sachs disease; phenylketonuria)
        b. Single gene abnormalities (Tuberous sclerosis)
        c. Chromosomal aberrations (translocation Down syndrome, Fragile X syndrome)
    2. Early alterations of embryonic development (30%)
        a. Maternal alcohol consumption causing prenatal damage due to toxins
    3. Pregnancy and perinatal problems (10%)
        a. Fetal malnutrition, prematurity, or hypoxia
        b. Maternal trauma—pregnant women are at higher risk for injury due to family violence than non-pregnant women.
    4. Physical disorders acquired in childhood
- Biochemical Approaches
    1. Concomitant mental disorder must be specifically treated with antidepressants for depression, or stimulants for ADHD.
    2. Agitation, aggression, and tantrumming may respond to antipsychotics—high dosage, low potency drugs more cognitively dulling than low dosage, high potency ones.
    3. Aggressive or self-abusive behaviors may be helped by Lithium (see Stereotypy Habit Disorder).
    4. Tantrumming and aggression may be helped by
        a. Carbamazepine (Tegretol)
            (1) 10-20 mg/kg/day in 2-3 divided doses
            (2) Side effects—drowsiness, nausea, vertigo, psychosis.
            (3) Blood and hepatic studies for blood dyscrasias and hepatotoxicity.
        b. Propranolol (Inderal) up to 2 mg/kg/day
            (1) Side effects—dizziness, fatigue, insomnia, depression, nausea, diarrhea, bronchospasm

- Intrapersonal Origins
    1. Psychosocial deprivation
    2. Lack of stimulation
- Psychotherapeutic Interventions
    1. Behavior modification specific for acting-out behaviors
    2. Supportive treatment that raises self-esteem
- Family Dynamics/Family Therapy
    1. Dysfunctional family processes, such as abusive and chemically dependent families, generate certain types of mental retardation, as do families who undernurture and understimulate the child.
    2. Therapy needs to be geared to correcting dysfunctional processes without pathologizing the family.
    3. The deficits of the mentally retarded child create severe stress for the family. A pattern of overprotection and overcompensation may develop.
    4. Families need both respite care and help in focusing on the child's strengths.
    5. Psychoeducational approaches are essential to engender family cooperation with programs.
    6. Family group therapy decreases the family's sense of isolation and stress, and provides a forum for sharing effective management strategies.
- Group Approaches
    1. Traditional, insight-oriented group not indicated
    2. Behavior modification, educational group may be helpful.
    3. Socialization groups useful
- Milieu Interventions
    1. Interventions should be designed to address specific problematic behaviors.
    2. Aggressive behaviors are in response to the overwhelming powerlessness experienced by these children. Child needs help in coping with teasing and needs protection from harm by others.

3. Mental retardation, per se, is no longer generally considered criteria for admission to a psychiatric inpatient setting.
4. Community meetings in day care, group home, or sheltered workshop settings helpful.

- Community Resources
  1. Numerous resources in larger metropolitan areas
  2. Rural and suburban areas have extremely limited resources.
  3. Steady decline in services in the last twenty years
  4. Retarded adults have demonstrated their capacity to be reliable and effective workers for routine tasks under supervision.

Learning Disorders

These disorders are currently arranged in four groups in DSM IV (APA, 1993). These disorders are often associated with each other or with other disorders. There is a great deal of controversy over the inclusion of these as mental disorders. Often there is no sign of psychopathology with these children, and detection and treatment takes place within the school system. However, there may be an association with other Axis I disorders.

Mathematics Disorder

- Signs and Symptoms
  1. Arithmetic skills, as measured by standardized individually administered tests, are markedly below the level expected, given the person's schooling and IQ (as determined by an individually administered IQ test).
  2. The disturbance significantly interferes with academic achievement or activities of daily living that require mathematical ability.
  3. If a sensory deficit is present, the learning difficulties are in excess of those usually associated with it.

Disorder of Written Expression

- Signs and Symptoms
  1. Marked impairment in writing skills, as measured by a standardized,

individually administered test, given the person's schooling and intellectual capacity.

2. The disturbance significantly interferes with academic achievement or activities of daily living that require the composition of written texts.
3. If a sensory deficit is present, the learning difficulties are in excess of those usually associated with it.

Reading Disorder

- Signs and Symptoms
    1. Reading achievement, as measured by an individually administered standardized test of reading accuracy or comprehension, is substantially below that expected given the person's chronological age, measured intelligence and age-appropriate education.
    2. The disturbance significantly interferes with academic achievement or activities of daily living that require reading skills.
    3. If a sensory deficit is present, the learning difficulties are in excess of those usually associated with it.

Learning Disorder Not Otherwise Specified

(This category is for disorders that do not meet criteria for any specific learning disorder—for example, a disorder in which spelling skills are substantially below that expected given the person's chronological age, measured intelligence, and age-appropriate education.)

Motor Skills Disorder

Developmental Coordination Disorder

- Signs and Symptoms
    1. Performance in daily activities that require motor coordination is substantially below that expected given the person's chronological age and measured intelligence
    2. Marked delays in achieving motor milestones
    3. Clumsiness
    4. Poor sports performance

5. Poor handwriting
6. The disturbance significantly interferes with academic achievement or activities of daily living.
7. Not due to a general medical condition.

The following information refers to Motor Skills and Learning Disorders

- Differential Diagnosis
  1. Mental Retardation
  2. Neurological disorders
  3. Pervasive Developmental Disorders
  4. ADHD
  5. Inadequate schooling
  6. Impaired vision or hearing
  7. PTSD induced regression and loss of recently acquired skills
- Mental Status Variations
  1. Determined by history, observation
  2. Teacher report/checklists essential
  3. Performance on standardized tests
- Nursing Diagnoses
  1. Growth and development, altered
  2. Ineffective individual coping
  3. Self-concept, disturbance in
  4. Communication, impaired, verbal
- Genetic/Biological Origins
  1. Perinatal injury of various kinds
  2. No information on sex ratio for the arithmetic and coordination disorders. The others are from two to four times more common in males than females. The prevalence rate is 2-10% of the population.
  3. Some show a history in first-degree biologic relatives.
  4. May have other neurological "soft signs."

- Biochemical Approaches

  No evidence that medication directly benefits children with these disorders; may be used for associated conditions.

- Intrapersonal Origins/Psychotherapeutic Interventions
  1. Intrapersonal origins not identified
  2. Psychotherapy may be helpful with issues of low self-esteem and school failure.
  3. School counseling and collaboration with the school guidance counselor may be helpful.
- Family Therapy
  1. Families may need assistance in behavior management strategies and psychoeducational approaches may be in order.
- Group Approaches
  1. Helpful in self-esteem issues and to overcome feelings of differentness.
- Milieu Interventions
  1. Do not meet criteria for admission to inpatient settings.
- Community Resources
  1. Educational intervention depends upon degree of impairment.
  2. Special education

Communication Disorders

The Communication Disorders are diagnosed by psychologists and speech and hearing therapists and scores on standardized measures of nonverbal intellectual capacity and receptive language development.

These disorders interfere with academic achievement and social relationships or activities of daily living that require the expression or comprehension of verbal or sign language.

Phonological Disorder

- Signs and Symptoms
  1. Consistent failure to make correct articulation of speech sounds

2. Frequent substitutions or omissions of speech sounds, giving the impression of baby talk

Expressive Language Disorder

- Signs and Symptoms
  1. Marked impairment in the development of expressive language.

Mixed Receptive/Expressive Language Disorder

- Signs and Symptoms
  1. Marked impairment in the development of language comprehension

Stuttering

- Signs and Symptoms— marked impairment in speech fluency with frequent repetitions or prolongations of sound or syllables.

The following refers to all Communication Disorders

- Differential Diagnosis
  1. Normal childhood dysfluency—an intermittent speech dysfluency which occurs before age three
  2. Spastic dysphonia—a speech disorder similar to stuttering distinguished by an abnormal breathing pattern.
- Mental Status Variations
  1. Often causes the speaker great anxiety and fearfulness of speaking. Certain associated features may be noted:
     a. Linguistic mechanisms such as altering speech rate
     b. Motor movements frequently accompanying stuttering such as eye blinks, tics, tremors of the face and head, fist clenching
  2. Severity of symptoms may increase under pressure to communicate, such as during an interview.
- Nursing Diagnoses
  1. Impaired verbal communication
  2. Anxiety
- Genetic/Biological Origins

1. Familial pattern noted in Communication Disorders
2. Stuttering—research supports genetic evidence for the origin of stuttering.
    a. Male to female ratio is three to one.
    b. Fifty percent of first degree biological relatives affected.
3. May have generalized neurological soft signs
4. No factors have been shown to be clearly associated with recovery.
5. Approximately 80% recover before age 16.
6. Females more commonly recover than males.

- Psychotherapeutic Interventions
    1. Therapy would focus on overcoming the associated anxiety and frustration.
    2. Relaxation training and stress management may help provide a sense of mastery and self control.
- Family Therapy
    1. Family may help raise child's self esteem
    2. Assisting the parents to understand and be empathetic with the patient would be of benefit.
    3. Contributory family dysfunctional patterns need to be addressed.
- Group Approaches
    1. To overcome low self-esteem and impairment of social functioning
- Milieu Interventions
    1. Communication disorders do not meet criteria for admission to inpatient settings.
- Community Resources
    1. Speech and hearing therapy—usually not covered by third party payers
    2. School systems may have diagnostic and treatment service available

Pervasive Developmental Disorders (PDD)

These are extreme neuropsychiatric disorders that primarily affect verbal and nonverbal communication, social skills, and imaginative activity. Basic psychological functions are profoundly affected. Often there is an accompanying diagnosis of mental retardation.

Autistic Disorder

- Signs and Symptoms—includes a total of at least six items from 1, 2, and 3, with at least two from 1, and one each from 2 and 3.
  1. Qualitative impairment in social interaction as manifested by at least 2 of the following:
     a. Marked impairment in the use of multiple nonverbal behaviors, such as eye-to-eye gaze, facial expression, body postures, and gestures to regulate social interaction
     b. Failure to develop peer relationships appropriate to developmental level
     c. Markedly impaired expression of pleasure in other people's happiness
     d. Lack of social or emotional reciprocity
  2. Qualitative impairments in communication as manifested by at least one of the following:
     a. Delay in, or total lack of, the development of spoken language (not accompanied by an attempt to compensate through alternative modes of communication such as gesture or mime)
     b. In individuals with adequate speech, marked impairment in the ability to initiate or sustain a conversation with others
     c. Stereotyped and repetitive use of language or idiosyncratic language
     d. Lack of varied spontaneous make-believe play or social imitative play appropriate to developmental level
  3. Restricted repetitive and stereotyped patterns of behavior, interests, and activities, as manifested by at least one of the following:
     a. Encompassing preoccupation with one or more stereotyped and

restricted patterns of interest that is abnormal either in intensity or focus

   b. Apparently compulsive adherence to specific, nonfunctional routines and rituals

   c. Stereotyped and repetitive motor mannerisms (e.g., hand or finger flapping or twisting, or complex whole body movements)

   d. Persistent preoccupation with parts of objects

4. Delays or abnormal functioning in at least one of the following areas, with onset prior to age three

   a. Social interaction

   b. Language as used in social communication

   c. Symbolic or imaginative play

- Associated features—the younger the child and the more severe the impairment, the higher the number of associated features.

  1. Abnormal development of cognitive skills

  2. Abnormal posture and motor behavior

  3. Odd response to sensory input such as oblivion to pain or cold but hypersensitivity to benign sounds, such as birds chirping. There may be a fascination with some sensations of touch, such as a velvet pillow.

  4. Abnormalities in eating, drinking, or sleeping

  5. Abnormalities of mood

  6. Self-injurious behavior, such as head-banging, finger-biting, gouging skin

- Differential Diagnosis

  1. Mental retardation—MR people, even seriously impaired, can socialize and communicate in some way.

  2. Schizophrenia is rare in childhood, and the additional diagnosis should be made only if delusions or hallucinations meeting the criteria for schizophrenia can be made.

  3. Hearing impairments and specific developmental language and speech disorders can be differentiated by the presence of social interaction and a desire for communication.

4. Tic Disorders and Stereotypy/Habit disorder—have stereotyped body movements, but no impaired reciprocal social interaction.
5. The category of "Pervasive Developmental Disorder Not Otherwise Specified" is used where there is
   a. Qualitative impairment in the development of reciprocal social interaction and communication skills
   b. Criteria not met for Autistic Disorder, Schizophrenia, Schizotypal, or Schizoid Personality Disorder
6. Avoidant Personality Disorder
7. Schizotypal Personalty Disorder

- Mental Status Variations
  1. Severe impairment in reciprocal social interaction
  2. Communication deficits
- Nursing Diagnoses
  1. Social interaction, impaired
  2. Communication, impaired verbal
  3. Violence, potential for, self-directed
  4. Self-concept, disturbance in personal identity
  5. Coping, ineffective family: compromised/disabling
- Biological Origins Autism is considered an organic syndrome today and not a deficit in parent-child relations
  1. Male to female ratio 3:1-4:1
  2. Tuberous sclerosis
  3. Maternal rubella
  4. Untreated phenylketonuria
  5. Encephalitis
  6. Fragile X syndrome
  7. EEG studies show nonfocal abnormality.
  8. Brain computed tomography (CT) scan is abnormal in 25% with ventricular dilatation a frequent finding.

9. Cerebellar abnormalities found on some magnetic resonance imaging (MRI) tests and some post-mortem exams
10. Increased frontal lobe glucose metabolism has been noted in position emission tomography (PET) scan.
11. Abnormal levels of neurotransmitters or their metabolites have been found in blood or cerebrospinal fluid.
12. Autistic individuals have more seizures as they age, as opposed to the general population.

- Biochemical Approaches
  1. Pharmacologic intervention has little impact on core features but may help to control secondary symptoms and may help families continue home care.
  2. Intervention includes:
     a. Haloperidol in nonsedating doses
     b. Fenfluramine (Pondimin) lowers blood serotonin
     c. Opiate antagonists are being explored to reduce interpersonal withdrawal by blocking exogenous opioids.
     d. Lithium may help aggressive or self-injurious behaviors.
- Interpersonal Approaches
  1. Individual psychotherapy is futile given the profound neuropsychiatric, cognitive, and language deficits.
  2. Special education is necessary, and parents may decide to institutionalize these children.
  3. Parents need support when coping with these decisions.
  4. In the event that the client is hospitalized, predictability of routine is essential.
- Family Dynamics/Family Therapy
  1. A former view of PDDs was that certain parental personalities produced this disorder along with particular child-rearing practices. Parents need help overcoming this bias and any associated guilt.
  2. Parents must be given accurate information about this disorder.
  3. Siblings of children with these disorders need support.

4. Behavioral management strategies are important and need rigorous reinforcement outside of the institution.

- Group Approaches
  1. Not indicated for clients
  2. Family support groups indicated
- Milieu Interventions
  1. Enhance communication and interaction.
  2. Behavioral control if necessary.
  3. Increase repertoire of activities and interests.
  4. Increase self-care within level of capabilities.
  5. Provide reinforcement for appropriate behaviors.
  6. Provide psychoeducational support for family.
  7. Maintain seizure precautions as this group is at high risk for seizures.
- Community Resources
  - a. Autism Society of America—national group with local chapters
  - b. Community mental health centers may provide family support groups or respite care. Knowledge about the validity and definition of these other PDDs remains quite limited. Continued research is needed to establish their validity.

Rett's Disorder

- Signs and Symptoms
  1. Normal development for at least the first six months as manifested by all of the following:
     - a. Apparently normal perinatal development
     - b. Apparently normal psychomotor development
     - c. Normal head circumference at birth
  2. Onset of all of the following between 5 and 48 months
     - a. Deceleration of head growth

b. Loss of previously acquired purposeful hand movements, with the development of stereotyped hand movements such as wringing or washing

c. Loss of social engagement early (although social interaction often develops later)

d. Appearance of poorly coordinated gait or trunk movements

e. Marked delay and impairment of expressive and receptive language with severe psychomotor retardation

- Differential Diagnosis

1. Autistic disorder
2. Childhood disintegrative disorder,
3. Mental retardation

Childhood Disintegrative Disorder

- Signs and Symptoms (APA, 1993)

1. Apparently normal development for at least the first two years as manifested by the presence of age-appropriate verbal and non-verbal communication, social relationships, play and adaptive behavior.
2. There is clinically significant loss of previously acquired skills in at least two of the following areas

   a. Expressive or receptive language

   b. Social skills or adaptive behavior

   c. Bowel or bladder control

   d. Play

   e. Motor skills

3. There are abnormalities of functioning in at least two of the following areas:

   a. Qualitative impairment in social interaction, as manifested by at least two of the following:

      (1) Marked impairment in the use of multiple nonverbal behaviors such as eye-to-eye gaze, facial expression, body postures, and gestures to regulate social interaction

(2) Failure to develop peer relationships appropriate to developmental level

(3) Markedly impaired expression of pleasure in other people's happiness

(4) Lack of social or emotional reciprocity

b. Qualitative impairments in communication as manifested by at least one of the following:

(1) Delay in, or total lack of, the development of spoken language (not accompanied by an attempt to compensate through alternative modes of communication such as gesture or mime)

(2) In individuals with adequate speech, marked impairment in the ability to initiate or sustain conversation with others

(3) Stereotyped and repetitive use of language or idiosyncratic language

(4) Lack of varied spontaneous make-believe play or social imitative play appropriate to developmental level

c. Restricted, repetitive, and stereotyped patterns of behavior, interests, and activities, including motor stereotypes and mannerisms

- Differential Diagnosis

1. Other Pervasive Developmental Disorders
2. Schizophrenia

Asperger's Disorder

- Signs and Symptoms (APA, 1993)

1. Qualitative impairment in social interaction, as manifested by at least two of the following:

a. Marked impairment in use of multiple nonverbal behaviors such as eye-to-eye gaze, facial expression, body postures, and gestures to regulate social interaction

b. Failure to develop peer relationships appropriate to developmental level

c. Markedly impaired expression of pleasure in other people's happiness

d. Lack of social or emotional reciprocity

2. Restricted, repetitive, and stereotyped patterns of behavior, interests, and activities

3. Lack of any clinically significant delay in cognitive development as manifested by the development of age-appropriate self-help skills, adaptive behavior, and curiosity about the environment

4. Lack of any clinically significant general delay in language

- Differential Diagnosis—other Pervasive Developmental Disorders

Pervasive Developmental Disorder Not Otherwise Specified (including Atypical Autism)

- Signs and Symptoms (APA, 1993)—severe and pervasive impairment in the development of reciprocal social interaction, verbal and nonverbal communication skills, or the development of stereotyped behavior, interests and activities

Disruptive Behavior and Attention Deficit Disorder

Manifested by behaviors that are disturbing to others and often socially disruptive. The behaviors are referred to as ''externalizing'' symptoms. They interfere with the child's social functioning and learning.

Attention-Deficit Hyperactivity Disorder (ADHD), (APA, 1993) Includes either symptoms of inattention (1) or hyperactivity (2)

- Signs and Symptoms

1. Inattention—at least six of the following symptoms of inattention have persisted for at least six months to a degree that is maladaptive and inconsistent with developmental level

a. Often fails to give close attention to details or makes careless mistakes in schoolwork, work, or other activities

b. Often has difficulty sustaining attention in tasks or play activities

c. Often doesn't seem to listen to what is being said to him or her

d. Often does not follow through on instructions, fails to finish schoolwork, chores or duties in the workplace (not due to oppositional behavior or failure to understand instructions)

e. Often has difficulties organizing tasks and activities

f. Often avoids, expresses reluctance about, or has difficulties engaging in tasks requiring sustained mental effort (such as schoolwork or homework)

g. Often loses things necessary for tasks or activities

h. Often forgetful in daily activities

2. Hyperactivity Impulsivity—at least five of the following symptoms have persisted for at least six months to a degree that is maladaptive and inconsistent with developmental level

   a. Often fidgets with hands or feet or squirms in seat

   b. Leaves seat in classroom or in other situations in which remaining seated is expected

   c. Often runs about or climbs excessively in situations where it is inappropriate (in adolescents or adults, may be limited to subjective feelings of restlessness)

   d. Often has difficulty playing or engaging in leisure activities quietly

   e. Is always "on the go" or acts as if "driven by a motor"

   f. Often talks excessively

   g. Often blurts out answers to questions before the questions have been completed

   h. Often has difficulty waiting in lines or waiting turn in games or group situations

   i. Often interrupts or intrudes on others

   j. Scores outside of normal values on parent-teacher checklists, such as the Connor's Parent Teacher Scales and the Rutter's Rating Scales.

- Differential Diagnosis

   1. Response to a chaotic environment, including parenting problems.

   2. Specific learning disabilities

3. Acute situational reactions
4. Adjustment Disorders
5. Conduct Disorder and Oppositional Defiant Disorder may be coded on Axis I
6. Mental Retardation
7. Pervasive Developmental Disorders
8. Mood Disorders

- Mental Status
  1. Emotional lability
  2. Disruptive behavior in classroom
- Nursing Diagnoses
  1. Coping individual, ineffective
  2. Social interaction, impaired
  3. Self-concept, disturbance in self esteem
  4. Coping, ineffective family—compromised/disabling
- Biological Origins
  1. May be sex-linked—more males than females
  2. Fathers may be alcoholic or have Antisocial Personality Disorders
  3. Conduct disorder and specific developmental disorders more frequent in relatives
  4. CNS abnormalities
  5. Noradrenergic, dopaminergic, and serotonergic abnormalities
  6. Hyper/hypothyroid may be contributory.
- Biochemical Approaches: Decision to use stimulants based on symptoms.
  1. Between 70 and 80% of children with ADHD respond to medication.
  2. Methylphenidate hydrochloride (Ritalin) (prescribed most frequently)
     a. Begin with 5 mg 1-2 times/day
     b. Dosage raised 5-10 mg/week

c. Maximum daily dosage 60 mg

d. Important to enlist cooperation of school to administer lunch time dose

3. Dextroamphetamine Sulfate (Dexedrine)

   a. Approved for children 3 to 5 years

      (1) Dosage—begin 2.5 mg daily, by tablet; daily dosage may be raised in increments of 2.5 mg at weekly intervals

   b. 6 years and older

      (1) Dosage—begin 5 mg once or twice daily; daily dosage may be increased in increments of 5 mg at weekly intervals until optimal response is obtained; maximum dose less than 40 mg/day

4. Magnesium Pemoline (Cylert)

   a. Not recommended for children under 6

   b. Persons over 6

      (1) Initial dosage 37.5 mg daily

      (2) Increased weekly by 18.75 until satisfactory clinical benefit

      (3) Maximum dosage 112.5 mg/daily

   c. Has a delayed therapeutic response of 3 weeks

5. Beneficial effects of stimulants

   a. Improved cooperation with adults: parents, and teachers note behavioral improvement

   b. Improved family functioning

   c. Increased socialization

   d. Child becomes more goal oriented

   e. Improvement noted on cognitive tasks possibly due to better attention, better inhibitory control and increased motivation

6. Side effects for stimulants include

   a. Reduced appetite

b. Insomnia

c. Growth retardation noted in some studies, but Ritalin has the fewest side effects of the stimulants.

- Intrapersonal Origins
  1. Retarded ego development
  2. Low self esteem
- Psychotherapeutic Approaches
  1. Play therapy—structured, one-to-one with frequent reinforcement and incentives for evidence of self control, ''point system'' and other behavioral interventions for positive reinforcement
  2. Careful environmental control—tasks and chores should be broken down into short, manageable components and homework should also be done in short periods with opportunities for breaks
  3. Convey unconditional positive regard as these children often have low self-esteem and respond to positive reinforcement.
  4. Avoid teasing.
  5. Assist with organization and planning.
  6. Approach the child with firmness, consistency and limit-setting as well as patience.
- Family Dynamics
  1. Dysfunctional family system
  2. Sociopathic, alcoholic, conduct-disordered relatives
  3. Chaotic environment
- Family Therapy
  1. Promote consistency and schedule.
  2. Involve siblings.
  3. Bibliotherapy
  4. Behavioral reinforcement from family therapist
  5. '' Time out'' vs. physical punishment
  6. Offer diversions, such as tapes and stories to counteract the ADHD child's constant chatter.

- Group Approaches
  1. Parent support group
  2. Systematic Training for Effective Parenting (STEP) and Parent Effectiveness Training (PET) classes
  3. Sports activities using large muscle groups, such as soccer and swimming can be helpful.
- Milieu Interventions
  1. Children with a primary diagnosis of ADHD usually do not meet criteria for hospitalization although ADHD may be comorbid with other diagnoses, such as Major Depression and Post Traumatic Stress Disorder.
  2. Parents need information on structuring and planning the child's milieu at home.
     a. Point system
     b. Behavioral charts and schedules
     c. Decrease external stimuli
     d. Provide for large muscle activity to discharge energies
     e. Limit setting on disruptive behavior
     f. Clear explanation of expectations
     g. Encourage positive peer activities.
     h. Multidisciplinary coordination involving child's teachers
     i. Provide opportunities and incentives for success.
- Community Resources
  1. Support groups such as Attention Deficit Disorder Association (ADDA), Attention Deficit Information Network (AD-IN), and Children with ADD (CHADD)

Conduct Disorder

- Definition:
  1. A persistent pattern of conduct in which the basic rights of others and major norms and rules are violated.
  2. Behavior may include

a. Physical aggression
b. Cruelty to people and animals
c. Property destruction, including fire-setting
d. Stealing (overt and covert)
e. Lying, cheating
f. School truancy and runaway

3. Associated with early use of tobacco, alcohol, nonprescribed drugs
4. The child lacks empathy, guilt or remorse, and often blames others.
5. Low self esteem covered by bravado with low frustration tolerance, irritability, and recklessness are common.
6. Poor academic achievement is usual.

- Differential Diagnosis (Not diagnosed by single acts of antisocial behavior, but by persistent and repetitive patterns)
  1. Oppositional Defiant Disorder—the rights of others are violated as well as major age-appropriate social norms.
  2. Bipolar Disorder usually represents brief manic episodes.
- Associated Conditions
  1. Anxiety
  2. Depression
  3. Specific Developmental Disorder
  4. ADHD
  5. Adolescent chemical dependency and substance abuse
  6. Antisocial Personality (Axis II) not used for children, but may be diagnosed at age 15
- Mental Status
  1. May present as angry or superficially friendly
  2. Self-centered and entitled
  3. Major defenses include denial, projection, and tendency to blame or implicate others.
  4. Poor insight

5. May attempt to bully examiner and behave in coercive or threatening ways

- Nursing Diagnoses
  1. Coping, ineffective individual
  2. Violence, potential for, self directed or directed toward others
  3. Anxiety
  4. Adjustment, impaired
  5. Self-concept, disturbance in body image, self-esteem, role performance; personal identity
  6. Coping, ineffective family: compromised/disabling
  7. Social interaction, impaired
- Biological Origins-common in children of antisocial and alcoholic parents
- Biochemical Approaches
  1. Associated conditions, such as ADHD, depression or post-traumatic stress disorder may be treated pharmacologically.
  2. Drug screens to identify drug use and abuse
- Intrapersonal Origins
  1. Fixed in separation-individuation phase
  2. Retarded ego development; id driven
  3. May have been a victim of physical or sexual abuse, or both; behavior is attempt to master anxiety (Burgess, 1990)
- Psychotherapeutic Interventions
  1. Security and trust provided climate for growth
  2. Foster behavioral change to raise self-esteem
  3. Assist to understand dynamics of anger to establish locus of control.
  4. Increase autonomy to raise self-esteem.
  5. Recognize and express feelings to eliminate dysfunctional defenses.
  6. Help to process grief and loss.

7. Computer-assisted self evaluation and provision of alternatives helpful due to massive use of denial to cover vulnerability.

- Family Dynamics
  1. Multiple moves or schools
  2. Inconsistent management/harsh discipline
  3. History of parental rejection
  4. Shifting of parent figures
  5. Paternal absence or alcoholism
  6. Large family size
  7. Early institutional living
  8. Association with delinquent sub-group
  9. Isolates self in family
  10. Court involvement/Child Protective Services, often known to multiple agencies
- Family Therapy
  1. Foster self-responsibility, differentiation of self.
  2. Decrease blaming communication.
  3. Allow for expression of grief and tenderness.
  4. Multiple family therapy approaches may be beneficial.
- Group approaches
  1. Allow for confrontation.
  2. Test new ways of relating.
  3. Model effective coping.
  4. Form healthy relationships.
  5. Refer to Alateen or Children of Alcoholics (COA) group.
  6. Chemical dependency assessment and referral to appropriate 12-Step program if indicated
  7. Utilize exercises designed to deal with feelings, facilitate trust and develop healthy coping.
- Milieu Interventions

1. Residential treatment indicated for severe cases
2. Milieu may be part of group home or detention facility.
3. Provide for physical safety of patient and others.
4. Promote regulation of impulse control.
5. Promote positive problem-solving abilities.
6. Promote healthy expression of anger, such as providing safe place; gymnasium.
7. Provide structured mechanisms for learning trust, such as Ropes Program, Escape to Reality, etc.
8. Disseminate accurate information about staff changes, turnover, etc since changes may reawaken old abandonment issues.
9. Primary nursing promotes bonding with adult

- Community Resources
  1. Appropriate 12-Step Program
  2. Big Brother, Big Sister programs
  3. CASA (Court Appointed Special Advocates)
  4. Promote sports, fitness activities.
  5. Outward Bound therapeutic programs
  6. Parents Involved Network
  7. Federation of Families for Children's Mental Health
  8. Case management may be essential due to multiple agency involvement and family tendency to seek help only in crisis times.

Oppositional Defiant Disorder (ODD)

- Signs and Symptoms
  1. A pattern of negativistic, hostile, and defiant behavior without the serious violation of other people's basic rights
  2. Diagnosis made only if behavior is more common than that of other children of the same age.
  3. Usually the defiance is seen only with adults and peers the child knows well and is justified by the child.
  4. Examples of disruptive behavior include:

   a. Frequent arguing and losing temper
   b. Refusal to cooperate with chores and tasks
   c. Deliberately annoying others
   d. Spitefulness
5. Onset by age 8 years and not later than early adolescence

- Differential Diagnosis
  1. Conduct disorder preempts this diagnosis.
  2. Psychotic disorder preempts this diagnosis.
  3. Features of ODD are often seen in dysthymia, manic, hypomanic, or major depression.
  4. Passive Aggressive Personality Disorder may be diagnosed if patient is under 18 and does not meet all criteria for ODD.
  5. Chemical dependency may co-exist or preempt.
- Mental Status
  1. Few signs of the disorder are seen on mental status.
  2. When confronted with behavior, the client often utilizes projection and blames others.
  3. Associated features include labile mood, bad temper, and low frustration tolerance.
  4. Associated use of psychoactive substances
- Nursing Diagnoses
  1. Coping, ineffective, individual
  2. Violence, potential for, self directed or directed toward others
  3. Anxiety
  4. Adjustment, impaired
  5. Self-concept, disturbance in body image, self-esteem, role performance; personal identity
  6. Coping, ineffective family—compromised/disabling
  7. Social interaction, impaired
- Biological Approaches

1. Stimulant medication to treat associated ADHD
2. Antidepressants for associated depression
   a. Imipramine (Tofranil) may be utilized with children over 12.
      (1) A dose of 2.5 mg/kg/day should not be exceeded.
      (2) ECG changes of unknown significance have been reported in pediatric patients with doses twice this amount (PDR, 1994)
      (3) An ECG recording should be taken prior to the initiation of larger-than-usual doses and at appropriate intervals thereafter
   b. Lithium carbonate has been shown to be effective in some studies of aggressive children (Lewis, 1991).
   f. Intrapersonal Origins—may be related to physical or sexual abuse or both
   g. Psychotherapeutic Approaches
1. Promote self esteem and self worth.
2. Skill building in interpersonal relationships
3. Play therapy to encourage awareness of feelings, facilitate disclosure of issues, learn new ways of effective coping
   a. Board games
   b. Talking, Feeling, Doing game (Richard Gardner)
   c. The Ungame
4. Art Therapy—drawing, modeling, sand tray to process unconscious issues

- Family Therapy
  1. Utilize family therapy to promote healthy family interaction and decrease tendency to pathologize child
  2. Support parental hierarchy
  3. Explore alternate ways of coping, especially assisting parents to avoid playing into oppositional tendencies.
- Group Therapy

1. Encourage verbalization of feelings and develop positive social support mechanisms.
2. Learn alternate ways of coping.
3. Psychodrama encourages trying out new behaviors.
4. Provide positive reinforcement.

- Milieu Interventions—(Children with this diagnosis are rarely admitted to inpatient settings, although they may have a dual diagnosis with a major mental health problem.)
  1. Environmental activities and group process are necessary, as well as those mentioned under conduct disorder.
- Community Resources
  1. Parenting classes, such as STEP and PET
  2. Sports and team activities
  3. Wilderness and Outward Bound type programs
  4. Camps, YMCA, YWCA programs

Eating Disorders of Infancy or Early Childhood

Pica

- Signs and Symptoms
  1. Persistent consumption of non-nutritive substances such as dirt, plaster, hair, bugs, pebbles.
  2. Behavior not part of a culturally sanctioned practice
  3. Duration of at least one month
- Differential Diagnosis
  1. Autistic disorder
  2. Schizophrenia
  3. Kleine-Levin Syndrome
- Group—Parenting Support Groups
- Milieu Interventions—Environmental Interventions
  a. Establish safe environment.

b. Provide adequate supervision.

- Community Resources
  1. Public health nurses
  2. Well child clinics
  3. Lead poisoning prevention programs
  4. Social services

Rumination Disorder of Infancy

- Signs and Symptoms
  1. Well-defined syndrome characterized by partially digested food being brought up into the mouth and ejected, or chewed and reswallowed
  2. Repeated regurgitation, without nausea or associated gastrointestinal illness, for at least one month following a period of normal functioning
  3. Weight loss or failure to make expected weight gain
  4. The condition has a 25% mortality rate.
  5. There may be associated parenting problems due to the caretaker's frustration with the child.
- Differential Diagnosis
  1. Congenital anomalies, such as pyloric stenosis or GI infections.
  2. Esophageal reflux
- Nursing Diagnoses:
  1. Altered nutrition, less than body requirements
  2. Ineffective family coping
  3. Altered family process
- Biological Origins

  No information; spontaneous remissions are common.
- Family Dynamics/Family Therapy
  1. Parents may become frustrated and alienated from the infant due to his/her failure to respond.

2. The noxious odor of the regurgitate may cause the parent to avoid holding the infant.

- Community Resources
    1. Public health nursing—health teaching regarding the nature of the illness and suggestions for coping are essential.

Tic Disorders

Tics are defined as sudden, repetitive movements, gestures or utterances that mimic some aspect of normal behavior (Leckman and Cohen, 1991). Tics cannot be controlled, but can be suppressed for varying lengths of time. They are worsened by stress and diminished during sleep. Examples of tics are:

1. Simple motor tics—eye blinking, facial grimacing
2. Simple vocal tics—coughing, throat-clearing, sniffing, snorting, barking
3. Complex motor tics—facial gestures, grooming behaviors, touching
4. Complex vocal tics
    a. Repeating words and phrases out of context
    b. Coprolalia—compulsive, stereotyped use of obscene language
    c. Palilalia—repetition of a phrase or word with increasing rapidity
    d. Echolalia—stereotyped repitition of another person's words or phrases
    e. Echokinesis—imitation of the movements of another person

Tourette's Disorder

Essential features are multiple motor and one or more vocal tics.

- Signs and Symptoms
    1. Tics appear simultaneously or at different periods throughout the illness.
    2. Can occur many times a day to intermittently with as much as a symptom-free period of a year or more.
    3. The anatomic location, number, frequency, complexity, and severity change over time.

4. Onset is prior to age 21.

- Differential Diagnosis

1. Psychoactive substance intoxication
2. Central nervous system disease, such as Huntington's Chorea and viral encephalitis
3. Abnormal motor movements may be present in many neurologic disorders, organic mental disorders, and schizophrenia. None of these disorders involve the peculiar vocalizations such as clicks, grunts, yelps, barks, hisses, and sniffs of Tourette's disorder.

Chronic Motor or Vocal Tic Disorder

1. Either motor or vocal tics, but not both as in Tourette's Disorder
2. Symptom severity and functional impairment less than Tourette's

Transient Tic Disorder

1. Single or multiple motor and/or vocal tics that occur many times a day, nearly every day for at least two weeks, but for no longer than twelve consecutive months.
2. Diagnosis not made if there is a history of Tourette's, Chronic Motor or Vocal Tic Disorder, which requires a duration of at least one year.

Tic Disorder Not Otherwise Specified

1. Tics that do not meet criteria for a specific Tic disorder

The following information is true for all Tic Disorders

- Mental Status

1. There may be associated anxiety due to social situation embarrassment.
2. Depressed mood is common, especially in Tourette's

- Nursing Diagnosis for Tic Disorders

1. Impaired social interaction due to communication barriers
2. Impaired verbal communication
3. Powerlessness

4. Anxiety related to unexpected manifestation of tics
5. Ineffective individual coping related to anxiety
6. Chronic low self-esteem
7. Altered sensory/perception kinesthetic

- Biological Origins for Tic Disorders
    1. Familial patterns reported for all cases of tic disorders—more common in first degree biological relatives of people with Tourette's.
    2. Positively associated with ADHD and Obsessive-Compulsive Disorder in clinical samples. OCD more common in first-degree biological relatives of those with Tourette Syndrome.
    3. At least three times more common in males than females
    4. Controversy over association with
        a. Taking phenothiazines
        b. Head trauma
        c. Taking CNS stimulants
        d. Intrauterine environment
            (1) Maternal life stress
            (2) Complications of pregnancy
            (3) First trimester nausea
    6. EEG abnormalities in 50%

- Biochemical Approaches for Tic Disorders
    1. Medication used only in very severe cases of chronic motor or vocal tic disorder.
    2. Haloperidol (Haldol) effective in chronic tic disorders and Tourette's
        a. Not recommended for under 3 years old
        b. Age 3-12 years: 0.05-0.075 mg/kg/day
        c. Over 12: 0.5—5 mg 2 to 3 times daily. Low incidence of sedation and autonomic effects, high incidence of extrapyramidal reactions.

3. Pimozide (Orap)
    a. Dopaminergic blocking activity, like Haldol
    b. Over age 12 up to 10 mg/day
4. Clonidine (Catapres) 0.05 mg to 45 mg daily
    a. Not as effective as Orap or Haldol, but no tardive dyskinesia risk. Useful for patients who cannot tolerate Haldol.

- Psychotherapeutic Interventions
    1. Behavioral therapy is effective in symptom modulation.
    2. Autogenic relaxation and stress management may be useful in helping the patient to self-regulate as symptoms may be exacerbated by stress
    3. Massed practice—a behavioral technique in which the patient intentionally practices the undesired behavior.
    4. Acceptance by the therapist is key in treatment.
- Family Therapy
    1. Parents need guidance in understanding the biological determinants of this disorder and in recognizing the compulsive nature.
    2. Punishment may reinforce the symptom.
    3. Efforts to help the child overcome socialization problems should be emphasized.
- Group Approaches
    1. The child may benefit from inclusion in a diverse group with opportunity to receive support from other members
- Milieu—Patients would rarely be hospitalized for this disorder.
    1. Care planning would focus on associated depression if present, or ADHD.
    2. Opportunity to process feelings of differentness in the milieu as an extension of normal adolescent growth and development should be provided.
- Community Resources

1. Gilles de la Tourette Foundation
2. Self-help groups available in larger metropolitan areas

Elimination Disorders

Enuresis

- Signs and Symptoms (APA, 1993)
  1. Continued pattern of involuntary or intentional voiding of urine not accounted for by physical disorder
  2. Occurring after the age when continence is expected
  3. Age criterion
     a. Five and six year old two times per month
     b. Older children one time per month
     c. Mental age at least four
  4. Wetting may be involuntary or intentional
  5. Primary enuresis—not preceded by a period of urinary continence lasting at least one year
  6. Secondary enuresis—preceded by a period of urinary continence lasting at least one year
- Differential Diagnosis
  1. Physical disorders, such as diabetes, or seizure disorder
  2. Urinary tract infections
- Associated Conditions
  1. The incidence of major mental illness is greater among those with Functional Enuresis than in the general population.
  2. Associated with other behavioral disorders and psychopathology, however, associated disorders may stem from the enuresis.
  3. Secondary enuretics have the same rate of emotional or behavioral problems as primary enuretics.
  4. Functional Encopresis, Functional Enuresis, Sleepwalking Disorder and Sleep Terror

- Mental Status
    1. Child may have low self-esteem due to caretaker rejection or social ostracism by peers.
- Nursing Diagnoses
    1. Urinary incontinence, functional
- Biological Origins
    1. Low functional bladder volume
    2. More males than females
    3. Seventy-five percent have first-degree biological relative with the disorder.
- Biochemical Approaches
    1. Imipramine (Tofranil) 1.5 mg/kg/day to no more than 2.5 mg/kg/day. Side effects include:
        a. Dry mouth
        b. Constipation
        c. Tachycardia
        d. Sleep disorders
        e. Drowsiness
        f. Postural hypotension
        g. Cardiac conduction slowing
    2. ECG changes of unknown significance have been reported in pediatric patients with doses twice this amount (PDR, 1994)
    3. An ECG recording should be taken prior to the initiation of larger-than-usual doses and at appropriate intervals thereafter
- Psychotherapeutic Interventions
    1. Psychotherapy alone is not an effective treatment, but may be helpful with associated psychiatric conditions such as PTSD, Depression, ADHD, Anxiety
    2. Hypnotherapy may be effective, although the duration of recovery has not been substantiated.

3. Behavioral techniques (Conditioning)
    a. Mowrer apparatus (bell and pad), awakens child upon wetting and works by a combination of Pavlovian conditioning, avoidance learning, and placebo effect.
    b. Intermittent reinforcement and overlearning reduce relapse.
    c. Retention control training
    d. Rapid awakening training
    e. Reinforcement for daytime micturation

Encopresis

- Signs and Symptoms (APA, 1993)
    1. Repeated passage of feces into places not appropriate for that purpose, such as clothing or bedding
    2. Age criterion—chronological and mental age at least four years
    3. Event occurs at least once a month for at least 3 months
    4. May be involuntary or intentional
- Differential Diagnosis- physical disorder, such as aganglionic megacolon
- Mental Status
    1. Poor self-esteem
- Associated Conditions
    1. Enuresis
    2. Sleep walking disorder
    3. Sleep terror
- Nursing Diagnoses
    1. Altered elimination, bowel
    2. Bowel incontinence
- Biological Origins
    1. Twelve percent of fathers of encopretics are encopretic.

2. Ratio of male to female encopretics ranges from 66% to 88% of samples.
3. Encopresis occurring with mental retardation is common but poorly defined.
4. Inadequate physiological functioning of defecation

- Intrapersonal Origins
  1. Social learning theory attributes disordered learning or insufficient learning
  2. Secondary encopresis involves learned avoidant behavior, reinforced by delay of painful defecation.
  3. Psychogenic theories formulated by Freud—compliance vs. opposition (''anal period'')
- Psychotherapeutic Interventions Treatment determined by thorough assessment
  1. Toilet training needed if appropriate training has not taken place
  2. Positive behavioral reinforcement of appropriate toileting behavior
  3. Secondary encopresis related to more serious psychopathology—need to treat high levels of anxiety, anger, or depression
  4. If encopresis is response to severe environmental stress, modifying the stressor brings relief.
- Family Therapy
  1. Orient family counseling to supporting behavioral techniques.
  2. Treat family psychopathology if present; some theorists postulate issues of paternal distance and maternal anxiety, as well as parental absence.
  3. Support and management alternatives lessen parental pressure on child, enabling learning to take place.
- Group Therapy-generally not indicated for Enuresis and Encopresis
- Milieu Interventions
  1. Not usually admitted for elimination disorders

2. Behavioral techniques to reward appropriate behavior and eliminate unwanted behavior

Other Disorders of Infancy, Childhood, or Adolescence

This section includes several disorders with little in common other than their development during childhood and adolescence. Some have similarities to previously discussed syndromes.

Separation Anxiety Disorder

Concerning separation from those to whom the child is attached

- Signs and Symptoms
    1. Essential feature is excessive anxiety.
    2. May experience anxiety to the point of panic following separation, beyond that expected of the child's developmental level.
    3. Diagnosis made by the presence of three of the following for more than two weeks:
        a. Unrealistic worry about harm to major attachment figures
        b. Unrealistic, persistent worry that calamity will cause separation, e.g., kidnapping, accident
        c. School refusal or reluctance in order to stay with major attachment figure
        d. Refusal to sleep away from a major attachment figure or sleep away from home
        e. Avoidance of being alone, including clinging to and shadowing attachment figure
        f. Nightmares involving theme of separation
        g. Complaints of physical symptoms upon anticipation of separation
        h. Complaints of excessive distress in anticipation of separation, e.g., temper tantrums, crying, pleading
        i. Complaints or distress when separated, e.g., wants to return home or needs to call parents
- Differential Diagnosis

1. Medical problems
2. Developmentally appropriately separation anxiety
3. Pervasive Developmental Disorder and Schizophrenia

- Mental Status
  1. May refuse to separate from parent
  2. May cling, cry and fuss if parent tries to leave
  3. If separates, checks frequently in spite of reassurances and knowledge that parent is close by.
- Nursing Diagnoses
  1. Anxiety: mild, moderate, severe
  2. Coping, ineffective individual
  3. Powerlessness
  4. Self-esteem, situational, low
  5. Social interaction, impaired
  6. Social isolation
  7. Fear
- Biological Origins
  1. Specific Developmental Disorder involving language may predispose to this condition
  2. Mothers with anxiety disorders more common in this population according to some studies
  3. More common in females than males
- Intrapersonal Origins
  1. Moderate to catastrophic stressor as defined on Axis IV
  2. More research needed on genetic vs. environmental transmission
- Psychotherapeutic Interventions
  1. Brief, symptom focused therapy approaches
     a. Emphasis on symptom reduction, empowerment, mastery and control

b. Goal is to decrease symptoms quickly to enhance functioning, avoid permanent dysfunction

2. Psychodrama
3. Art work
4. Play therapy utilizing role play, doll house, sand box, puppets
5. Therapeutic games, storytelling
6. Relaxation training may be helpful.

- Family Therapy
  1. Calm down parental system by decreasing anxiety and rigidity.
  2. Decrease conflict and increase problem-solving.
  3. Clarify communication.
  4. Increase individual autonomy and decrease fusion.
  5. Take focus off child as symptom-bearer.
- Group Approaches
  1. Self-esteem group
  2. Play therapy group
  3. Theraplay
  4. Organized and informal play/sports opportunities
- Milieu Interventions
  1. Treatment is best done in outpatient setting.
  2. Organization and predictability helpful
  3. Gradually foster child's independence and self-reliance.
- Community Resources
  1. Educational programs for parents
  2. Church and sports activities

Selective Mutism (Elective Mutism)

- Signs and Symptoms
  1. Rare disorder similar to oppositional disorder in that child is persistently uncooperative with authority figures.

2. Child is uncooperative in verbal communication with persons other than immediate family members.
    a. The child or adolescent persistently refuses to talk in one or more major social situations (including school) but usually speaks at home.
    b. There is an ability to comprehend spoken language and to speak.
    c. The child may communicate by gestures, nodding or shaking the head, or by short, monotone utterances.

- Differential Diagnosis
    1. Severe or Profound Mental Retardation, Pervasive Developmental Disorder, and Developmental Expressive Language Disorder. Persons with these disorders may have an inability to speak, not refusal to do so.
    2. Children in families who have recently emigrated to a country of a different language may refuse to speak the new language. If comprehension of the new language is adequate but the refusal to speak persists, the diagnosis should be made.
- Mental Status
    1. Attempts to engage the patient in conversation are futile, although the presence of adequate receptive language is apparent.
- Nursing Diagnoses
    1. Impaired communication
    2. Altered Socialization
    3. Altered Family Process
    4. Ineffective individual coping
    5. Parental role conflict
- Biological Origins/Biochemical Approaches
    1. No information on familial pattern
    2. No biochemical approaches known
- Intrapersonal Origins
    a. Associated with shyness and other oppositional behavioral problems

b. Case histories report symptoms developed following reprimand for saying something

- Psychotherapeutic Interventions
  1. Challenging to treat since these patients don't talk to the therapist and often passively refuse nonverbal communication
  2. Psychoanalysis reportedly is beneficial
  3. Behavior therapy may be beneficial
- Family Dynamics/Family Therapy
  1. Maternal overprotection
  2. Major personality or psychiatric conflict or a combination of these
  3. Families seen as vulnerable to a hostile world
  4. Symptom is seen as an expression of family conflict and anxiety about revealing family secrets.
  5. Silence used as manipulation
  6. Increased rate of psychiatrically ill parents/abnormal family dynamics
  7. Family therapy and school counseling essential
- Group Approaches
  1. Not indicated
- Milieu Interventions
  1. Mutism does not meet criteria for inpatient admission.
  2. If accompanied by other disorder, provide reinforcement for verbal responses.
- Community Resources
  1. Parenting classes
  2. Socialization and sports activities

Reactive Attachment Disorder of Infancy or Early Childhood

- Signs and Symptoms (APA, 1993)
  1. Presence of grossly disturbed caretaking resulting in profoundly disturbed social relatedness and failure to thrive.

2. Markedly disturbed social relatedness in most contexts, beginning before age 5, as evidenced by either a. or b.
    a. Persistent failure to initiate or respond to most social interactions
    b. Indiscriminate sociability, e.g., excess familiarity with relative strangers by making requests and displaying affection
3. Grossly pathogenic care, as evidenced by at least one of the following:
    a. Persistent disregard of the child's basic emotional needs for comfort, stimulation, or affection, e.g., overly harsh punishment or consistent neglect by caregiver
    b. Persistent disregard of the child's basic physical needs, including nutrition, adequate housing, and protection from physical danger and assault (including sexual abuse)
    c. Repeated change of primary caregiver so that stable attachments are not possible, e.g., frequent changes in foster parents
    d. The presumption is that the care in 3 is responsible for the disturbed behavior in 1.

- Differential Diagnosis
    1. Mental Retardation or Pervasive Developmental Disorder, such as Autistic Disorder
    2. Children with severe neurologic abnormalities, including deafness, blindness, profound multisensory defects, major central nervous system disease, or severe chronic physical illness may have many needs that they are unable to fill, and may have minor secondary attachment disturbances, without markedly disturbed social relatedness.
- Mental Status
    1. Observation of the child indicates lack of developmentally appropriate social responsiveness.
    2. Apathy and lack of interest in the environment may be noted.
    3. Child may stare, have a weak cry and poor muscle tone, as well as low motility.

4. Home visit often required to document the evidence of neglect or abuse, as caregiver reports often extremely unreliable.

- Nursing Diagnosis
  1. Altered role performance, parenting
  2. Altered family processes
  3. Altered comfort
  4. Ineffective family coping (disabled)
  5. Potential for injury
  6. Altered communication
  7. Unilateral neglect
  8. Altered growth and development
- Intrapersonal Origins
  1. Response to neglect
- Psychotherapeutic Approaches
  1. Provision of adequate caretaking
- Family Dynamics
  1. Parental severe character pathology
  2. Severe depression, isolation, and lack of support systems
  3. Lack of bonding in first weeks of life
  4. Transgenerational pattern of dysfunctional parenting, abuse, neglect, and mental illness
  5. Overwhelming psychosocial stresses in parents with emotional deficits
- Family Therapy
  1. Engage relevant family members in treatment.
  2. Identify family stresses.
  3. Assess family resources.
  4. Assess and intervene in dysfunctional conflicts affecting child's well being
  5. Supervise care.

6. Recommend out-of-home placement if necessary.

- Group Approaches—not indicated
- Milieu Approaches
  1. Does not meet criteria for psychiatric hospitalization
  2. Patient may be placed in infant home or pediatric unit to treat other conditions or awaiting placement; cuddling and stimulation essential; staff may model appropriate behavior to parents.
- Community Resources
  1. Community mental health parent support groups
  2. Parenting classes
  3. Public health nursing
  4. Pediatric/family-centered outpatient program
  5. Child protective services
  6. Child abuse prevention services
  7. Case management and coordination of care essential among agencies interfacing with family
  8. Multidisciplinary team approach consisting of team members essential

Stereotypic Movement Disorder

- Signs and Symptoms
  1. Intentional, repetitive, nonfunctional behaviors such as hand-shaking or waving, body-rocking, head banging, mouthing of objects, nail-biting, nose or skin-picking
  2. The disorder either causes physical injury to the child or markedly interferes with normal activities.
- Differential Diagnosis
  1. Rocking and thumb-sucking are common in normal infants and young children.
  2. Pervasive Developmental Disorder, Tic Disorder and Obsessive Compulsive Disorder.

3. Stereotyped behavior of Tic Disorder is involuntary, even though it can be suppressed for a period of time.

- Mental Status
  1. Behaviors appear compulsive and involuntary
- Nursing Diagnoses
  1. Physical mobility, impaired
  2. Potential for injury
- Biological Origins
  1. Common in mental retardation
  2. Associated with congenital deafness and blindness
  3. Associated with degenerative and CNS disorders
  4. Temporal-lobe epilepsy and severe Schizophrenia may be associated.
  5. May be induced by certain psychoactive substances such as amphetamine, in which case the diagnosis of Psychoactive Substance-Induced Organic Mental Disorder should also be made
- Biochemical Treatment
  1. Haloperidol 0.5-16 mg/day. Side effects include sedation, headache, extrapyramidal symptoms, tardive dyskinesia, neuroleptic malignant syndrome, orthostatic hypotension, photosensitivity, anorexia, constipation, paralytic ileus, impaired liver function, hypersalivation, agranulocytosis, anemia, leukopenia, cough reflex suppression, laryngeal edema, bronchospasm, diaphoresis
  2. Lithium Carbonate (Lithium) 600-2100 mg in 2-3 divided doses, Keep blood levels to 0.4–1.2 mEq/L. Adverse reactions include nausea vomiting, headache, tremor, weight gain.
  3. Opiate antagonists are presently under study.
- Family Dynamics/Family Therapy
  1. Provide family support and information re: management and pharmacology
- Group Approaches—Not indicated
- Milieu Approaches

1. Prevent physical injury by observation, restraint or promoting activities that interfere with self-injury
2. Observe for infection of wounds
3. Prevent and treat neuroleptic side effects

- Community Resources
  1. Respite programs
  2. Public health nursing

Diagnosis Commonly Applied to Children and Adolescents

Although not listed in DSM IV under child and adolescent disorders, several diagnoses are frequently utilized by clinicians who provide care for children and adolescents. While many of the theories, treatment interventions, resources will be the same as for the adults in these categories, information that is different for children and adolescents will be presented in this section.

Post Traumatic Stress Disorder

- Signs and Symptoms
  1. Repetitive play in which themes or aspects of trauma are expressed and re-experienced.
  2. Sexualized play indicative of sexual knowledge greater than would be expected of a child's developmental age may be an indicator of suspected abuse.
  3. Loss of recently acquired developmental skills or language skills is often a way the avoidant criteria are expressed.
- Differential Diagnosis
  1. Assessment of suspected sexual abuse, including the use of anatomical dolls in evaluation, is a specialized skill and should not be attempted by those untrained in such evaluations (APSAC).
  2. A physical examination including colposcopy (if indicated) by pediatricians or nurse practitioners specially trained in evaluating reports of sexual abuse.
- Psychotherapeutic Interventions
  1. Specific interventions include art therapy, sand tray, play therapy, psychodrama, group work, and relaxation training.

- Family Therapy
    1. Parent counseling about child behaviors and sexual abuse dynamics is essential. V codes including physical abuse of child, sexual abuse of child, and neglect of child may also be used when abuse is the focus of clinical attention.
- Community Resources
    1. Nurses, along with other professionals are mandated reporters of suspected physical or sexual abuse.
    2. Multidisciplinary coordination is essential.

Bipolar Disorders

Although depression and mania have been reported in children and adolescents for years, many clinicians believed that children did not experience mood extremes (Weller & Weller, 1991).

- Signs and Symptoms:
    1. Diagnostic criteria are the same as for adults.
    2. Manic adolescents present similarly to adults.
    3. Manic children less than 9 years present with irritability and emotional lability
    4. Older children present with euphoria, elation, paranoia, and grandiose delusions.
    5. Excitement/depression extremes more common with puberty (Weller, 1991)
- Differential Diagnosis
    1. The following conditions must be ruled out:
        a. Drugs
            (1) Amphetamines
            (2) Corticosteroids
            (3) Sympathomimetics
            (4) Isoniazid
        b. Endocrine disorders, such as hyperthyroidism

c. Neurologic conditions, such as head trauma and seizure disorders, tumors

d. Infections-encephalitis, influenza, syphilis, AIDS

2. The following psychiatric conditions must be ruled out:

    a. Attention Deficit Hyperactivity Disorder

    b. Conduct Disorder is often a comorbid condition, but ''pure'' conduct disorder does not include pressured speech, flight of ideas, or grandiosity (Lewis, 1991)

3. Schizophrenia

4. Psychological testing may be utilized in diagnostic evaluation

    a. Rating scales include:

        (1) Children's Depression Inventory(CDI)

        (2) School Age Depression Listed Inventory (SADLI)

        (3) Bellevue Index of Depression (BID)

        (4) Children's Depression Rating Scale-Revised

        (5) Mania Rating Scale

- Mental Status (presentation similar to manic adults)
- Nursing Diagnoses

    1. Same as for adult bipolar disorders

    2. Alterations in parenting

- Genetic/Biologic Origins (same as adult)

    1. When onset of illness prepubertal, rate of bipolar disorder in family members three times that of those with postpubertal onset

    2. Detailed chromosomal studies lacking (Lewis, 1991)

- Biochemical Approaches

    1. Complete physical examinations, baseline laboratory studies and ECG must be done prior to initiating Lithium.

    2. Children and adolescents often tolerate Lithium better than adults, although its use with children must still be considered investigational.

3. Dosages range from 600 mg daily for a weight of 15-25 (kg) to 1500 mg per day for a weight range of 50-60 kg.
4. Carbamazepine (Tegretol) is frequently given in doses of 15-30 mg/kg/day for rapid cycling mania. It is still investigational.
5. Valproic acid (Depakene) is given to those who are non-responsive to Lithium or Tegretol. The dose is 25-60 mg/kg/day.

- Intrapersonal Origins
  1. Mania runs in families
  2. Bipolar parents may exercise inadequate parenting techniques.
  3. Cohort effect indicates increased incidence of bipolar illness in individuals born after 1940.
- Psychotherapeutic Interventions
  1. Hospitalization often indicated
  2. Age specific psychotherapy/play therapy
- Family Dynamics/Family Therapy
  1. Psychoeducational approaches essential
  2. Support and empathy
  3. Biological origins of this disorder must be taken into account (therapist may be dealing with several bipolar persons in the family).
- Group Approaches
  1. Play group
  2. Self esteem group
  3. Therapist needs to be able to provide ''time out'' to protect other group members.
- Milieu Interventions
  1. Same milieu approaches as adults, but modified for developmental levels
  2. Nursing staff need to be able to provide safe environment for other patients as well.

Depressive Disorders

Much attention has been given in the last 15 years to depression in children and adolescents. In addition, there are numerous ''extrinsic conditions,'' such as living in conditions of poverty or experiencing violence and abuse which create a higher risk (Krauss, 1993).

- Signs and Symptoms (Same as adults with the following modifications)
    1. More difficult to diagnose melancholic subtype as many children have not had previous episodes and therefore have not manifested complete recovery (Lewis, 1991)
    2. Seasonal disorders difficult to diagnose because of back to school stressors
    3. Dysthymia has a one-year duration rather than two years as in adults (APA,1993).
    4. Failure to gain weight substitutes for weight loss.
    5. School performance may deteriorate.
    6. Somatic complaints are common.
    7. Irritability is common.
    8. Favorite activities may be avoided.
    9. Adolescent clinical picture may be complicated by alcohol or drug use and abuse.
    10. Increase of suicide attempts with puberty
    11. Dexamethasone suppression test (DST)
- Differential Diagnosis
    1. Psychiatric conditions
        a. Disruptive Behavior Disorders
        b. Adjustment Disorder with Depressed Mood
        c. Post Traumatic Stress Disorder
    2. Medical conditions
        a. Infections, such as mononucleosis and subacute bacterial endocarditis

b. Neurological Disorders or tumors, such as epilepsy and post concussion

c. Endocrine disorders including diabetes and thyroid problems

d. Medications

e. Other disorders, such as alcohol abuse, anemia, and electrolyte abnormality (Lewis, 1991)

- Associated Conditions with Adolescent Depression

  (1) 75% have anxiety

  (2) 50% have an Oppositional Disorder

  (3) 33% have a Conduct Disorder

- Mental Status (may have similar presentation as adult)

  1. Clinically depressed children look sad, and often describe themselves in negative terms.
  2. Concentration is often problematic.
  3. Lack of energy may be apparent.
  4. Anhedonia most common symptom
  5. Morbid ideation may be present.

- Nursing Diagnoses (same as adult depression)
- Genetic/Biologic Origins (same as adult)
- Biochemical Approaches (Informed consent necessary as many drugs not approved for use in children under age 18)

  1. Tricyclic antidepressants most commonly used

     a. Imipramine (Tofranil) 5 mg/kg/day—Baseline EKG studies must be done because of the higher risk of cardiotoxicity in children and the cardiac monitoring should continue.

     b. Nortriptyline 30 mg-50 mg/day is approved for adolescent use.

  2. Selective serotonin-reuptake inhibitors are not yet approved for use in children, although they are increasingly prescribed, but usually not to children under 8. Of these, fluoxetine (Prozac) is the most commonly used, with an initial dosage of 10 mg/day.
  3. MAOIs are used sparingly as the dietary restrictions make their use problematic in children and adolescents.

- Intrapersonal Origins (Review section on adult depression)
- Psychotherapeutic Interventions
    1. Determined by the child's cognitive and emotional development.
    2. Assess child's self-perception of competence skills training: behavioral therapy may be necessary for youngsters whose low self-competence perception is accurate. Erroneous self-perceptions can be mitigated by Cognitive Therapy (Lewis, 1991).
    3. Play therapy allows opportunity for fantasy work and success, and also identification and expression of feelings.
    4. Behavioral therapy allows for development of skills.
    5. Life stress focus helps child to accept reality of change, for example, the "Changing Family Game" allows children to problem-solve and process feelings through the various stages of parental conflict, separation, life with one parent, and parents' dating and forming blended families.
    6. Bibliotherapy is also helpful, as are scaling and identifying feelings.
- Family Dynamics/Family Therapy
    1. Many family factors are extrinsic risk factors to the child:
        a. Substance abusing/mentally ill parents
        b. Foster care
        c. Native American children from certain tribes have two to three times the suicide rate of other U.S. youngsters their age.
        d. Poverty, homelessness, and inner-city living
        e. Lack of consistent caretakers
        f. Prolonged parent/child separation
        g. Physical or sexual abuse
        h. Catastrophic events
        i. Marital discord and instability in the family environment (Krauss, 1993); emotional and physical neglect are considered by some experts to be the most damaging of all forms of abuse (deTriquet, 1994)
        j. Review adult antecedents of depression

2. Family therapy necessary in enhancing family and child functioning—clinicians differ on whether the same therapist should see both the child and the family or whether a modified version of family consultation is in order. Usually determined by the background and experience of the therapist, the resources and philosophy of the agency, and the treatment locale.

- Group Approaches
  1. Modified for child's emotional and developmental level
  2. Self-esteem groups
  3. Children of alcoholics/Alanon
  4. Problem-solving
  5. Trauma groups
- Milieu Interventions
  1. Safe environment
  2. ''Copycat'' self-destructive behavior problematic with adolescents
  3. Comorbidity complicates inpatient treatment
- Community Resources
  1. Community health home visiting of at-risk families
  2. Crisis lines (suicide major cause of death among adolescents)

Questions
Select the best answer

1. A 7-year-old girl discloses to the school nurse that her stepfather has been rubbing her genitals. The girl makes this accusation after seeing a sexual abuse prevention program in her family life education class. Which is the most appropriate first action by the nurse?
   a. Ask the girl to draw a picture of what happens to her at home.
   b. Call the girl's family and schedule an appointment so that she can confront her accuser
   c. Obtain anatomically correct dolls to evaluate the girl's disclosure more fully
   d. Report the allegations to child protective services

2. Six- year-old Zack is referred by his teacher. He is inattentive, squirms in his seat, butts in other children's games and conversations, has difficulty following directions, and was noted by the school bus driver to run in front of the bus when it approached. A tentative diagnosis for Zack would be:
   a. Parent-child problem
   b. COA syndrome
   c. Attention Deficit Hyperactivity Disorder
   d. Developmental Coordination Disorder

3. Zack's symptoms are referred to as:
   a. ''Internalizing''
   b. Antisocial
   c. Aggressive
   d. ''Externalizing''

4. In evaluating Zack's behavior, it would be most important to obtain:
   a. His prenatal record
   b. His report card
   c. A teacher behavioral checklist
   d. The school nurses' health record

5. Zack's mother is convinced that her son is immature and that her problems with him stem from her inability to ''get him to listen.'' ''I've tried everything with him. . . . I take his toys away . . . I spank him . . . I've even threatened to

send him to live with his father.'' Zack's mother needs help in providing which of the following for her son ?

a. Consistency and structure
b. Love
c. Discipline and structure
d. Flexibility

6. The most accurate evidence of Attention-Deficit Disorder would occur during:

a. Observation in a free space, such as a playroom
b. Mental status examination
c. A checkers game
d. Parent interview

7. The class of pharmacologicals utilized in treating ADHD are:

a. Antidepressants
b. Anxiolytics
c. Serotonin reuptake inhibitors
d. Stimulants

8. A standard dose of methylphenidate would be up to:

a. 5-15 g/day
b. 10-60 mg/day
c. 55-100 mg tid
d. 1 mg/kg/day

9. Which of the following does not apply to ADHD:

a. Conduct Disorder and Specific Developmental Disorders are more frequent in relatives
b. Inconsistent discipline and limit setting
c. No sex link theory has been postulated
d. Higher incidence of fathers with alcohol disorders

10. Ten-year-old David has been admitted to the children's unit since he has shown poor impulse control and serious risk taking behavior. He persists in walking into the nurses' station, grabbing other children's clothing, and interrupting during community meetings. An important nursing intervention to help David learn self-control would be:

a. Having David participate in reviewing the behavioral chart and point system developed for him
b. Serving David his meals in his room
c. Gradually increasing ‘‘chair time’’when his behavior is disruptive
d. Sending David to the adult unit so he can receive the attention he misses from his family

11. David’s mother tells the clinical specialist leading the multi-family therapy sessions on the unit that her husband refuses to attend the meetings due to his heavy drinking, which has increased since David was admitted. She becomes tearful and discusses her feelings of being overwhelmed due to her many problems. In addition to encouraging her to continue attending the scheduled sessions, it would be helpful to:

    a. Refer her to a divorce attorney
    b. Say ‘‘He probably isn’t ready to obtain any benefit from the session’’
    c. Explain the function of Alanon family groups and provide her with a meeting list
    d. Offer to call David’s father and urge him to attend

12. All of the following are common manifestations of the child with a conduct disorder **except:**

    a. Violates basic rights of others
    b. High tolerance for frustration
    c. Poor academic achievement
    d. Reckless behavior

13. Which of the following is true of conduct disorders?

    a. Often diagnosed by single acts of antisocial behavior
    b. Respects rights of others
    c. Persistent and repetitive patterns of antisocial behavior
    d. Brief episodes of manic behavior

14. The major defenses utilized by the child with a Conduct Disorder are:

    a. Somatization
    b. Denial and projection
    c. Dissociation
    d. Sublimation

15. The goals of short-term psychotherapy with a child with a Conduct Disorder would include:

    a. Establishing a locus of control
    b. Increase dependence on others to facilitate cooperation
    c. Differentiate from the family of origin
    d. Sublimate problematic feelings

16. All of the following may be seen in families with a child with a Conduct Disorder **except:**

    a. Shifting of parent figures
    b. Small family size
    c. Association with delinquent sub-group
    d. History of parental rejection

17. The multidisciplinary child team in a residential facility for children develops a care plan for a child with a Disruptive Behavior Disorder. The plan calls for provision of physical safety, promoting regulation of impulse control, promoting **healthy** expression of anger. What else would be important for this child:

    a. Encouraging dependence on key staff figures
    b. Developing independence from peer group
    c. Promoting positive problem solving
    d. Encouraging gender role identity

18. Ada Williams, RN,CS, is leaving the children's unit where young Ron Smith, a child with a Conduct Disorder, has been hospitalized for three weeks. The best way for the team to handle Ada's leaving is to:

    a. Say nothing and hope the children will think she is on vacation
    b. Let the parents know and encourage them to keep it secret from the children
    c. Process Ada's leaving the unit during several community meetings
    d. Have the new RN announce that Ada has left

19. Eleven-year-old Ricky is brought to therapy by his parents. His mother says that he has been disobedient and resistant to various attempts to manage his behavior. He argues about rules and is often late coming in for dinner. He has a labile mood and blames his behavior on his parents' ''strictness''. Ricky most likely meets criteria for:

    a. Overanxious disorder
    b. Conduct disorder

c. Oppositional-Defiant disorder
d. Attention Deficit Hyperactivity Disorder

20. The symptoms of Oppositional Defiant Disorder are most evident in which setting:

    a. Unfamiliar settings
    b. School
    c. Sports activities
    d. Clinicians offices

21. Disorders associated with Oppositional Defiant Disorder include all of the following **except:**

    a. Depression
    b. Hyperactivity
    c. Pervasive Developmental Disorder
    d. Psychoactive substance use

22. Children with Oppositional Defiant Disorder are admitted to inpatient settings:

    a. Increasingly, in order to stop the spread of juvenile delinquency
    b. Rarely
    c. For associated Axis I Disorders
    d. In order to try out new behaviors.

23. The major features of Separation Anxiety Disorders include all of the following **except:**

    a. Mood swings
    b. Fear of separation
    c. Social avoidance
    d. Persistent worry

24. Four-year-old Jessica has been following her mother around the house constantly for the last month. She refuses to visit her grandparents, throwing a tantrum when her mother tries to leave her with them. Before the anticipated visit, she complains of earaches. A tentative diagnosis for Jessica would be:

    a. Dysthymia
    b. Psychological factors affecting physical condition
    c. Pervasive developmental disorder
    d. Separation Anxiety Disorder

25. An underlying worry of children with Jessica's diagnosis is

    a. Abandonment due to loss of major attachment figures
    b. Castration anxiety
    c. Unfulfilled Oedipal yearnings
    d. Sexual abuse

26. Jessica will be evaluated in the clinical specialist's office. She refuses to leave her mother in the waiting room. The best intervention for the nurse would be to:

    a. Carry Jessica into her office
    b. Reschedule the appointment until Jessica is ready
    c. Refer Jessica to the child psychologist for testing
    d. Invite both Jessica and her mother into the office

27. The clinical specialist gives Jessica the nursing diagnosis of social interaction, impaired, and moderate anxiety. Additional family history that she may likely discover in her work with this child and her mother may be:

    a. Jessica's mother was sexually abused as a child
    b. Jessica's mother was previously treated for an anxiety disorder
    c. Jessica's father has Obsessive-Compulsive Disorder
    d. Jessica's father meets criteria for antisocial personality

28. Treatment modalities indicated for Jessica would include:

    a. Antidepressants
    b. Anxiolytics
    c. Play therapy
    d. Serotonin reuptake inhibitors

29. All of the following would be appropriate goals for family therapy with Jessica's family **except:**

    a. Emphasize Jessica's role as symptom bearer
    b. Clarify communication
    c. Decrease family conflict
    d. Decrease anxiety and rigidity

30. The clinical nurse specialist is intake coordinator in a managed mental health care setting. A clinician wants to admit a child with Separation Anxiety Disorder to a children's unit. Which would be the most likely response of the intake coordinator:

a. Arranging immediate admission
b. Informing the clinician that the diagnosis would not normally meet criteria for inpatient treatment
c. Arranging for a partial hospitalization admission
d. Having the clinician contact the primary care physician for referral to inpatient care

31. An anxiety disorder commonly diagnosed in children who have experienced sexual abuse is:

    a. Overanxious disorder
    b. Separation Anxiety Disorder
    c. Avoidant Disorder of childhood or adolescence
    d. Post Traumatic Stress Disorder

32. Traumatic events are often re-experienced by children through:

    a. Avoiding places that remind them of the event
    b. Art therapy
    c. Psychodrama
    d. Repetitive play

33. Which of the following would be the **most effective** family intervention for a family in which one of the children is diagnosed with Pica:

    a. Transgenerational family therapy
    b. Marital therapy
    c. Systematic family therapy
    d. Parenting classes and education

34. Six-month-old Charles is diagnosed by his pediatrician as having Rumination Disorder of Infancy. Which of the following is **not true** in the presentation of this syndrome:

    a. Fully digested food is brought up into the mouth with no associated nausea or retching
    b. The condition is potentially fatal
    c. There are associated parenting problems
    d. The regurgitated food is ejected or reswallowed

35. Differential diagnosis requires ruling out several other conditions. All of the following problems may have characteristics that mimic this disorder **except:**

    a. Pyloric stenosis

b. Congenital anomalies of the upper GI tract
c. Pica
d. Gastroenteritis

36. Related family problems in response to Rumination Disorder of Infancy include all of the following except:

    a. Parents may become frustrated
    b. Parents become closer to the infant because of his illness
    c. Parents may reject the infant due to the noxious odor of the regurgitate
    d. Parents may begin to feel alienated from the infant

37. The school nurse is asked to evaluate a seven-year-old boy who clears his throat repetitively. In the absence of any definitive physiological problem, this behavior might be diagnosed as which of the following:

    a. Attention Seeking Disorder
    b. A simple vocal tic
    c. A simple motor tic
    d. Pathognomonic of ADHD

38. All of the following are characteristics of tic disorders **except:**

    a. Sudden
    b. Rapid
    c. Deliberate
    d. Recurrent

39. Echolalia and coprolalia are examples of:

    a. Simple vocal tics
    b. Simple motor tics
    c. Complex vocal tics
    d. Complex motor tics

40. Tourette's disorder is characterized by which of the following:

    a. Onset after age 21
    b. Multiple motor and one or more vocal tics
    c. Location of tics remains constant
    d. Daily occurrence for less than six months

41. Little Charlie is referred for head banging. The movements appear voluntary

and nonspasmodic, and he does not appear distressed by the activity. Charlie may have a condition known as:

a. Stereotypic Movement Disorder
b. Chronic Motor Tic
c. Transient Tic Disorder
d. Tourette's Disorder

42. Six-year-old Cynthia is noticed by her first grade teacher because of a pattern of clenching and unclenching her hands in front of her face. She almost certainly exhibits signs of:

a. Anxiety
b. Mental Retardation
c. Stereotypic Disorder
d. Diagnosis cannot be determined by the information presented

43. Variations in the mental status of children with Tic Disorders may include all of the following **except:**

a. Manifestations of the disorder may be noted during assessment
b. A caretaker may report that another family member has the disorder
c. Anxiety is rarely noted
d. There may be associated depression

44. An appropriate nursing diagnosis for a child with a Tic Disorder would be:

a. Impaired elimination
b. Alteration in comfort
c. Injury, potential for
d. Impaired social interaction due to communication barriers

45. The typical dosage of Haloperidol for a 14 year old boy with Tourette's Disorder would be which of the following?

a. 1.0 to 15 mg per day in divided doses
b. 0.1 mg to 0.5 mg once per day
c. 0.5 to 1.5 mg. daily
d. 0.5 to 5 mg 2 to 3 times a day

46. A therapeutic intervention for Tic Disorders might include intentionally performing the undesired behavior. This is termed:

a. Behavior therapy

b. Massed practice
c. Autogenic training
d. Flooding

47. Key points in counselling parents of children with Tic Disorders would include all of the following **except:**

   a. Assist them to understand the biogenetic determinants of the disorder
   b. Help them to tailor punishments to fit the unwanted behavior
   c. Encourage the parents to help the child overcome socialization deficits
   d. Informing them that symptoms may be exacerbated by stress

48. The family of a child with a Tic Disorder asks the clinical nurse specialist about a good inpatient program for their child. The best response from the nurse would be:

   a. Arrange for admission after changing the diagnosis to Major Depression
   b. Refer the family to a child psychiatrist
   c. Explain that she would only recommend hospitalization if the insurance would cover the stay
   d. After ruling out any associated depression, explain to the family that outpatient care is the treatment of choice and help them articulate with community resources.

49. One-and-one-half-year-old Jamie is brought to the psychiatric intake center by his parents because he soils his pants once a day. Functional encopresis would not be diagnosed because:

   a. Soiling is only once a day
   b. The child has not yet reached the age of continence
   c. The soiling is involuntary
   d. Soiling never occurs with enuresis

50. Michael, age six, was completely toilet trained by age three and one half. He has recently begun wetting the bed every night. There is no organic cause for the wetting. His diagnosis would be:

   a. Functional enuresis
   b. Primary enuresis
   c. Secondary enuresis
   d. Functional encopresis

51. All of the following may be causes of enuresis **except:**

a. Diabetes
b. Urinary tract infection
c. Seizure disorder
d. Low self-esteem

52. There are a number of genetic/biological factors related to the genesis of enuresis. All of the following are relevant **except:**

a. Low functional bladder volume
b. More females have this disorder than males
c. 75% have first degree biological relatives with this disorder
d. Urinary tract infections should be ruled out

53. Imipramine is often used in the treatment of enuresis. All of the following are potential side effects except:

a. Agitation
b. Tachycardia
c. Cardiac conduction slowing
d. Postural hypotension

54. All of the following are effective techniques used in treating enuresis **except:**

a. Mowrer apparatus training
b. Retention control training
c. Rapid awakening training
d. Negative reinforcement for failure

55. The Mowrer apparatus is an example of which of the following:

a. Intermittent reinforcement and overlearning to reduce relapse
b. Positive reinforcement
c. Combined Pavlovian conditioning, avoidance learning and placebo effect
d. Negative reinforcement

56. Treatment for encopresis might be based on a variety of theories. The **most realistic** approach would be to base treatment considerations on which of the following:

a. Social learning theory
b. Learned avoidant behavior theory
c. Psychogenic compliance vs. opposition
d. Comprehensive assessment

57. All of the following are helpful therapies/interventions for comprehensive care of the encopretic child **except:**

    a. Family therapy
    b. Behavior therapy
    c. Group treatment
    d. Parenting classes

58. The clinical specialist implementing the family therapy for a family with an encopretic child should do which of the following:

    a. Emphasize the function of the symptom
    b. Encourage the parents to apply parental pressure to reinforce the symptom
    c. Confront the family with their behavior in reinforcing the symptom:
    d. Orient the treatment to supporting the behavioral interventions

59. All of the following would be helpful interventions for stuttering except:

    a. Ritalin 10 mg bid
    b. Psychotherapy focusing on overcoming the associated anxiety and frustration
    c. Relaxation training and stress management to help provide a sense of mastery and self control
    d. Family therapy approaches to help raise the child's self esteem

60. Speech disorders would be effectively treated by all of the following interventions **except:**

    a. Family therapy to address dysfunctional patterns
    b. Group therapy to improve self esteem and social functioning
    c. Milieu therapy to provide a corrective environment
    d. Speech and hearing therapy

61. All of the following may be seen in a child or adolescent who has Elective Mutism **except:**

    a. Persistent refusal to talk in one or more major social situations
    b. Ability to comprehend spoken language
    c. Physical ability to speak
    d. Refusal to communicate even with gestures or monotone utterances

62. Reactive Attachment Disorder is characterized by all of the following **except:**

    a. Markedly disturbed social relatedness

b. Indiscriminate sociability
c. Mental Retardation or Pervasive Developmental Disorder
d. Grossly pathogenic care

63. Stereotypic Movement Disorder is characterized by behaviors that are:

a. Intentional, repetitive,injurious
b. Unintentional, repetitive, injurious
c. Intentional, repetitive, non-injurious
d. Unintentional, repetitive, noninjurious

64. Elective mutism is a relatively rare condition that must be differentiated from all of the following **except:**

a. Mental retardation
b. Pervasive Developmental Disorder
c. Developmental Expressive Disorder
d. Identity Disorder

65. Ten-month-old Melissa is frequently seen rocking herself to sleep with her thumb in her mouth, rubbing her face. This behavior is:

a. Typical of Pervasive Developmental Disorder
b. Normal in infants and little children
c. Indicative of Mental Retardation
d. Indicative of Stereotypy Habit Disorder

66. The following are all common findings of Stereotypic Movement Disorder **except:**

a. Mental Retardation is almost never present
b. Intentional repetitive non-functional behaviors are present
c. Behaviors appear compulsive
d. Behaviors appear involuntary

67. A possible nursing diagnosis for Elective Mutism is:

a. Personal Identity Disturbance
b. Altered self concept
c. Impaired communication
d. Decisional Conflict

68. Which of the following would be an appropriate pharmacological intervention for Elective Mutism:

a. Ritalin
b. Zoloft
c. Elavil
d. No biochemical intervention has been proven to be effective

69. One appropriate psychopharmacological treatment of Stereotypic Movement Disorder would include:

a. Tricyclic antidepressants
b. Benzodiazepines
c. Hydroxyzine pamoate
d. Lithium Carbonate or Haloperidol

70. Provision of adequate caretaking is the treatment of choice for:

a. Major depression
b. Elective Mutism
c. Reactive Attachment Disorder
d. Undifferentiated ADHD

71. Ten-year-old Andrew is seen by the staff nurse in the mental health clinic because of temper outbursts at home. His record indicates that he has a full scale IQ of 68; reads at a first grade level and is sociable and pleasant until frustrated. Andrew's medical diagnosis would most likely be:

a. Attention Deficit Hyperactivity Disorder
b. Avoidant disorder
c. Mild mental retardation
d. Moderate mental retardation

72. Which of the following is **not true** of persons with moderated mental retardation:

a. Former designation was "trainable"
b. Can successfully live independently in the community
c. IQ ranges from 35 to 55
d. May have difficulties with social conventions

73. Leonard has an IQ of 25, can "sight read" several words, can do simple tasks if closely supervised, such as sweeping and wiping counters, and has basic hygiene skills. Leonard meets criteria for which of the following:

a. Pervasive Developmental Disorder
b. Severely mentally retarded

c. Moderately mentally retarded
d. Profoundly mentally retarded

74. There are often other associated disorders with children who are mentally retarded. All of the following disorders are three to four times more prevalent among the mentally retarded, **except:**

a. Pervasive Developmental Disorder
b. ADHD
c. Stereotypy/Habit Disorder
d. Identity Disorder

75. A useful nursing diagnosis to use in planning care for mentally retarded children would be:

a. Ineffective individual coping
b. Parenting, alteration in, potential
c. Sleep pattern disturbance
d. Self care deficit

76. Tantrumming and aggression in mentally retarded children may be helped by:

a. Ativan
b. Ritalin
c. Tegretol or Inderal
d. Lithium

77. Agitation, aggression, and tantrumming may respond to antipsychotics. It is important to remember cognitive dulling will be increased more with:

a. High dosage, low potency drugs
b. Low dosage, low potency drugs
c. High dosage, high potency drugs
d. Low dosage, high potency drugs

78. Characteristics of Pervasive Developmental Disorders include all of the following **except:**

a. Basic psychological functions are seldom affected
b. Verbal and nonverbal communication are primarily affected
c. Social skills are usually affected
d. Imaginative activity is almost always affected

79. Odd response to sensory input such as oblivion to painful stimuli and hypersensitivity to benign stimuli is associated with:

    a. Mental retardation
    b. Bipolar Disorder
    c. Attention Deficit Hyperactivity Disorder
    d. Pervasive Developmental Disorder

80. Inability to communicate or socialize with others is a distinguishing characteristic of which disorder:

    a. Narcissistic Personality Disorder
    b. Profound Mental Retardation
    c. Disruptive Behavior Disorder
    d. Pervasive Developmental Disorder

81. An outdated theory of the genesis of Pervasive Developmental Disorder was that it was caused by:

    a. Dysfunctional mother-child interaction
    b. Poor levels of emotional differentiation
    c. Biological phenomena
    d. Codependency in caregivers

82. Families need particular support in dealing with a child who has Pervasive Developmental Disorder. One of the **most important** interventions for parents of such children would be:

    a. Referring them for Family Planning counselling
    b. Assisting them in dealing with guilt and self-blame
    c. Uncovering transgenerational patterns of abuse
    d. Providing legal assistance

83. Pharmacological intervention may be used to control secondary symptoms of Pervasive Developmental Disorder. Which of the following medications may be helpful:

    a. Anxiolytics
    b. Tricyclic antidepressants
    c. Serum serotonin reuptake inhibitors
    d. Lithium carbonate

84. Frank has been diagnosed with Developmental Reading Disorder. This disorder can be most accurately described as:

a. Mild mental retardation
b. Prevalent in substandard school systems
c. Impairment in the development of word recognition skills and reading comprehension
d. Common among children of dysfunctional families

85. Seven-year-old Tony has marked difficulty forming coherent speech. His vocalizations sound like baby talk. He has particular difficulty with r, sh, th, f, z, and l. The most likely diagnosis for Tony after a thorough evaluation would be:

a. Developmental reading disorder
b. Developmental articulation disorder
c. Phonological Disorder
d. Developmental Expressive Language Disorder

86. Developmental Disorders are more likely to be found in which segment of the population:

a. Two to four times more common in males than females
b. Two to four times more common in white males than black males
c. More common in rural than urban children
d. More common in urban than rural children

87. Research presently substantiates which of the following possible origins of Developmental Disorders:

a. Maternal understimulation
b. Lack of parental knowledge of psychosocial growth and development
c. Paternal alcohol abuse
d. Perinatal injury

88. The clinical specialist is an intake coordinator who case manages mental health providers for a large insurance company. A psychologist wants to admit a seven-year-old boy to the children's psychiatric unit. The child's diagnosis is Developmental Disorder Not Otherwise Specified. Specific reasons for admission stated by the psychologist include starting a medication trial in an inpatient setting. There is no other associated diagnosis. Which of the following is **true** about the use of medication with developmental disorders:

a. Tricyclic antidepressants have been found to be beneficial
b. Serotonin reuptake inhibitors may help a limited number of cases

c. Muscle relaxants help overcome the anxiety associated with developmental disorders
d. There is no evidence that medication directly benefits these conditions.

89. Which of the following symptoms do clinicians find in bipolar youngsters?
    a. The younger the child, the more developed are symptoms of elation and euphoria.
    b. Older children have few symptoms of grandiosity.
    c. Irritability and emotional lability is more commonly seen with children under age nine.
    d. Extremes of excitement and depression become less common with puberty.

90. Which of the following medications would not mimic mania in children?
    a. Insulin
    b. Amphetamines
    c. Isoniazid
    d. Corticosteroids

91. Although Conduct Disorder is often a comorbid condition with Bipolar Disorder, Bipolar Disorders would be diagnosed if which of the following were present?
    a. Substance abuse and chemical dependency
    b. Risk taking behavior
    c. Inattention and behavior problems at school by teacher reports
    d. Speech push, flight of ideas and grandiosity

92. Sam is a thirteen year old boy who is admitted to the adolescent unit with an initial diagnosis of Bipolar Disorder. Sam weighs 50 kg (110 lb). Which of the following would not be appropriate in planning for Sam's care?
    a. Initiate Lithium immediately upon admission to rapidly interrupt the symptoms.
    b. Arrange for a complete physical examination, including baseline laboratory studies.
    c. Orient Sam to the unit rules and ''point''system upon admission.
    d. Provide Sam with an information sheet about the unit daily activities.

93. The dosage range of Lithium ordered for Sam would be:
    a. Titrated initially

b. No greater than 600 mg daily
c. Closer to 1500 mg/day in divided doses
d. Dependent on whether he was being treated with chlorpromazine

94. The clinical nurse specialist on the unit makes contact with Sam's family to arrange for family treatment. Which of the following should be considered in arranging these sessions?

a. The family will probably be uncooperative and disruptive, as Bipolar Disorders commonly have familial origins.
b. The unit social worker will become enraged if the nurse does any work with the family
c. Shortened length of stay means that Sam will probably not have family treatment due to managed care regulations
d. Psychoeducational approaches are very critical in working with this family

95. Children and adolescents who are exposed to certain "extrinsic factors"are at greater risk for developing emotional mental disorders, such as depression. examples of extrinsic factors include all of the following except:

a. Poverty
b. Violence
c. Exposure to TV violence
d. Abusive situations

96. Which of the following is not true of the diagnosis of Depressive Disorders in children?

a. It is easier to diagnose melancholic subtype
b. Dysthymia has a one year duration
c. Failure to gain weight substitutes for weight loss
d. Irritability is common

97. A number of different clinical syndromes may be comorbid with depression in adolescents. Which of the following is most likely to be found?

a. Alcohol abuse
b. Conduct Disorder
c. Oppositional Disorder
d. Anxiety

98. Melissa is a clinically depressed 14 year old girl whose parents have recently

divorced after a long history of family violence and substance abuse. Melissa's father is in the military, and requested a transfer to another duty station following the finalization of the divorce. Melissa has exhibited suicidal ideation, poor school performance, and isolative behavior. She is admitted to the adolescent unit. Which is the most likely initial order(s) that will be written for Melissa's care?

a. Prozac, 20 mg., at breakfast
b. Complete physical examination, including baseline laboratory tests, pregnancy tests, and ECG
c. Begin Ropes program
d. Begin COA group

99. The medication management most likely to be initiated for Melissa would be:

a. Fluoxetine
b. Imipramine
c. Methylphenidate
d. Carbamazepine

100. Which of the following is considered by some experts to be the most damaging form of abuse?

a. Emotional and physical neglect
b. Marital discord
c. Sexual abuse
d. Physical abuse

101. Native american children of certain tribes have a suicide rate:

a. Less than that of white youngsters
b. Two to three times the rate of other Americans their age
c. Four to five times the national average
d. Fifty percent of urban African-American children

Answers

1. d
2. c
3. d
4. c
5. c
6. a
7. d
8. b
9. b
10. a
11. c
12. b
13. c
14. b
15. a
16. b
17. c
18. c
19. c
20. b
21. c
22. b
23. a
24. d
25. a
26. d
27. b
28. c
29. a
30. b
31. d
32. d
33. d
34. a
35. c
36. b
37. b
38. c
39. c
40. b
41. a
42. d
43. c
44. d
45. d
46. b
47. b
48. d
49. b
50. c
51. d
52. b
53. a
54. d
55. c
56. d
57. c
58. d
59. a
60. c
61. d
62. c
63. a
64. d
65. b
66. a
67. c
68. d
69. d
70. c
71. c
72. b
73. b
74. d
75. d
76. c
77. a
78. a
79. d
80. d
81. a
82. b
83. d
84. c
85. c
86. a
87. d
88. d
89. c
90. a
91. d
92. b
93. c
94. d
95. c
96. a
97. d
98. b
99. b
100. a
101. b

Bibliography

American Nurses' Association.(1985). *Standards of Child and Adolescent Psychiatric and Mental Health Nursing Practice*. St. Louis: American Nurses' Association.

American Professional Society on the Abuse of Children (1990). *Guidelines for psychosocial evaluation of suspected sexual abuse in children*. Chicago: APSAC.

American Nurses' Association. (1994). *Statement on Psychiatric-Mental Health Clinical Nursing Practice and Standards of Psychiatric-Mental Health Nursing Practice*. Washington, DC: American Nurses' Association.

Burgess, A. W., Hartman, C. R., & Kelley, S. J. (1990). Assessing child abuse: The TRIADS checklist. *Journal of Psychosocial Nursing and Mental Health Services. 28*(4), 7–14.

deTriquet, J. (1994). *Child abuse: A community perspective.* Plenary address in the Eastern Virginia Medical School conference on child abuse. Norfolk, VA.

First, M. B. (1991). *DSM-IV options book: Work in progress.* Washington, DC: American Psychiatric Association.

Fortinash, K. M., & Holaday-Worret, P. A. (1991). *Psychiatric nursing care plans.* St. Louis: Mosby Year Book.

Haber, J., McMahon, A. L., Price-Hoskins,P., & Sideleau, B. F. (1992). *Comprehensive psychiatric nursing*. St. Louis: Mosby Year Book.

Herman, J. L. (1992). *Trauma and recovery*. NY: Basic Books.

Kaplan, H. I., & Sadock, B. J. (1990). *Pocket handbook of clinical psychiatry*. Baltimore: Williams & Wilkins.

Kestenbaum, C. J., & Williams, D. T. (1988). *Handbook of clinical assessment of children and adolescents*. NY: New York University Press.

Krauss, J. (1993). *Health care reform: Essential mental health service*. Washington, DC: American Nurses Publishing.

Lechman, J. F., & Cohen, D. J. (1991). Clonadine treatment of Tourette's syndrome. *Archives of General Psychiatry, 48,* 324–328.

Lewis, M. (1991). *Child and adolescent psychiatry: A comprehensive textbook*. Baltimore: Williams & Wilkins.

McFarland, G. K. & Thomas, M. D. (1991). *Psychiatric mental health nursing*. Philadelphia: Lippincott.

Noshpitz, J. D., Call, J. D., Cohen, R. L., Harrison, S. I., Berlin, I. N., & Stone, L. A. (Eds). (1987). *Basic handbook of child psychiatry: Advances and New Directions.*Vol. V. NY: Basic Books.

Othmer, E., & Othmer, S. C. (1989). *The clinical interview using DSM III-R.* Washington, DC: American Psychiatric Association Press.

Paquette, M., Neal, M. C., & Rodemich, C. (1991). *Psychiatric nursing care plans for DSM III-R.* Boston:Jones and Bartlett.

Physician desk reference. (1994).(48th ed.). Montvale, NJ: Medical Economics Data Production.

Pothier, P. (1988). Graduate preparation in child and adolescent psychiatric and mental health nursing. *Archives of Psychiatric Nursing. 2*(3), 170–172.

Rapoport, J. L., & Ismond, D. R. (1990). *DSM III-R Training guide for diagnosis of childhood disorders.* NY: Brunner/Mazel.

Stuart, G. W., & Sundeen, S. J. (1991). *Principles and practice of psychiatric nursing.* St. Louis: Mosby Year Book.

Weller, E. B., & Weller, R. A. (1991). Mood disorders. In M. Lewis, *Child and adolescent psychiatry: A comprehensive textbook.* (pp. 646–663). Baltimore, MD: Williams & Wilkins.

Williams, J. W. (1987). *Diagnostic and statistical manual of mental disorders.* DSM-III-R. Washington, DC: American Psychiatric Association.

Wilson, H. S., & Kneisl, C. R. (1992). *Psychiatric nursing.* Redwood City, CA: Addison-Wesley.

The Larger Mental Health Environment

Sherrill Marshall

Contemporary Issues in Psychiatric Mental Health Nursing

- Recent Changes in Mental Health:
    1. Increased numbers of individuals are being diagnosed as mentally ill.
    2. Psychiatric diagnoses have become more inclusive.
    3. Shift from psychosocial interpretation of mental illness to neurochemical and biological interpretation
    4. Changes in third-party payment patterns are shifting treatment towards treating more acutely ill patients in shorter periods of time.
- Psychiatric/Mental Health Nursing
    1. Although cost of all health care has increased, cost of mental health treatment has increased at a greater rate. As a result, treatment has been restricted in most settings.
    2. Treatment is being moved from inpatient to outpatient community-based models.
    3. Psychiatric nursing recruitment has decreased
        a. Reasons for decrease
            (1) Significantly less federal money currently available for education than 20 years ago
            (2) Psychiatric Nursing is not taught as a separate, distinct specialty content in many nursing schools.
            (3) Women are entering other, non-traditional professions.
            (4) Adverse stigma associated with psychiatric patients
            (5) Fewer job opportunities as for-profit hospitals use increased numbers of non-nursing personnel.
    4. Professional development tasks for Psychiatric/ Mental Health Nursing in the 1990s:
        a. Support educational programs which prepare psychiatric mental health nurses to provide primary mental health care in a variety of settings
        b. Differentiate specialty content of graduate curriculum from general psychosocial emphasis in undergraduate areas

c. Clinical practice must demonstrate clear areas of expertise that differentiate psychiatric nursing from other mental health professions and the basic psychosocial skills of generalist nurses.

d. Psychiatric nursing/mental health research must reflect current national priorities such as funding reform.

e. Professional organizations and individual nurses must work to improve reimbursement mechanisms for mental health treatment.

f. Professional organizations and individual nurses must influence legislation to provide legal recognition of advanced nursing practice.

g. Educational institutions must increase educational emphasis on biopsychosocial and pharmacological integration.

5. Recommendations for the future

   a. Come to a professional consensus on content of psychiatric nursing curriculum.

   b. Practice, licensure, and certification standards should reflect the holistic aspects and flexibility of nursing knowledge.

   c. Certification activities should reflect current changes in clinical practice.

   d. Practice environments should allow nurses to focus on their abilities and skills rather than specific practice settings.

Conflict Resolution

- Key Issues

1. Interpersonal conflict is a common phenomenon.

   a. Nurses often encounter conflicts between

      (1) Clients and their families

      (2) Clients and their care-givers

2. Psychiatric clients may present with a history of ineffective, conflict laden, interpersonal relationships.

3. In the complex health care environment, conflict is often unavoidable.

a. High stress work areas may decrease individuals' ability to cope effectively with difficult interpersonal situations.

(1) The ability to resolve conflicting situations is key to the delivery of nursing care.

(2) Conflict resolution is a process, and skills in conflict resolution can be learned.

4. Consequences of interpersonal conflict and adverse effects of professional conflict include:

a. Deterioration in client care

b. Job dissatisfaction leading to increased employment turnover rates

c. Decreased productivity

5. Common responses to interpersonal conflict

a. Denial-avoidance

b. Overpowering

c. Accommodation

d. Compromise

d. Collaboration

- Strategies to resolve conflicts are functions of the assertiveness and cooperativeness of individuals.

1. Authoritarian styles are the result of high assertiveness and low cooperativeness. The conflict resolution styles are competition and force.

a. Supervisory personnel make decisions and tell parties the solution.

2. Collaboration occurs when individuals are highly assertive and highly cooperative.

a. Participants are involved in a problem-solving process of resolution.

3. Negotiation and compromise are the results of moderate levels of assertiveness and cooperativeness.

a. A process of striving for a win-win solution

   b. Usually most effective with a neutral third-party present
   c. May result in neither party being satisfied
4. Withdrawal and avoidance occur when assertiveness and cooperativeness are low.
   a. The lack of assertiveness and cooperativeness may result in passive/aggressive behaviors.
5. Accommodation occurs when assertiveness is low but cooperativeness is high.
6. Helpful techniques
   a. Keep a positive approach.
   b. Attempt to resolve conflict when parties are calm and receptive.
   c. All communication must be clearly understood by all parties.
   d. Communicate with respect.
   e. Give positive feedback whenever possible.
   f. Avoid quick judgments.
   g. Do not hold grudges.

Contracting Process

- Mental health services are often subject to contracting processes.
  1. Some services offered by health care providers are subject to contracting procedures.
  2. Facilities and organizations offering mental health services are always involved in contracting processes.
     a. Hospitals
     b. Treatment centers
     c. Outpatient and ambulatory care centers
     d. Day treatment and partial hospitalization centers
  3. Managed Care and Utilization Review organizations seek to contract with:
     a. Hospitals and alternative care facilities

b. Mental health professionals with all levels of licensure, expertise, and specialization

c. Referral sources

d. Suppliers and providers of medical supplies and equipment

4. Insurance companies and third-party payers contract with:

a. Facilities

b. Health care professionals

c. Managed care firms for services

d. Individual subscribers and health plan participants

- Reasons promoting contractual liaisons

1. To promote and protect market share

a. Contracting can define a particular market

(1) Geographic purposes—for example, a group practice may be capitated to provide mental health services to people in a certain ZIP code.

(2) Population purposes—for example, all members of an HMO must be treated by a certain facility.

(3) To refine site locations and utilization patterns

2. To increase profitability for both the selected health care professionals and facilities

a. Contracting by market sectors promotes profitability by eliminating the consumers (patients) ability to select their providers.

b. A defined population allows for more effective marketing-focused specifically on the contracted populations.

3. To lower costs for third-party payers and facilities

a. Contracting offers payers discount fees and may commit providers to predetermined utilization targets.

b. Facilities and providers can experience lowered costs of operation because

(1) Physical space (buildings, offices, etc.) developed only as needed

(2) Contracted sectors can do group purchasing, improve materials management, avoid duplicate purchases of machinery and equipment.

(3) Advertising and marketing activities can be specific to the contracted population.

c. At-risk-type contracts can be priced according to the risk factors of the population

- The Process

1. Needs analysis—every participant in the mental health market has a specific set of needs.

   a. Hospitals need to promote utilization and increase census and utilization of patient days.

   b. Health care professionals need to increase their earnings and profitability.

   c. The Managed Care firms need to control utilization and cost of delivery.

   d. The consumer needs accessibility to care and reasonable costs.

2. Once the need has been determined, a plan must be developed as to how those needs must be met via:

   a. Cost/profit proforma

   b. Feasibility studies

   c. Competition in the local market

   d. Legal issues

3. Contracts may be effected by outside specialists

   a. Third Party Administrators (TPAs) often act as the liaison between contracting parties

   b. Many contract lawyers practice in medical law specialties

4. Contracts may be effected directly between the CEOs of the provider organization and the subscriber

   a. Direct contracting more accurately represents participant interests.

   b. Direct contracting lowers cost of contracting by not utilizing third-party participants.

5. Other participants in the contracting process
    a. Outside agents and specialists
        (1) Law firms specializing in contract law
        (2) Third Party Administrators (TPAs)
        (3) Employer groups
            (a) Union organizations
            (b) Small business liaisons
        (4) Provider groups
            (a) Corporate hospital chains
            (b) Small independent and/or rural facilities bonding together for contractual strength
        (5) Consumer groups
            (a) Common interest populations
                - Aged communities
                - Special medical need communities like diabetics, HIV, handicapped
            (b) Self-employed groups seeking group rate considerations

Consultation

- Consultation practice is based upon theory
    1. Theorists
        a. Gerald Caplan—consultation with a mental health professional is a means of coping with and correcting problems in society (Caplan, 1964).
            (1) Consultation is a three-way process involving
                (a) The consultant—the mental health professional
                (b) The consultee—the person or entity purchasing the consultation service, and
                (c) The client—the person or group of people expected to benefit from the consultee's increase in knowledge or expertise

(2) Consultation is an expert service that occurs between professionals.

b. Client-Centered Consultation was developed by Carl Rogers.

(1) Concerned with the client's view of situation

(2) The consultant directly assesses the client and assists the consultee to develop a plan to meet the client's needs.

c. Consultee-Centered Consultation

(1) Concerned with the consultee's ability to manage the current situation as well as similar future situations

(2) The consultant assesses the consultee's responses and assists the consultee to develop new behaviors.

d. Program-Centered Consultation

(1) Concerned with program design and implementation

(2) The consultant makes recommendations to the administrator based on analysis of presented data.

d. Kurt Lewin applied small group dynamics to consultation theory.

(1) Two methods to solving interpersonal problems:

(a) Direct intervention

(b) Consultation

- Indirectly change variables, structure.
- Involve people in decisions about relevant issues.

f. Schein (1990)

(1) Coined term ''process consultation''

(2) Consultant attempts to assist client to understand the process between himself/herself and others.

(3) Client's own actions and their impact on others are of particular importance.

2. Structural stages of consultation

a. Entry

b. Goal setting
c. Problem solving
d. Decision making
e. Termination

Delivery of Mental Health Care

- Public or Community Mental Health system

1. Community mental health nurses hold the principles of primary, secondary, and tertiary prevention as central to their work (Wilson and Kneisl, 1992).
    a. Examples of primary prevention
        (1) Identifying high-risk populations
        (2) Providing mental health education
    b. Examples of secondary prevention
        (1) Providing brief psychotherapy to individuals, families, and groups
        (2) Providing emergency mental health services
    c. Examples of tertiary prevention
        (1) Plan for client's discharge from the hospital.
        (2) Serve as a client advocate.
2. Current issues in community mental health
    a. Historical background
        (1) In 1963 President Kennedy proposed the Community Mental Health Centers Act.
        (2) In 1980 President Carter introduced the Community Mental Health Systems Act.
        (3) The result of these two acts was deinstitutionalization or the shift of thousands of mentally ill people from hospitals to the community and often to the street.
    b. Current situation of community mental health

(1) Wilson (1992) described the community mental health system as a ''clearinghouse where dispatching and processing clients has replaced storing them.''

(2) Talbot (1979) declared deinstitutionalization a misnomer, explaining that transinstitutionalization was what occurred when the mentally ill were shifted from ''a single lousy institution to multiple wretched ones.''

c. Nurses are often the case managers for clients of the community mental health system. The case manager is expected to be the care giver, the connection between the client and the system, and the client advocate. Case managers are expected to arrange housing, food, and health care for this disenfranchised powerless group for whom there are meager resources.

- Private Mental Health Care

Delivery systems for mental health care are influenced by the trends in employer-offered health insurance. Managed care has become a major element in the delivery of American health care

1. Managed care may involve a variety of delivery systems including HMOs and PPOs. Both of these types of plans use utilization review systems as do many indemnity plans

   a. Utilization review systems

      (1) Many types of utilization review systems have been implemented with various degrees of control.

         (a) Pre-admission requirements

         (b) Concurrent review systems

         (c) Retrospective review systems

         (d) Bill review systems

   b. Goals of managed care

      (1) Management of revenue

      (2) Control of cash flow

      (3) Control of staffing expenses

      (4) Improved purchasing control of equipment and resources

c. Reasons for participation in HMOs and managed care plans
   (1) Lower cost and more predictable costs than traditional indemnity plans
   (2) Accessibility of services
   (3) Emphasis on health promotion/illness prevention

d. Criticisms of managed care
   (1) Not making significant progress in cost containment
      (a) Most managed care programs have been blamed for increased provider costs secondary to increased administrative costs.
      (b) Most managed care programs have shown increased co-payments and employee contributions.
      (c) The most successful, in terms of cost containment, managed care plans are those whose criteria for treatment are **rigidly** diagnosis based.
   (2) Limited accessibility of care
      (a) Managed care programs require utilization of member providers.
         - May pose geographic restriction to members
         - Participants often object to being unable to utilize providers of their choice.
   (3) Consumers' opinions of managed care impact on the delivery of mental health care
      (a) Limited support for the effectiveness of psychiatric concurrent review programs
      (b) No support for programs requiring prior approval

2. Employer issues in the delivery of care
   a. Predominant focus is cost containment.
      (1) Some employers report they would sacrifice worker's freedom of choice for purpose of cost containment.

b. Many employers who recognize that employees' mental health can increase productivity are active sponsors of Employee Assisted Programs (EAP). Under most EAPs, employees are not charged for the first through fourth visits to an employer selected EAP clinician.

c. Conservative utilization patterns by selected providers help employers limit time out of work by employees and perhaps more importantly to self-insured employers, limit benefit costs.

d. Delivery of health care is changing

   (1) Moving away from traditional physician-provider-hospital arrangements

   (2) Moving toward an integration of clinical services

   (3) Objectives of changing delivery systems

      (a) Reduce costs.

      (b) Improve quality.

      (c) Increase focus on health promotion and illness prevention.

3. Private practice and primary mental health care

   a. According to Haber and Billings (1993) "Primary mental health care may begin prior to or at the first point of contact with the mental health system and is continuous and comprehensive. The scope of primary mental health care is broad because it looks at the needs of the whole person. Addressing a broad range of mental health concerns, it includes all services necessary for promotion of optimal mental health, prevention of mental illness, and health maintenance, such as parenting classes, assertiveness training, stress management, bereavement groups, and health teaching."

   b. According to Krauss (1993), "studies of primary care practices find a substantial amount of psychiatric morbidity among individuals who consult their providers for non-psychiatric health services. Such studies find rates of diagnosable psychiatric disorders that range from 11 percent to 36 percent."

      (1) Nurses are extremely well qualified to provide treatment and case management for clients who are seriously mentally ill (Krauss, 1993).

(2) PMH nurses combine scientific knowledge and holistic vision to assist clients to face the challenges of daily living (Krauss, 1993).

(3) ''At the specialists level, direct care functions, including psychotherapy, continue to expand in response to society's need for a broader more flexible range of mental health services'' (Haber and Billings, 1993).

- Private Practice Considerations (Lego, 1984)

1. Advantages of private practice
   a. Control of the scope of practice
   b. Flexibility of hours
   c. Financial rewards
2. Disadvantages of private practice
   a. The nurse is solely responsible for the practice.
   b. Professional isolation—in a solo practice there may be no back-up for professional judgment and decision making.
   c. ''On-call''—the nurse in a 1:1 contractual relationship with a client must be available.
   d. There are no adjunct therapists or other assistive personnel.
   e. Competition for a limited ''pool'' of patients
3. Qualifications—''The psychiatric-mental health advanced practice nurse (APRN) is a licensed RN who is educationally prepared at the masters' level, at a minimum, and is nationally certified as a clinical nurse specialist in psychiatric and mental health nursing. The psychiatric mental health APRN has the ability to apply knowledge, skills, and experience autonomously to complex mental health problems'' (ANA, 1994).
4. Starting the practice
   a. Initial start-up expenses
      (1) Furniture for office and waiting room
      (2) Office equipment
      (3) Newspaper announcements
      (5) ''Yellow Pages'' advertisement

(6) Stationary, billing forms, and file supplies

(7) Legal fees for incorporation

b. Ongoing operating expenses

(1) Office rent

(2) Utilities

(3) Answering service, voice mail and pagers

(4) Insurance, including:

(a) Health and life

(b) Malpractice

(c) Disability

(d) Property and casualty

(5) Accountant fees

5. Fees and third-party reimbursement

a. Psychiatric mental health APRN (CNS) are clearly eligible for reimbursement under CHAMPUS and FEHBP (Federal Employee Health Benefit Plan). However "the battle for equitable reimbursement in the cost formula is not over. The ANA position is that if a service is covered by federal or private health benefit plan and a nurse is legally authorized to deliver the service, then nurses should be reimbursed for the service" (Billings, 1993, p. 179).

b. Fees for 50-minute sessions range between \$50 to \$90.

c. Reimbursement by insurance category

(1) Most managed care plans do contract with APRNs for psychotherapy; however, the fee maximums may be less than other providers.

(2) Private indemnity plans—9 states mandate direct payment to APRNs, 20 states have legislation that allows direct reimbursement (McCloskey and Grace, 1994).

(3) Medicaid—four states offer medicaid reimbursement to psychiatric mental health APRNs, although 28 states offer this reimbursement to nurse practitioners (McCloskey and Grace, 1994)

(4) Medicare—APRNs are eligible for Medicare Part B only in some rural areas.

6. Collaboration with a psychiatrist

   When clients need hospitalization or medications, they may require referral to a psychiatrist. It is important that APRNs have good working relationships with psychiatrists who share similar views of appropriate care.

7. Accountability

   Advanced practice psychiatric mental health nurses are accountable to their clients and to the profession as delineated in *Statement on Psychiatric-Mental Health Clinical Nursing Practice and Standards of Psychiatric-Mental Health Nursing Practice* (ANA, 1994)

- Home Care Delivery Systems (continue to increase although there are few in mental health)

  1. Hospitals are entering the home care market.
     a. Popularity and acceptance of home care delivery has been evidenced by continued growth of private home care agencies.
  2. Home care delivery systems allow improved discharge planning.
     a. Lengths of stay can be kept to minimum and still assure quality follow-up with home care services.
     b. Clients respond better to home-based care.

Empowerment through Specialization (Styles, 1989)

- Conditions for Power

  1. Legitimacy
     a. Legitimacy is defined as "accordance with law or accepted rules."
     b. Nursing, unlike other professions, has no single source of sanction.
  2. Homogeneity
     a. Defined as consistency, equality, and parity
     b. Requires
        (1) Definition and differentiation

(2) Demand for service individuals

(3) Quality

(4) Sanction

(5) Stature

(6) Representation and advocacy

(7) Connectedness to other parts of the system

3. Unity

a. Defined as oneness, accord, harmony

b. To be powerful a system must have a high degree of unity—in purpose, in standards, and in vision.

- Indications of Power

1. Professional identification
2. Title and practice entitlement
3. Institutional privileges
4. Compensation
5. Third-party reimbursement
6. Quality control
7. Career advancement and recognition

- Empowerment for Nurses

1. Education

a. Raise awareness of nurses, other professionals, and consumers

2. Specialization

a. Specialization can be traced to the craft guilds of the Middle Ages.

b. According to Styles (1989) specialization improves professional competence, quality of services, cost of services, and professional satisfaction.

(1) Professional competence is improved because specialization enables nurses to concentrate on one area of knowledge and technique.

(2) Quality is improved through external control, for example, third party payment tied to specialty certification.

(3) Cost is reduced because specialists can achieve economies of scale and cost reductions because their practice is focused to one area.

(4) Professional satisfaction often increases due to mastery of a service area and the ability to concentrate interest and energies as well as close association with peers.

Leadership and Management

- Leadership and Management Theories

1. Dictionary definitions of leadership are ''to guide, to influence, to direct''; management is defined in stronger terms—''to direct, to control,to make submissive''

2. Leadership can also be defined as an interaction between the variables of situation, communication, and the group.

3. Ohio State Research

a. Two types of leadership structures

(1) Initiating structure

(a) Concerned with the task at hand

(2) Consideration structure

(a) Concerned with establishing an environment and positive relationship with the employee

(3) Research concluded that neither type of leadership is preferable

b. Trait theories are attempts to determine which personality traits result in effective leadership

(1) See leadership as dependent on personality traits in the following areas:

(a) Physical and social makeup

(b) Intelligence

(c) Personality

(d) Task relations

(e) Social characteristics

c. Situational theories look at the interactions between the leader and members of a group in particular situations

(1) Addresses the appropriateness of the match given the circumstance.

(2) Identifies three leadership styles

(a) Democratic verses autocratic

(b) Participatory verses directive

(c) Laissez-faire verses motivational

- First-line Managers

1. First-line managers (head nurses, unit managers, program or project directors) have a key role in the maintenance of the structure of the working environment.

2. First-line managers provide the link between upper administration and the delivery of patient care.

3. Three key areas where the first-line manager must demonstrate competency are:

a. Structuring a harmonious, effective work place through management of:

(1) Budget

(2) Equipment

(a) Identify resources

(b) Assure continued availability of equipment

(3) Staffing

(a) Recruitment, interview, selection process

(b) Determining staff mix versus patient workload

(4) Leadership

(a) Determining goals and organization of the unit

(b) Building work teams

(c) Resolving conflicts

(d) Ensuring communication

            (e) Motivating professional growth
        (5) Assisting nursing staff
            (a) Developing and upholding performance standards
            (b) Determining and meeting staff development needs
        (6) Demonstrating excellence as a practitioner
            (a) Performing in stressful circumstances
            (b) Continuing professional growth and development
            (c) Maintaining professional competence

- Leadership Behavior Affects Employee Performance
    1. Recent research reveals that employee behavior is determined by the type of leadership that employees receive.
        a. Most effective leadership behaviors
            (1) Encouraging teamwork
            (2) Empowering staff
            (3) Fostering collaboration and cooperation
            (4) Providing support
            (5) Setting high standards
            (6) Providing an example
    2. Pagonis (1992) described leadership in terms of traits, process, and work.
        a. Leader must demonstrate two traits
            (1) Expertise
            (2) Empathy
        b. Steps of leadership
            (1) Know yourself
            (2) Learn how and what to communicate
            (3) Know your mission
        c. Work within the organization
            (1) Delegate

(2) Maintain relationships within system

(3) Techniques:

(a) Shape the vision

- Establish first priority
- Define the objectives

(b) Educate

- Give and get feedback
- Formal communication following chain of command

3. Stivers (1991) discussed women as leaders:

a. Nurses, as women leaders, may have some difficulty with self-definition.

b. Stivers described two approaches to leadership

(1) Mainstream—''masculine''—women should be taught to lead as well as men and display ''masculine'' leadership characteristics:

(a) Tough

(b) Bold

(c) Decisive

(d) Masterful

(e) Risk criticism for being unfeminine

(2) Woman's approach—women's characteristics are significant. Female leaders do not have to imitate men to be effective. Positive ''feminine'' leadership characteristics include the following:

(a) Caring

(b) Collaboration

(c) Quality oriented

(d) Run the risk of being criticized as ineffective

(3) The reality is probably a balancing act between the two styles.

- Stiver's Recommendations
  1. Graduate education for nurse administrators that integrates two approaches to management
     a. Women's issues at center of curriculum
     b. Teaching advantages/disadvantages of both styles is empowering to nurse administrators.
     c. Include ''big picture'' focus that includes political, economic, governmental context of the organization.
     d. Teaching negotiating, critical thinking, communication skills.
- Problem Solving—A Key Leadership Task
  1. Key issues
     a. Psychiatric nurses encounter multiple complex problems.
     b. Good problem solving skills and a systematic method of solving problems is an efficient way to arrive at viable solutions.
     b. Problem solving format used by work teams assures all members input, assists all team members in coming to the solution within the same time frame, and insures greater acceptance of the solution(s) reached.
  2. Steps in problem solving process
     a. Define the problem accurately
        (1) Make sure the focus isn't a problem symptom or the most bothersome aspect of the problem.
     b. Define the objectives.
        (1) All problems have multiple solutions.
           (a) What does the problem solver want to get from the solution?
           (b) Must all parts of the problem be solved or would narrower objectives be acceptable under the circumstances?
     c. Identify possible causes for the problem.
        (1) Identification of causes often leads to solutions.
     d. Formulate multiple solutions to the problem.

(1) This is very effective in a group setting

e. Methods of generating solutions

   (1) Group discussion

   (2) Brainstorming

   (3) Multi-voting

   (4) Blind balloting

f. Select the most preferable solution(s) to the problem.

g. Formulate an action plan.

   (1) Plans should be specific.

   (2) Include specific steps to take.

   (3) Assign responsibility.

   (4) Set deadlines/target dates.

h. Implement the action plan.

i. Reassess the status of the problem.

j. Review problem solving steps again, if necessary.

Legal and Ethical Issues

- Definitions

  1. Law is established and standardized rules of human conduct enforced by society.
  2. Nursing law is not a unique entity, but subject to existing structures of the laws, which vary from state to state.
  3. The increased demands on the professional nurse require nurses to be aware of their legal responsibilities.

- Torts

  1. A tort is a civil wrong.
  2. It is a violation of an individual's rights that entitles the wronged individual to seek damages from the wrongdoer.
  3. Tort liability has impacts on psychiatric-mental health nursing in two areas: negligence (unintentional torts) and intentional torts.

a. Negligence—in order to recover damages, four elements of negligence must have been present.
   (1) The nurse must have the duty of care.
   (2) The nurse must breach that duty.
   (3) The patient must have been harmed.
   (4) The nurse's breach of duty must have caused the harm.
b. Duty of care depends on conditions of employment or the establishment of nurse-patient relationship.
c. A psychiatric-mental health nurse breaches the duty of care if the nursing care provided fails to meet the accepted standards of psychiatric-mental health clinical practice. A standard of care is generally measured by comparing the behavior of the nurse with the behavior of a reasonable and prudent nurse in similar circumstances.
d. Common negligence actions include failure to monitor a patient's condition, medication errors, abandonment, and failure to provide a safe environment.

4. Intentional torts—unlike negligence a patient does not have to prove harm or damages. Actions for intentional torts usually arise from:
   a. Lack of informed consent
   b. Battery or false imprisonment in relation to seclusion and restraint procedures
   c. Breach of confidentiality

- Other types of laws that impact the rights and responsibilities of nurses
   a. Statutory law
      (1) Federal and/or state laws prohibiting or demanding some code of behavior, for example, Nurse Practice Acts
   b. Criminal law
      (1) Stipulates punishment for offenders and includes acts such as homicide or robbery
- Nursing licensure
   1. The American Nurses' Association (ANA) became concerned about

licensure and moved for governmental intervention in the early 1900s.

2. By 1952 all states and territories had established laws related to the practice of nursing.
3. By 1958 the ANA had developed a model nurse practice act.
   a. Nursing laws, licensing requirement, and nurse practice acts vary from state to state.
4. Basic licensing requirements generally include
   a. Completion of a state-approved school
   b. Payment of a fee
   c. Passing an examination prepared by the National Council of State Boards of Nursing
5. Advanced practice licensing requirements generally include:
   a. Completion of a post-graduate program, either a degree program or a certificate program
   b. National or specialty certification
   c. Payment of a fee
6. License renewal is usually required every two years
   a. Most states require a renewal fee.
   b. Many states require board approval and/or continuing education.

- The Nurse Practice Acts
  1. Designed to meet the needs of individual states and establish standards of professionalism; formulated to protect public by establishing minimum competency levels for nurses
  2. Components of most nurse practice acts
     a. Definition of nursing
        (1) Scope of practice
            (a) General practice
            (b) Advanced practice, including prescriptive authority where applicable

b. Requirements for licensure
   (1) Basic or general practice
   (2) Advanced practice including:
      (a) CRNAs
      (b) CNS or ARNP
      (c) Nurse practitioners
c. Exemption from licensure
d. Conditions for revocation of licensure
e. Provision for reciprocity for licenses from other states
f. Description of the board of nurse examiners
g. Board responsibilities
h. Penalties for practicing without a license

3. Board of nurse examiners
   a. Generally appointed by the governor, although in some states they are elected.
   b. May be composed of all nurses, however, most states include lay members
   c. Responsible to ensure that the nurse practice act is carried out
4. Disciplinary actions may be invoked by the state board of nurse examiners:
   a. Formal reprimands
   b. Probation
   c. Denial of renewal of licensure
   d. Suspension of licensure
   e. Revocation of licensure
5. The most common reasons for review by a board
   a. Practicing nursing while under the influence of drugs or alcohol
   b. Addiction or dependency on alcohol or other addictive drugs

- Malpractice insurance for nurses

1. Generally provided by the employer
    a. Nursing care provided under the supervision of an organization generally implicates the management.
    b. More cost effective to purchase group coverage
2. Every registered nurse should carry individual malpractice insurance.
    a. Due to the increase in lawsuits brought against individual nurse
    b. Policies available from professional service organizations
3. Methods to avoid lawsuits
    a. Proper documentation including specific and legible records that are signed
    b. Adhere to facility standards on the transcription of orders and verbal or phone orders
    c. In the case of errors, follow facility requirements.
    d. In the event of legal actions, pursue independent counsel.

- Ethical issues
    1. Ethics are principles of right or good conduct.
    2. The ANA first adopted an official code of ethics in 1950, the latest code in 1993.
    3. As explained in *Statement on Psychiatric-Mental Health Clinical Nursing Practice and Standards of Psychiatric-Mental Health Nursing Practice* (ANA, 1994) "The PMH nurse's decisions and actions on behalf of clients are determined in an ethical manner." Criteria for ethical behavior include:
        a. The PMH nurse's practice is guided by the *Code for Nurses.*
        b. The PMH nurse maintains a therapeutic and professional relationship with clients at all times.
        c. The PMH nurse maintains client confidentiality and appropriate boundaries.
        d. The PMH nurse functions as a client advocate.
        e. The PMH nurse delivers care in a nonjudgmental and nondiscriminatory manner sensitive to client diversity.

f. The PMH nurse identifies ethical dilemmas that occur in practice and seeks available resources to help formulate ethical decisions.

g. The PMH nurse reports abuse of clients' rights,and incompetent, unethical, and illegal practices.

h. The PMH nurse participates in obtaining the client's informed consent for procedures, treatments, and research, as appropriate.

i. The PMH nurse discusses with the client the roles and parameters of the relationship.

j. The PMH nurse carefully manages self disclosure.

k. The PMH nurse does not promote or engage in intimate or sexual relationships with current clients.

l. The PMH nurse avoids sexual relationships with clients or former clients and recognizes that to engage in such a relationship is unusual and an exception to accepted practice.

Organizational Theories

- Origin of organizational theories
    1. Organizational theories have their origins in cultures and civilizations dating back to 5000 B.C.
    2. Formalized theories were studied and documented during the Industrial Revolution.
    3. Established schools of thought of organizational theories were established in the early 1900s.
- Modern systems theory
    1. Based on the assumption that work organizations are a complex blend of characteristics
        a. Human comfort and environmental needs of workers
        b. Social and emotional needs of workers
        c. Variables based on the complexity of the task, and the availability of resources
    2. Modern organizational theory is based on an examination of variables of an organization conducted by various means:

a. Observation

b. Worker surveys

c. Experimentation

d. Objective analysis

4. Modern organizational theory is based on key questions.

    a. What are the most important parts of the system?

    b. What is the interrelationship of those key parts of the organization?

    c. What are the channels or processes that tie the key parts together?

    d. What are the performance goals and objectives of the organization?

5. Key components of the system

    a. The individual workers

    b. The division of labor and responsibilities

    c. Formal and informal relationships within the organization

    d. The physical environment

6. Management factors influence how the various components become integrated

    a. Communication

    b. Group problem solving

    c. Establishing feedback mechanisms

    d. Exercising control and management

Quality Management

- Purpose of quality management

    1. Accountability

        a. Legal precedents have demanded accountability of physicians, nurses, and institutions.

        b. The payers of health insurance costs are demanding proof of quality.

2. To improve quality
    a. Monitoring practice trends will reveal potential problem areas.
    b. Tracking the effectiveness of interventions will lead to improved quality.
3. To provide recognition
    a. To reinforce good employees
    b. To identify positive actions and trends

- The quality management process
    1. Set standards
        a. Establish the goals for the organization.
        b. Incorporate established standards from the professional community.
            (1) *Statement on Psychiatric-Mental Health Clinical Nursing Practice and Standards of Psychiatric-Mental Health Nursing Practice* (ANA, 1994)
            (2) The Joint Commission on the Accreditation of Healthcare Organizations (JCAHO)
            (3) State and Federal standards (HCFA)
            (4) Professional accreditation bodies
                (a) Committee on the Accreditation of Rehabilitation Facilities (CARF)
                (b) American Medical Association
                (c) Others specific to the facility and the composition of the professional staff
        c. In addition to generic standards, clinical practice guidelines should be developed for the specific client population being served.
        d. The standards provide the basis for all other measures of quality.
    2. Establish criteria.
        a. Criteria should specify measurable indicators of performance.
        b. Criteria should be realistic and meaningful.

3. Evaluate performance.
    a. Apply the criteria to the actual practice.
        (1) Employ varied methods in the evaluation process.
            (a) Peer review
            (b) Medical records audits
            (c) Direct monitoring and supervision.
            (d) Interview clients to determine their degree of satisfaction.
            (e) Measure the cost-benefit ratio.
        (2) Document findings.
            (a) Track findings and results.
            (b) Organize the findings into meaningful sequences of information and data.
            (c) Whenever possible, graph the data to aid in its interpretation and understanding.
        (3) Establish corrective actions.
            (a) Involve nurses in the corrective action process.
            (b) Empower staff to make decisions and implement corrective actions.
            (c) Make sure the corrective action addresses the identified problems.
            (d) Document the corrective action and the persons responsible for its implementation.
        (4) Follow-up
            (a) Establish a system for tracking and monitoring the impact and cost of the corrective actions.
            (b) Don't assume that because a corrective action has been implemented, that it will work.
            (c) Document the results of the corrective action, whether successful or not.
            (d) If a corrective action process is not effective at improving quality, it should be changed.

4. Many alternative methods of establishing quality assurance programs exist; research the system that will be most appropriate for your facility or organization.
    a. If the facility is accredited under the JCAHO, the quality assurance plan should be developed according to the "Ten Steps of Monitoring and Evaluation" as outlined in JCAHO publications.
    b. Many professional organizations have established quality assurance programs available.
    c. Involve staff in the entire quality assurance process.
        (1) Promotes acceptance
        (2) Helps clarify the goals and objectives of the program
        (3) Employees will take a greater ownership in the program.

- Audit Systems
    1. Types of audits
        a. Retrospective—conducted on closed records following discharge
            (1) Advantages
                (a) Does not impede delivery of care
                (b) Generally perceived as less threatening than concurrent review
                (c) Can be done by personnel as work load permits, i.e., during night shifts
            (2) Disadvantages
                (a) Does not permit opportunities to correct the care immediately
                (b) Findings are generally perceived as being less important than concurrent findings because the event has already passed.
        b. Concurrent—conducted during the hospital stay
            (1) Advantages

(a) Permits opportunities to immediately address identified concerns

(b) Promotes a sense of urgency or importance to the quality assurance process

(c) Can be used as a learning and supervisory tool for improved performance

2. Focuses of audits

a. Medical records audits

(1) Criteria may include

(a) Compliance of documentation to facility established standards

(b) Neatness and legibility of the documentation

(c) Compliance of documentation to treatment plan areas of concern

(d) Timeliness of documentation

(2) The audit process may be conducted by

(a) Unit nursing personnel

(b) Medical records and clerical personnel

(c) Supervisors and directors

- To provide valuative data of persons being supervised

b. Actual performance audits

(1) Monitoring and evaluation of important aspects of patient care

(a) Administration of medication

(b) Communication skills with patients and co-workers

(c) The delivery of therapy and hands-on elements of care

(2) Determination of client satisfaction

(a) By conducting interviews

(b) By the use of surveys

- Peer review systems
  1. Purpose
     a. Evaluation provided by peers is intended to promote acceptance of the findings.
        (1) Similarly skilled individuals under the same working conditions objectively evaluating each other
     b. Promotes a sense of teamwork
        (1) Peers rank each other in accordance to established criteria.
  2. Advantage of peer review
     a. Establishes a consistent threshold of performance for the individual, department, facility, or organization
        (1) Criteria is mutually agreed upon.
        (2) All members held to the same criteria.
     b. A cost effective means of maintaining quality
        (1) No additional personnel resources are utilized.
        (2) Can usually be done as part of the facility's existing structure of meetings and functions
     c. Provides a confidential evaluation
        (1) Records and findings remain proprietary to the facility.
  3. Disadvantages of peer review
     a. Small departments or groups of personnel may not be objective in their findings.
        (1) Attempts to protect one another
        (2) Small groups may work together to exclude others from their circle.
     b. It is often difficult to motivate participants.
        (1) Physicians often feel immune from criticism and fail to note significant findings.

(2) Review activities are sometimes viewed as tedious and meaningless.

c. Lack of new ideas

(1) Established peer groups often become stagnant and do not look for new criteria

(2) Constantly changing technologies often require new viewpoints from the outside which may be excluded from established groups

Questions
Select the best answer

1. The purpose of quality management programs is:
    a. Legal accountability
    b. To meet demands of insurance companies
    c. To improve quality
    d. All of the above

2. The first step in the development of a quality management program is:
    a. Determine who will be responsible for the program
    b. Establish schedules for the collection of data
    c. Set standards
    d. Allocate resources for the program

3. The establishment of quality management criteria should be based upon:
    a. Issues of interest to the department or service head
    b. Realistic and meaningful aspects of care
    c. Known areas of deficiency or need
    d. Known areas of excellence

4. Performance can be evaluated by means of:
    a. Supervision
    b. Records audits
    c. Interviews with patients
    d. All of the above

5. When establishing corrective actions it is important to:
    a. Penalize poor performance
    b. Involve staff in the development of corrective actions
    c. Make sure the corrective actions provide several alternatives
    d. Ensure all members of the staff are involved in the process

6. It is important to provide follow-up in a quality management program to ensure:
    a. A tracking mechanism to identify successful and unsuccessful actions
    b. That there is proof that the activities were completed
    c. Documentation to terminate ineffective staff

d. It is required by law

7. The advantages of retrospective audits are:

   a. They are easier and faster
   b. They are perceived as less threatening
   c. Everyone can participate in the process
   d. They yield high quality data

8. The disadvantages of retrospective audits are:

   a. They do not provide immediate opportunities to improve care
   b. It is a more costly process
   c. They impede the delivery of patient care
   d. The record keeping process is more complicated

9. Which of the following is not an advantage of concurrent quality assurance reviews:

   a. Permit immediate opportunities for correction
   b. It is a more expedient form of review
   c. Promote a sense of urgency
   d. Can be used as a supervisory tool

10. The focus of audits of medical records may include:

    a. Neatness and legibility
    b. Documentation to treatment plan issues
    c. Timeliness of documentation
    d. All of the above

11. The purpose of peer review systems is to:

    a. Save money by having workers do the review of themselves
    b. Heighten workers scrutiny of each other's work
    c. Promote a sense of teamwork
    d. Help reduce the workload of supervisors

12. To encourage acceptance of peer review programs, the established criteria should be:

    a. Representative of the highest possible standards of care
    b. Mutually agreed upon by all members of the department
    c. Easy enough to assure success

   d. Focused on poor performers in the department

13. Small departments or facilities may encounter problems with peer review systems because:
   a. The group may not be objective in their findings
   b. The additional work may be viewed as burdensome
   c. The group may alienate poor performers
   d. The group may not be competent to evaluate its own performance

14. Peer review systems may not yield objective data because:
   a. The sample size is too small
   b. The participants may attempt to protect each other
   c. The process will not be taken seriously
   d. A successful department may not have any need to improve

15. Identify recent trends in the psychiatric nursing field that impact nursing practice:
   a. Increased numbers of mentally ill people, decreased lengths of stay, increased biochemical focus of interpretations of mental illness
   b. More successful resolutions of mental illness diagnosis, decreased lengths of stay, increased community based treatment, less federal money for psychiatric nursing education
   c. Increased psychodynamic interpretation of psychiatric issues, decreased lengths of stay, proportionately less women entering the nursing field, increased levels of community based care
   d. Integration of psychiatric nursing content into other course offerings, decreased numbers of mentally ill individuals due to modern drugs, adverse stigma associated with mental illness, increased complexity necessary in psychiatric nursing skills

16. Which of the following is not a professional development task for the next decade?
   a. Differentiating the parts of the role that treat mental illness from those which enhance and support mental health
   b. Developing new biochemical models to serve as a basis for treating mental illness
   c. Relating psychiatric nursing research to current national psychiatric nursing delivery priorities

d. Enhancing clinical practice standards such that psychiatric nursing as a specialty is clearly differentiated from generalists level knowledge in psychosocial aspects of nursing care

17. Which of the following factors is not considered an advantage of empowering nurses?

    a. Greater utilization of non-nursing personnel
    b. Improved patient care
    c. Increased retention rates
    d. Enhancement in the individual nurses' professional self-image

18. The main tenet of the Trait theory of leadership is:

    a. Leadership traits can be developed with proper education and training
    b. Leadership traits are inborn and based on personality
    c. Leadership traits are best developed in small peer groups and, once developed, can be generalized to larger organizations
    d. Leadership traits are inherently masculine and women need conscientious and determined work to develop theirs to the masculine level

19. The Ohio State leadership studies postulated that there were two type of leadership patterns: those that dealt with structuring the task and those that focused on leading the workers.
    Research on this theory held that:

    a. Neither type of leadership structure was preferable
    b. The type of leadership structure that was preferable depended upon the situation and the degree of mechanization in the task at hand
    c. The Ohio studies only related to midwestern males and could not be generalized to females or males from other cultures
    d. A leadership structure that focused on motivating the worker was far superior to the task oriented structure

20. The reason that first line managers are so key to nursing leadership is:

    a. They provide the link between the patient and upper administration
    b. Future nursing administrators and leaders are developed from first-line managers
    c. They are frequently in the position of supervising and developing new nurses and, as such, are responsible for the retention of new graduates by the profession
    d. They have the ability and authority to speak for groups of staff

21. Three key areas where the first-line manager must develop competency are:
    a. Budgeting, staffing, and demonstrating continued professional growth
    b. Leading staff groups, compiling records, and meeting regulatory/accreditation standards
    c. Creating an effective work place, assisting nursing staff, and demonstrating excellent clinical skills
    d. Upholding performance standards, monitoring patient care, ensuring the provision and maintenance of equipment

22. Which of the following is **not** one of the primary functions of the first line manager's leadership role?
    a. Building work teams
    b. Motivating professional growth
    c. Determining the goals and organization of the unit
    d. Developing policies and procedures that guide staff behavior

23. The first-line manager demonstrates clinical excellence by:
    a. Speaking at conferences and publishing papers
    b. Meeting with all staff members to review their performance
    c. Conducting satisfaction surveys of the patients in her area
    d. Displaying excellent clinical skills under stressful circumstances

24. Which of the following is **not** an effective nursing leadership behavior?
    a. Encouraging teamwork
    b. Disciplining staff who make mistakes
    c. Empowering staff
    d. Fostering collaboration and cooperation

25. According to Pagonis, an important part of intraorganizational functioning is the ability to:
    a. Know and adhere to the organization's priorities and mission
    b. Translate subordinates' concerns to upper administration and communicate administrative decisions to the staff
    c. Educate the staff about the organization by giving feedback and following the chain of command
    d. Demonstrate how change can be effected when problems arise

26. Stivers states that there are two distinct approaches to leadership that are options for nurses. They are:

a. Directive vs. Non-directive
b. Mainstream vs. Women's
c. Authoritarian vs. Laissez faire
d. Medical model vs. Empowerment

27. Which of the following is **not** a positive female leadership value?

a. Collaboration
b. Caring
c. Decisiveness
d. Quality

28. Which of the following should be included in graduate nurse education in order to integrate the masculine and feminine approaches to leadership?

a. Teaching and fostering traditional masculine values such as toughness and competitiveness
b. Psychologically focused group sessions to ventilate feelings of powerlessness and oppression
c. Curriculum which teaches negotiating skills, critical thinking, and communication skills
d. Exposure to traditional male-dominated areas of health care and business

29. Which of the following groups of psychological theorists address consultation issues as a major focus?

a. Caplan, Rogers, Lewin, and Schein
b. Freud, Adler, Sullivan, and Maslow
c. Horney, W. A. White, Boszormenyi-Nagy, and Lidz
d. Erikson, Vroom, Herzberg, and Skinner

30. According to Rogers, which skill is the most critical in the consultation process?

a. Consultation entry skills
b. Problem solving
c. Relationship development
d. Outcome assessment

31. The focus in Schein's Process Consultation model is:

a. The interaction between the client and others in the consultation situation
b. The process by which the client comes to decisions
c. The leadership process and its impact on the client

d. A review of the stage of the consultation process

32. Which of the following is **not** one of the structural stages of the consultation process?

    a. Termination
    b. Relationship generation
    c. Goal setting
    d. Decision making

33. Which of the following is **not** true of interpersonal conflict?

    a. Conflict is a common consequence of interpersonal relationships.
    b. Conflict usually results from the failure to form a therapeutic or professional relationship.
    c. High stress work situations decrease individuals' ability to deal with conflict.
    d. Conflict is often unavoidable and, therefore, conflict resolution skills need to be acquired.

34. Which of the following is an adverse effect of interpersonal conflict in the hospital?

    a. Unionization
    b. Clique formation
    c. Decreased productivity
    d. Authoritarian leadership patterns

35. Which of the following is **not** a strategy for conflict resolution?

    a. Denial-Avoidance
    b. Arbitration
    c. Authoritarian
    d. Negotiation

36. Managed Care and Utilization Review organizations seek to contract with which of the following types of organizations?

    a. Hospitals and health care facilities
    b. Mental health professionals
    c. Referral sources
    d. All of the above

37. Which of the following is **not** usually a reason to develop contracts between parties in the mental health field?

   a. To promote a larger market share
   b. To increase profitability
   c. To provide additional levels of indigent care
   d. To lower overall costs

38. Three of the following parties are common participants in the contracting process. Which party below does not make health care contracts?

   a. Employer groups such as small businesses and unions
   b. Individual patients with specialized interest in a certain type of care
   c. Health care provider groups such as hospital chains or consortiums
   d. Groups of consumers with common interests

39. Mental health services are a frequently contracted service. This has proven to be cost effective and profitable. Another reason to contract for mental health services is:

   a. To assure the availability of services for those individuals who require them
   b. Mental health services are best delivered in areas that are physically separate from other general medical and surgical areas
   c. Mental health requires a degree of specialized expertise which isn't available within the general medical community
   d. These contracts assure and legally stipulate the availability of mental health services

40. Which of the following is *not* a common problem associated with Managed Care?

   a. Increased paperwork and documentation
   b. Increased staff to respond to demands of managed care
   c. Capital expenditures for data tracking
   d. Excess nursing staff levels due to managed care requirements

41. Which is the most important factor in influencing trends in the delivery of mental health care?

   a. New advances in psychotropic drugs
   b. Health Maintenance Organizations'(HMO) dominance of major market share
   c. Move towards community based care

d. Increased amount of service delivery by non-physician Mental Health professionals

42. For employers, a key element in the selection and delivery of health care plans is:

    a. Regulatory agency involvement
    b. Total overall costs
    c. Employee satisfaction
    d. The degree to which the plan meets comprehensive needs

43. Which of the following does *not* account for the increase in homecare delivery?

    a. Allowance for improved discharge planning opportunities.
    b. Rural patients have improved access to health care.
    c. Decreased hospital lengths of stay
    d. Patient preference for receiving care at home

44. All but one of the following is a common problem associated with managed care:

    a. Enrollees feel that their care options are limited.
    b. Providers may compromise the level of care in order to meet managed care requirements.
    c. Increased cost to patients
    d. Increased range of services available to enrollees

45. It is important that psychiatric nurses develop good problem solving skills because:

    a. Psychiatric patients almost always present with more complex issues and problems than those in the general hospital.
    b. Problem solving is an efficient, effective way of arriving at viable solutions.
    c. Other specialties within nursing look to mental health specialists for this ability and frequently consult with psychiatric nurses as an expert resource.
    d. Problem solving is a skill that psychiatric nurses need to teach their patients and will be unable to do this unless they are, themselves, experts.

46. The first step in the problem-solving process is to:

    a. Gather all interested parties and meet to discuss the problem

b. Formulate a list of possible solutions to the problems
c. Identify, in as precise a way as possible, the causes for the problem
d. Define the problem accurately

47. Laws related to the practice and profession of nursing

 a. Are specific to the field of nursing
 b. Pertain to the specialized duties and responsibilities of nurses
 c. Are not a unique entity, but subject to the existing structures of law
 d. Were designed to address the changing role of the nurse professional

48. Which of the following is not a type of law that impacts the rights and responsibilities of nurses?

 a. Criminal law
 b. Malpractice law
 c. Annuity law
 d. Liability law

49. With regard to the licensure rules and regulations for nurses:

 a. All states have the same requirements for the licensure of nurses
 b. The requirements for the licensure of nurses varies from state to state
 c. All states require that applicants pass the same test
 d. All states require that applicants pay the same fee

50. Which of the following is not true about the nurse practice act?

 a. The nurse practice act varies from state to state.
 b. The nurse practice act specifies requirements for licensure in the particular state.
 c. The nurse practice act does not specify requirements for licensure.
 d. The nurse practice act states conditions for revocation.

51. Which of the following is not considered a disciplinary action by a state board of nurse examiners?

 a. Probation
 b. Suspension of license
 c. Requirements for additional continuing education
 d. Formal reprimands

52. Which of the following is the most common reason for a nurse's review by the board of nursing?

a. Incompetence in clinical practice
b. Performance complaints leveled by supervisors
c. Failure to renew licensure requirements in a timely manner
d. Sequela of behaviors secondary to chemical dependency

53. The nurse should employ the following methods in avoiding lawsuits:

a. Proper, specific, and legible documentation
b. Adherence to facility standards for transcription of orders
c. Following facility's policies and procedures when errors occur
d. All of the above

54. Which of the following is not a characteristic of modern systems theories?

a. The structure of the chain of command impacts workers' abilities to function.
b. Human comforts impact workers abilities to perform
c. Social needs of workers impact their ability to perform.
d. The complexity of the task and the availability of resources effects the organizational efficiency.

55. Modern organization theory examines:

a. What are the important parts of the system?
b. What are the interrelationships of key parts of the organization?
c. What channels tie the organization together?
d. All of the above

56. A factor influencing system integration is:

a. How the manager is perceived by the work force
b. The availability and accessibility of the management
c. The management's communications with the work force
d. The process for evaluation of employees

57. Practice, licensure, and certification standards should reflect:

a. Specific practice settings
b. Reimbursement issues
c. Graduate nursing education, only
d. The holistic aspects of and flexibility of nursing

58. All of the following are helpful techniques in conflict resolution **except:**

a. Always seek resolution of conflicts at the time they occur
b. Communicate with respect
c. Keep a positive approach
d. Do not hold grudges

59. Accommodation to conflict occurs when:

a. Assertiveness and cooperativeness are low
b. Assertiveness is low but cooperativeness is high
c. Assertiveness and cooperativeness are high
d. Assertiveness is high; cooperativeness is low

60. Consultation practice is based on:

a. Experience
b. Reimbursement
c. Theory
d. Practice setting

61. Deinstitutionalization was a result of:

a. Changes in mental health laws
b. The lack of nurses in state mental hospitals
c. States refused to continue funding for public hospitals
d. The Community Mental Health Centers Act of 1963

62. Utilization review may involve all of the following except:

a. Patient interviews and questionnaires
b. Pre-admission reviews
c. Concurrent review
d. Retrospective review

63. Many employers sponsor EAPs because:

a. EAP clinicians understand business
b. EAPs are unlicensed so benefits cost less
c. They recognize improved employee mental health can improve productivity
d. EAPs share therapy issues with personnel office

64. All of the following are advantages to private practice except:

a. Flexible hours

b. There are no adjunct therapists
c. Control of scope of practice
d. Financial rewards

65. In the matter of third-party payment, it is ANA's position that:

a. Nurses should be directly reimbursed for services they provide
b. Nurses should be paid the same as physicians
c. Nurses should not contract with managed care companies
d. Nurses should not provide psychotherapy

66. All of the following are conditions necessary for power except:

a. Legitimacy
b. Unity
c. Diversity
d. Homogeneity

67. Specialization improves care because:

a. Specialists are not subject to external control
b. Specialist care is more expensive
c. Professional competence is improved by concentration on one area
d. Specialty practice allows providers to be more independent

68. A tort is a:

a. Type of malpractice
b. Criminal act
c. A misdemeanor
d. A civil wrong

69. Boards of nurse examiners are:

a. Never elected
b. Composed of all RNs
c. Give the nursing license exam
d. Are responsible for the implementation of the Nurse Practice Act

70. The **Standards of Psychiatric-Mental Health Clinical Nursing Practice** criteria for ethical conduct does **not** discuss:

a. Reimbursement issues
b. Sexual contact between nurses and clients

c. Self disclosure
d. Informed consent

71. All of the following are reasons for the decline in numbers of psychiatric-mental health nurses **except:**

a. Adverse stigma associated with psychiatric patients
b. Significantly less federal money available for education
c. Psychiatric nursing is taught as separate and distinct content in many nursing programs
d. Fewer jobs in for-profit hospitals

72. Client-centered consultation was developed by:

a. Gerald Caplan
b. William Glasser
c. E. H. Schein
d. Carl Rogers

73. Kurt Lewin is a consultation theorist who:

a. Coined the term ''process consultation''
b. Developed the model client centered consultation
c. Applied small group dynamics to the consultation process
d. Saw consultation as a model to cope with society's problems

74. In order for negligence to occur all of the following must be present **except:**

a. The nurse must have the duty of care
b. The nurse must intentionally breach that duty
c. The patient must have been harmed
d. The nurse's breach of duty must have caused the harm

Answers

1. d
2. c
3. b
4. d
5. b
6. a
7. b
8. a
9. b
10. d
11. c
12. b
13. a
14. b
15. a
16. b
17. a
18. b
19. a
20. a
21. c
22. d
23. d
24. b
25. c
26. b
27. c
28. c
29. a
30. a
31. a
32. b
33. b
34. c
35. a
36. d
37. c
38. b
39. a
40. d
41. c
42. b
43. b
44. d
45. b
46. d
47. c
48. c
49. b
50. c
51. c
52. d
53. d
54. a
55. d
56. c
57. d
58. a
59. b
60. c
61. d
62. a
63. c
64. b
65. a
66. c
67. c
68. d
69. d
70. a
71. c
72. d
73. c
74. b

Bibliography

American Nurses Association (1994). *Statement on psychiatric-mental health clinical nursing practice and standards of psychiatric-mental health nursing practice.* Washington, DC: ANA.

Backer, B. A. (1991). You can get there from here: Guide toproblem definition in policy development. *Journal of Psychosocial Nursing, 29,* 24–29.

Billings, C. V. (1993). Psychiatric mental health nursing professional progress notes. *Archives of Psychiatric Nursing, 7*(3), 174–181.

Brown, C. L., & Schultz, P. R. (1991). Outcomes of power development in work relationships. *Journal of Nursing Administration, 21,* 35–39.

Caplan, G. (1964). *Principles of preventive psychiatry.* NY: Harper.

Chandler, G. E. (1991). Creating an environment to empower nurses. *Nursing Management, 22,* 20–23.

Duffield, C. (1992). Role competencies of first-line managers. *Nursing Management, 23,* 49-52.

Haber, J, and Billings, C. (1993). Primary mental health care: A vision for the future of psychiatric-mental health nursing. *ANA Council Perspectives, 2*(2),1.

Kison, C. (1989). Leadership: How, who and what? *Nursing Management, 20,* 72–74.

Kramer, M., & Schmalenberg, C. (1993). Learning from success: Autonomy and empowerment. *Nursing Management, 24,* 58–64.

Krauss, J. B. (1993) *Health care reform: Essential mental health services.* Washington, DC: American Nurses Publishing,

Lange F. C. (1987). The nurse as an individual, group, or community consultant. Norwalk, CT: Appleton-Century-Crofts.

Lego, S. (1984). The American Handbook of Psychiatric Nursing. NY: J. B. Lippincott.

Lewin, K. (1948) *Resolving social conflicts: Selected papers on group dynamics.* NY: Harper.

McCloskey, J. B., & Grace, H. K. (1994). *Current issues in nursing.* St. Louis: Mosby.

McNeese-Smith, D. (1993). Leadership behavior and employee effectiveness. *Nursing Management, 24,* 38–39.

Pothier, P. C., Stuart, G. W., Puskar, K. & Babich, K. (1990).Dilemmas and directions for psychiatric nursing in the 1990s. *Archives of Psychiatric Nursing, 4,* 268–291.

Pagonis, W. G. (1992, November-December). The work of the leader. *Harvard Business Review.* (118–126).

Reed, J. F. (1992). Situational leadership. *Nursing Management, 23,* 63–64.

Schein, E. H. (1990). Models of consultation: What do organizations of the 1990's need? *Consultation: An International Journal, 9,* 261–275.

Stivers, C. (1991). Why can't a woman be less like a man?: Women's leadership dilemma. *Journal of Nursing Administration, 21,* 47–51.

Styles, M. M. (1989). *On specialization in nursing: Toward a new empowerment.* Kansas City: American Nurses Foundation

Talbott, J. A. (1979) Deinstitutionalization: Avoiding the disasters of the past. *Hospital and Community Psychiatry.* 30:621

Tobias, L. L. (1990). *Psychological consulting to management: A clinician's perspective.* NY: Brunner/Mazel,

Wilson, H. S., & Kneisl, C. R. (1992). *Psychiatric nursing.* Redwood City, CA: Addison Wesley.

INDEX

REVIEW BOOK/AUDIO CASSETTE ORDER FORM

HEALTH LEADERSHIP ASSOCIATES, INC.

Please Print or Type

NAME: ______________________________

ADDRESS: ______________________________
Street Apt. #

____
City State Zip Code

TELEPHONE: ____________ Home ____________ Work

SECTION 1: AUDIO CASSETTES

Review Courses are approximately 15 hours in length unless otherwise notated and include course handouts.

QTY	REVIEW COURSE	PRICE	
____	Ambulatory Womens Health Care Nursing	$150	____
____	Inpatient Obstetric Nursing	$150	____
____	Ob-Gyn Nurse Practitioner	$150	____
____	** Childbearing Management	$45	____
____	Generalist Community Health Nurse	$150	____
____	Rehabilitation Nurse	$150	____
____	* Generalist Pediatric Nurse	$75	____
____	Generalist Medical-Surgical Nurse	$150	____
____	* Generalist Psychiatric & Mental Health Nurse	$75	____
____	Clinical Specialist in Adult Psychiatric and Mental Health Nursing	$150	____
____	* Generalist Gerontological Nurse	$75	____
____	Gerontological Nurse Practitioner	$150	____
____	Adult Nurse Practitioner	$150	____
____	Pediatric Nurse Practitioner	$150	____
____	Family Nurse Practitioner (consists of ANP, PNP & Childbearing Management courses)	$330	____
____	** Test Taking Strategies and Techniques	$30	____

* 8 hour course ** 2–4 hour course

SUB TOTAL: ____________

Maryland Residents add 5% sales tax: ____________

Shipping and Handling (2–4 hour course) $4.00 ____________

All other courses $10.00 ____________

TOTAL: ____________

SECTION 2: REVIEW BOOKS

QUANTITY	BOOK TITLE	PRICE	
____	Generalist Pediatric Nurse	$43.95	____
____	Gerontological Nursing	$43.95	____
____	Psychiatric Nursing	$43.95	____
____	* Adult Nurse Practitioner ❑ 2nd Edition	$43.95	____
____	Ob/Gyn Nurse Practitioner	$43.95	____
____	* Pediatric Nurse Practitioner ❑ 2nd Edition	$43.95	____
____	Family Nurse Practitioner Package (Includes ANP,Ob/Gyn,PNP Guides)	$112.00	____

***Orders received prior to July 1 will receive 1st Edition unless otherwise indicated**

SUB TOTAL: ____________

Maryland Residents add 5% sales tax: ____________

Shipping and Handling $4.95 one book: ____________

$2.00 for each additional book.: ____________

TOTAL: ____________

For orders of 10 or greater call 1-800-435-4775.
All prices subject to change without notice.

SECTION 3: REVIEW BOOK/AUDIO CASSETTE DISCOUNT PACKAGES

A discounted rate is available when purchasing Review Book(s) and Audio Cassettes together. When purchasing packages, indicate Book/Audio Cassette selections in sections 1 & 2. Calculate amount due in this section

QUANTITY	PACKAGE SELECTION	PRICE	
____	8 Hour Course/1 Review Guide	$115.00	____
____	15 Hour Course/1 Review Guide	$185.00	____
____	FNP Package	$405.00	____

FNP Package (consists of ANP,PNP,Ob/Gyn Guides & Audio Cassettes of the ANP, PNP and Childbearing Management courses)

SUB TOTAL: ____________

Maryland Residents add 5% sales tax: ____________

Shipping and Handling included in package rate.

TOTAL: ____________

PAYMENT DUE

Return mail orders to: Health Leadership Associates, Inc. P.O. Box 59153 - Potomac, MD 20859

For MasterCard and VISA Orders Only: Call Toll Free 1-800-435-4775

❑ My Check or money order is enclosed (US funds, payable to Health Leadership Associates, Inc.)

❑ Purchase Order is attached, P.O. # ____________

Please Charge My ❑ **Visa** ❑ **MC** Expiration Date ____________

Credit Card # ____________

Print Name ____________

Signature ____________

REVIEW GUIDES & AUDIOCASSETTES

1) Section 1 Total	$	____________
2) Section 2 Total	$	____________
3) Section 3 Total	$	____________
TOTAL PAYMENT DUE	$	____________